ATLAS OF REAL TIME 3D TRANSESOPHAGEAL ECHOCARDIOGRAPHY

ATLAS OF REAL TIME 3D TRANSESOPHAGEAL ECHOCARDIOGRAPHY

Dr. Francesco F. Faletra
Fondazione Cardiocentro Ticino Via Tesserete 48 6900 Lugano Switzerland

Dr. Stefano de Castro
Università di Roma - Dipartimento di Scienze cardiovascolari e Respiratorie, Piliclinico Umberto I, Università "La Sapienza" Viale del Policlinico 155, 00166 Roma, Italy

Dr. Natesa G. Pandian
Tufts University, School of Medicine, New England Medical Center, 750 Washington St., Boston MA 02111, Box 32, USA

Dr. Itzhak Kronzon
New York University School of Medicine, Leon H. Charney Div. Cardiology, 560 First Ave., New York NY 10016, USA

Dr. Hans-Joachim Nesser
Krankenhaus der Elisabethinen Linz, Fadinger Str. 1, 4010 Linz, Austria

Dr. Siew Yen Ho
National Heart & Lung Institute, Royal Brompton Hospital, Sydney Street, London, United Kingdom SW3 6NP

With 289 Illustrations, 284 in Full Color

Springer

Dr. Francesco F. Faletra
Fondazione Cardiocentro Ticino
Via Tesserete 48 6900
Lugano Switzerland
francesco.faletra@cardiocentro.org

Dr. Stefano De Castro
Dipartimento di Scienze cardiovascolari e Respiratorie, Piliclinico Umberto I,
Università "La Sapienza"
Viale del Policlinico 155, 00166 Roma,
Italy

Dr. Natesa G. Pandian
Tufts University, School of Medicine
Tufts Medical Center
800 Washington Street
Boston, MA 02111, USA
npandian@tuftsmedicalcenter.org

Dr. Itzhak Kronzon
New York University School of Medicine
Leon H. Charney Div. Cardiology
560 First Ave.
New York NY 10016
USA
itzhak.kronzon@nyumc.org

Dr. Hans-Joachim Nesser
Krankenhaus der Elisabethinen Linz
Fadinger Str. 1
4010 Linz
Austria
hans-joachim.nesser@elisabethinen.or.at

Dr. Siew Yen Ho
Royal Brompton Hospital
Sydney Street, London
United Kingdom SW3 6NP
yen.ho@rbht.nhs.uk

Additional material to this book can be downloaded from http://extras.springer.com

ISBN 978-1-4471-6888-1 ISBN 978-1-84996-083-0 (eBook)
DOI: 10.1007/978-1-84996-083-0
Springer Dordrecht Heidelberg London New York

Softcover re-print of the Hardcover 1st edition 2010

Printed on acid-free paper.

Springer is part of Springer Science+Business Media (www.springer.com)

DEDICATION

To Stefano

We have known him for many years, worked with him on many scientific and educational endeavors, and met him several times a year in different countries and various continents. What a pleasure and fun it was always! His energy, humor, and wisdom always turn each meeting into an interesting, frequently funny, and memorable event. He was a superb doctor, an accomplished scientist, and a great teacher with thorough knowledge not only in cardiology but also in literature, poetry, politics, economy, or any other topic that could arise during a conversation. His warmth, eloquence, wisdom generosity, and friendship will be sorely missed, together with the spark in his eyes, his beautiful smile, the bursts of his laughter, and his "Ciao" when we left.

Ciao, Stefano. Rest in peace. You will never be forgotten.

Francesco, Natesa, Itzhak, and Joachim

PREFACE

The notions of pain and pleasure and generally of all sensations plainly have their source in the heart and find in it their ultimate termination.

Aristotle, fourth century BC

After almost three decades of research and clinical development, three-dimensional (3D) echocardiography has recently become a valuable tool in the diagnosis and management of cardiovascular disease. Initial attempts at 3D echocardiography were laborious with images assembled from multiple 2D images, each separated in time, and later processed into composite 3D representations. Current approaches achieve 3D imaging with the use of matrix array transducers that allow physicians to realistically visualize cardiac anatomy and pathology in real time. These advances have led to major improvements in the accuracy of chamber volumes and cardiac structure quantification, as well as in their functional analysis.

The miniaturization of beam-forming electronics has allowed engineers to build a real-time 3D transesophageal transducer. This breakthrough technology enables faster image acquisition and delivers images of internal cardiac structures that are of superior quality than that obtained through either real-time transthoracic echocardiography or reconstructed 3D transesophageal (TEE) imaging technology.

This atlas is intended to provide a comprehensive overview of the normal anatomy of the heart's interior structures (i.e., native valves, interatrial septum, left atrial appendage, left atrium) as seen by this new revolutionary ultrasound technique. Normal 3D TEE cardiac structures are presented and compared side-by-side with their corresponding anatomical specimens, focusing on both basic and detailed portrayals of the heart's anatomic structures. Anatomic specimens have been provided by two pathologists expert in cardiac anatomy: Prof. Sew Yen Ho, Head of Cardiac Morphology at the National Heart and Lung Institute, Imperial College in London with Royal Brompton Hospital in London (coeditor), and Dr. Edgardo Bonacina of Hospital Niguarda Ca' Granda in Milan. Examples of the most common diseases are illustrated for each chapter. Several clinical cases where 3D TEE examination has played a relevant role in the decision-making process, or in monitoring catheter-based procedures, are described in the last chapter. The atlas ends with a series of 3D TEE anatomical plates where the most significant structures are imaged from different perspectives. This atlas specially targets cardiologists involved in echocardiography, but we hope that general cardiologists may appreciate it as well, since it can offer a wider vision of living normal and pathological cardiac anatomy. We are indebted to all experts who contributed with their precious work and suggestions to produce 3D TEE images and chapters making this atlas a reality.

Lugano, Switzerland — *Dr. Francesco F. Faletra*

Rome, Italy — *Dr. Stefano de Castro*

Boston, MA — *Dr. Natesa G. Pandian*

New York, NY — *Dr. Itzhak Kronzon*

Linz, Austria — *Dr. Hans-Joachim Nesser*

London, UK — *Dr. Siew Yen Ho*

ACKNOWLEDGMENTS

"I have been lucky to be in the right place, at the right time and with the right people!" Thus, I wish to express my gratitude to Dr. Edgardo Bonacina for providing me with impressive images of anatomic specimens, and to Dr. Julija Klimusina for her dedication to this project and extraordinary support in the collection of 3D TEE images. To Dr. Ivette Petrova and to Henry Martin Slater for their assistance with the English language. A personal thank you goes to the entire staff of both the Anesthesiology and Cardiac Surgery Department at Fondazione Cardiocentro Ticino for their support in the collection of intra-operative images. I am deeply indebted to Prof. Tiziano Moccetti, Dr. Elena Pasotti, and Dr. Giovanni Pedrazzini for their daily encouragement and enthusiasm. Finally, this book would not have been possible without the engagement and profound friendship of Prof. Angelo Auricchio to whom I am most grateful.

Francesco Fulvio Faletra

My appreciations go to all the fellows, sonographers and collaborators who contributed to the evolution of 3D technology.

Drs. Pandian, Nesser, and Kronzon

I wish to thank the Cardiac Morphology team and colleagues at the Royal Brompton Hospital for their steadfast support.

Dr. Ho

CONTENTS

CHAPTER 1

Technological Issues

Echocardiography has been in use for over 50 years. During this time, many technical advances have led to the evolution of the discipline from A-mode to transesophageal echocardiography (TEE). However, all echocardiographic methods are intrinsically unidimensional (such as M-mode echocardiography) or two-dimensional. *Everything in nature is three-dimensional.* Desire for three-dimensional (3D) imaging existed in a few minds, and for a long time, 3D echocardiography was a reverie of all "romantic" cardiologists who spent most of their working time dealing with echocardiography (most of the editors are in this group). Earlier technological efforts, used for implementing 3D echocardiography in the clinical scenario, yielded coarse 3D images. Thus, after years of working in a "flat land" of 2D images, mounting frustration was prevalent among these romantic "imagers."

The main problems were related to data acquisition and reconstruction. These required a long, time-consuming procedure because of the spatial location of the image planes, temporal alignment of the image frames within the cardiac cycle, correction for respiratory motion of the heart, rapid data transfer, storage of large amounts of data, development of algorithms for reconstruction, and display of 3D data on a 2D screen.

Recent advances in computer and crystals technology have led to the introduction of the matrix array transducer for use in transthoracic echocardiography. This technology uses a greater number of crystals (3,000) and is capable of generating real-time 3D images. Moreover, the reduction in size of the transducer footprint has led to the introduction of real-time 3D transesophageal echocardiography (RT 3D TEE). The resulting image quality has been superb, and probably for the first time, we have images of cardiac structures as they are seen by pathologists and surgeons. In this chapter, we briefly discuss some of the technological advances that have made it possible to perform 3D TEE in real time.

1.1 PIEZOELECTRIC CRYSTALS

The first, and currently the only, clinically available RT 3D TEE is the X7-2t TEE transducer (Philips Medical Systems), which combines xMATRIX technology and a new generation of piezoelectric material named PureWave crystals. Piezoelectric crystals are responsible for the delivery of ultrasound energy into the scanned tissue and for converting ultrasound echoes into electric signals. The coupling efficiency in converting electrical to mechanical energy and vice versa is key to image quality. For many years, ultrasound machines have used transducers with piezoelectric crystals made by polycrystalline compounds (lead–zirconate–titanate composite or PZR composites).

To create an overall piezoelectric effect, PZT ceramics must be subjected to a poling process (i.e. the application of an external electric field) to align dipoles within polycrystalline materials. Because of the imperfect alignment of the individual dipoles and the constraint of the grain boundaries, PZT composites may achieve at best only 70% polarization with corresponding constraints in the electromechanical coupling efficiency. The new generation of piezoelectric crystals (PureWave crystals) are without grain boundaries, so when these crystals are poled, near perfect alignment of dipoles (~100%) can be obtained. This results in dramatically enhanced electromechanical properties (Fig. 1.1).

Compared with conventional transducer material, the PureWave crystals are more uniform, have lower signal loss, and are able to transfer energy with greater precision and efficiency(Fi g. 1.2).

PureWave crystals exhibit ten times the strain of conventional transducers (i.e., the ability to change thickness under an electrical field). Their efficiency in converting electrical energy to mechanical energy marks a 68–85% improvement over traditional polycrystalline PZT-type ceramics. Gain in bandwidth and sensitivity enables these

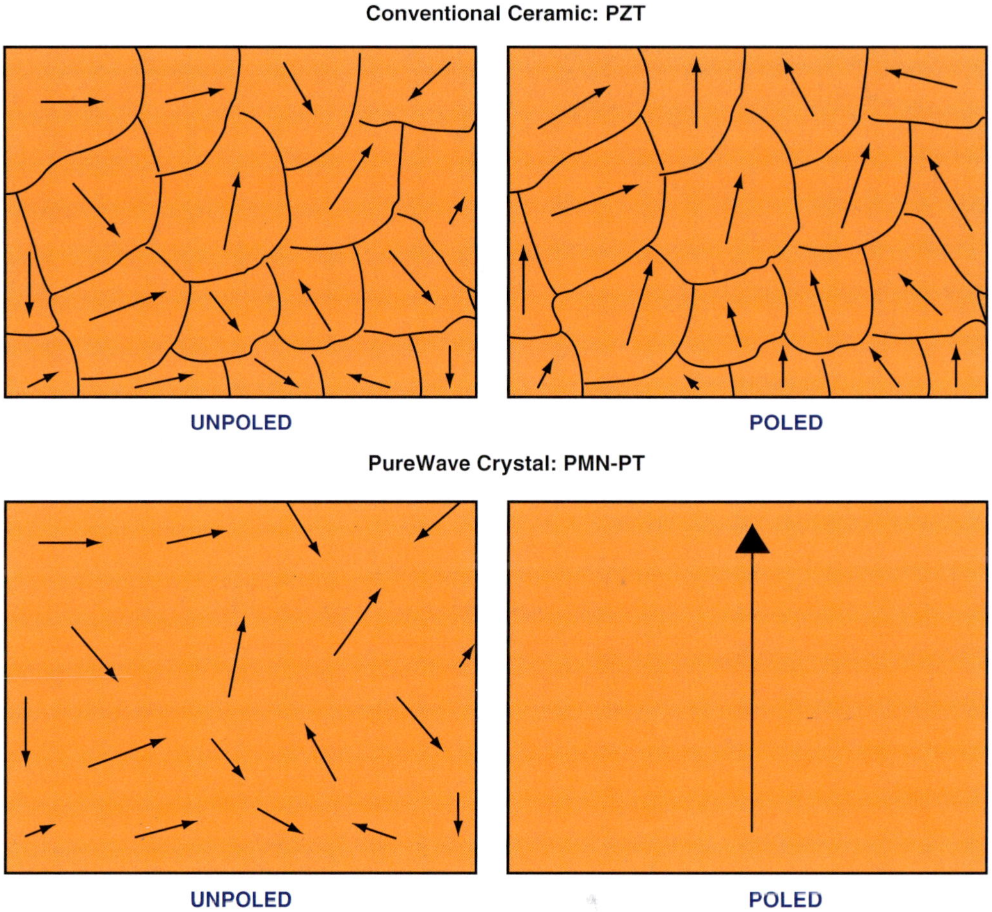

FIGURE 1.1 Application of electrical field on conventional ceramics and on PureWave crystal. A near perfect alignment can be achieved with PureWaveC rystal.

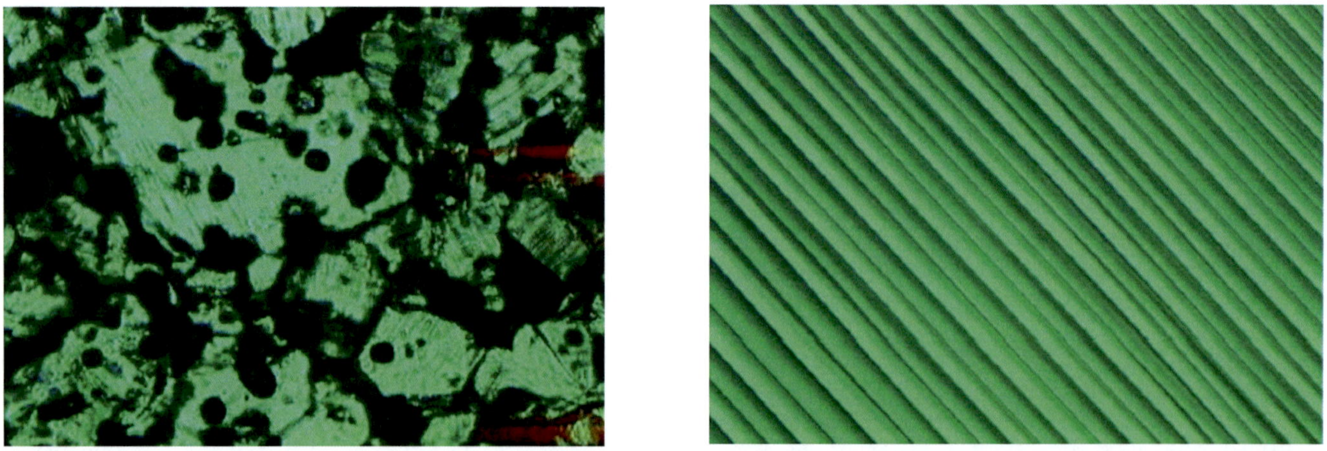

FIGURE 1.2 (a) The figure shows the imperfect, multicrystalline, randomly orientated grains of conventional transducer material; (b) This figure, however, shows the nearly perfect atomic level arrangement: uniform, with no grain boundaries of PureWave material.

crystals to cover the frequency range of two broadband transducers with a single probe. The greater sensitivity across a wider range of frequencies afforded by PureWave crystals provides the flexibility to transmit and receive harmonic frequencies at a full sensitivity level for enhanced harmonic performance. In other words, this technology leads to superior image quality by improving resolution, supporting advanced harmonics, and reducing artifacts.

1.2 3D TRANSESOPHAGEAL ECHOCARDIOGRAPHY

The biggest accomplishment, however, has been condensing the microelectronics into the tip of a transesophageal transducer probe. What technology has achieved successfully is to shrink the electronics from a system of over 150 front-end boards and package it into a transducer (Fig. 1.3). The new RT 3D TEE transducers contain 2,500 active piezoelectric PureWave crystals for fully sampled, high resolution 3D volumes, while maintaining a footprint as small as that of standard 2D TEE probes. (Fig. 1.4).

The 3D TEE system also provides all the conventional modalities such as 2D multiplane imaging, M-mode, pulse and continuous wave Doppler, and color Doppler imaging.

Real-time live 3D. A pyramidal set of 50×30° is displayed in real time. The 3D image changes as the transducer is moved just as in 2D TEE: manipulation of the TEE probe (i.e., rotation and change of position) leads to instantaneous changes in the image seen on the monitor. Theoretically, this modality can display any cardiac structure in a 3D format. In practice, it is very useful for capturing an image of the aortic valve in its entire volume. Other structures (e.g., mitral valve, atrial septum) are visualized only partially. One of the advantages of live 3D modality is the relatively high frame rate (20–40 Hz).

3D zoom modality. This modality can display a truncated but magnified pyramidal data set of variable size. When activated, a 2D preview image shows the original view and the orthogonal plane. After sizing the zoom sector over the region of interest, the RT 3D TEE is displayed. Minimizing sector width is important for increasing temporal resolution and image quality. This mode is preferred for displaying the mitral valve, the left atrial appendage, and the atrial septum. Both live and zoom modalities are devoid of artifacts commonly encountered with ECG-gated 3D acquisition.

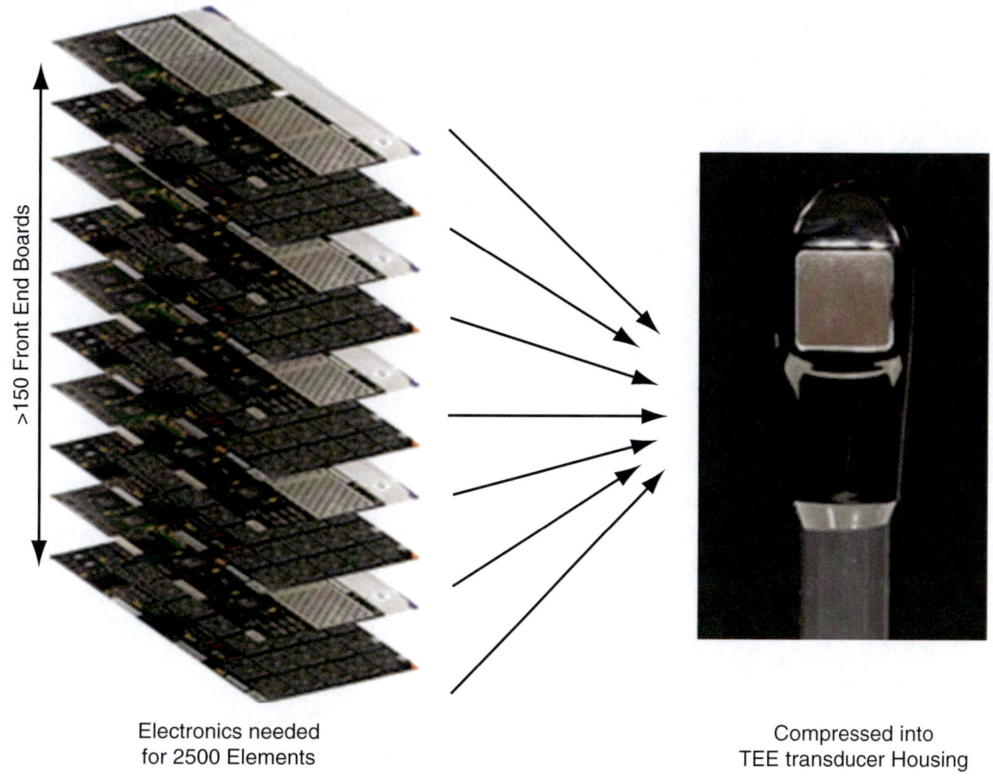

FIGURE 1.3 Shrinking beam-forming electronics.

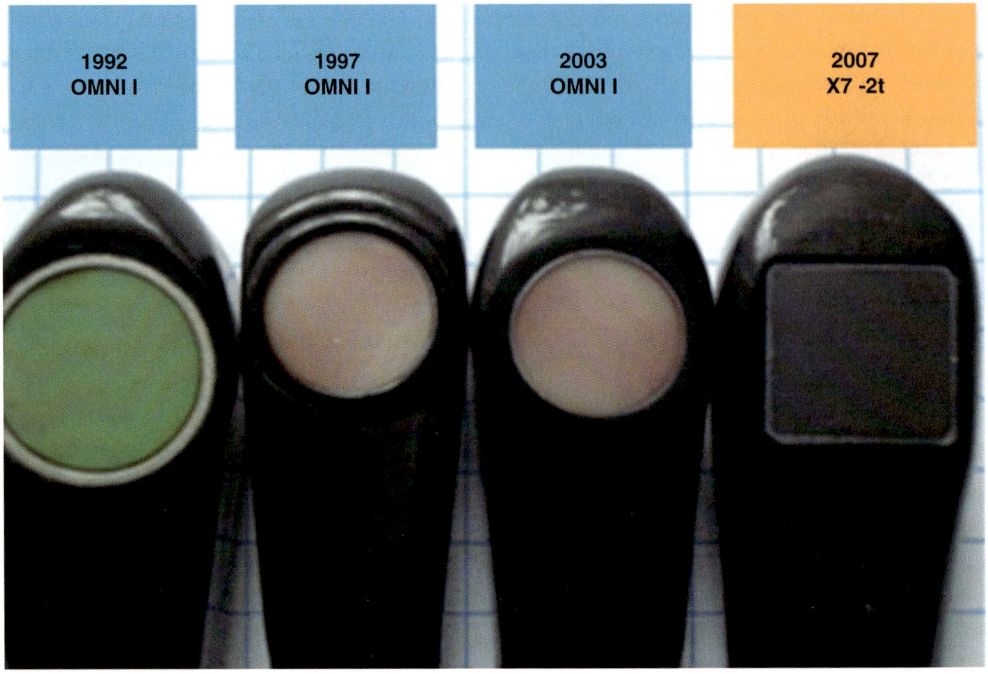

FIGURE 1.4 Comparative representation of Philips TEE probe. The x7-2t probe is a real-time 3D TEE transducer.

Full volume. A pyramidal volume of 60×60° up to 100×100° allows the inclusion of large cardiac volume. The full volume is constructed by merging 4–7 narrower segments of the pyramidal data set. This modality requires ECG gating. Thus, the full volume modality is not, in a strict sense, a real-time acquisition. Accordingly, it may suffer from artifacts due to the malapposition of the narrow pyramidal data set. Acquiring the data when the patient holds his breath can minimize such artifacts. In this modality the temporal resolution is higher when compared with zoom modality (up to 40 Hz). However, spatial resolution (particularly lateral resolution) deteriorates compared with real-time acquisition.

3D full volume for color Doppler. Similar to the full volume method described, this modality is constructed by merging 7–14 narrow pyramidal sets. The final representation, however, is a narrow pyramid, since two different modalities must be acquired – the anatomy and the flow. Thus it is essential to put the flow jet of interest in the center of the sector; otherwise part of the jet can be missed in the reconstruction. The temporal resolution obtained is up to 25 Hz.

CHAPTER2

General Concepts

"a picture is worth a thousand words...."

3D Echocardiography allows physicians to become a new kind of pathologist performing "electronic" dissections of the heart in living people rather than in cadavers"

Advances in computer technology, new generations of piezoelectric crystals (see Chap. 1) capable of converting mechanical into electric energy (and vice versa) with great efficiency, and miniaturization of electronic circuitries have made possible the development of a new matrix-array transducer so small that it can be inserted into the tip of a conventional transesophageal probe. As a result, in 2007, a new generation of real-time 3D transesophageal transducers (RT 3D TEE) with thousands of piezoelectric crystals became available for clinical use. Examinations with RT 3D TEE provide high quality images with close correlation to the actual anatomy (Figs. 2.1 and 2.2). Moreover, once a volumetric data set has been obtained, images can be rotated and angulated in any direction, allowing a better appraisal of the spatial relationship between structures (Fig. 2.3). Anatomical parts can be displayed from perspectives that can be shared with surgeons and pathologists (Fig. 2.4). The same volumetric data set can be cropped in any plane, revealing fine anatomical details (Fig. 2.5).

At first glance, some anatomical internal structures are not easily recognizable, when seen in "surface rendering" mode, especially for physicians who are used to dealing only with 2D images. In Fig. 2.6, the mitral valve and left atrial appendage are seen from an atrial perspective; however, the structure that abuts the atrial septum is not readily identifiable (arrow). By rotating the volumetric data set, this structure becomes easily identifiable as a bulge in the atrial wall caused by a slightly dilated noncoronary aortic sinus (Figs. 2.7 and 2.8).

One of the unique aspects of 3D RT TEE is its ability to image internal surfaces (the so called "en face" perspective). Sometimes, "en face" visualization may not help recognition of certain specific structures, especially when they are part of more extensive surface. In Fig. 2.9, the asterisk marks an area which is supposed to be the membranous septum. There is not a distinctive feature that identifies the septum from the "en face" perspective. However, the septum can be recognized on the basis of its spatial relationship with the surrounding structures (i.e. the inter-leaflet triangle between the noncoronary and the right aortic coronary leaflets). Conversely, "en face" images are very useful when a septal defect is present (see Chap. 6). The "en face" perspectives are also useful in defining the anatomical shape of structures. Figure 2.10 shows the anterior mitral leaflet imaged from an "en face" perspective after cropping the postero-lateral wall of the left ventricle. This is a unique view imaging the leaflet as it is and displaying it as a roughly triangular shaped structure. Another useful application of the "en face" perspective is the identification of the orifices of the vessels entering the heart's cavities. Figure 2.11 shows the entry of the coronary sinus into the right atrium (see Chap. 7).

Finally, the ability to visualize for long portions intracardiac catheters, including the tips, makes RT 3D TEE a suitable tool for monitoring percutaneous interventional procedures (see Chaps. 3 and 7). Figure 2.12 shows two catheters in the right atrium. Notably, the long curved segment of one of them can be easily followed. Figure 2.13 shows how appropriate cuts reveal nearly the entire course of a catheter into the right cavities.

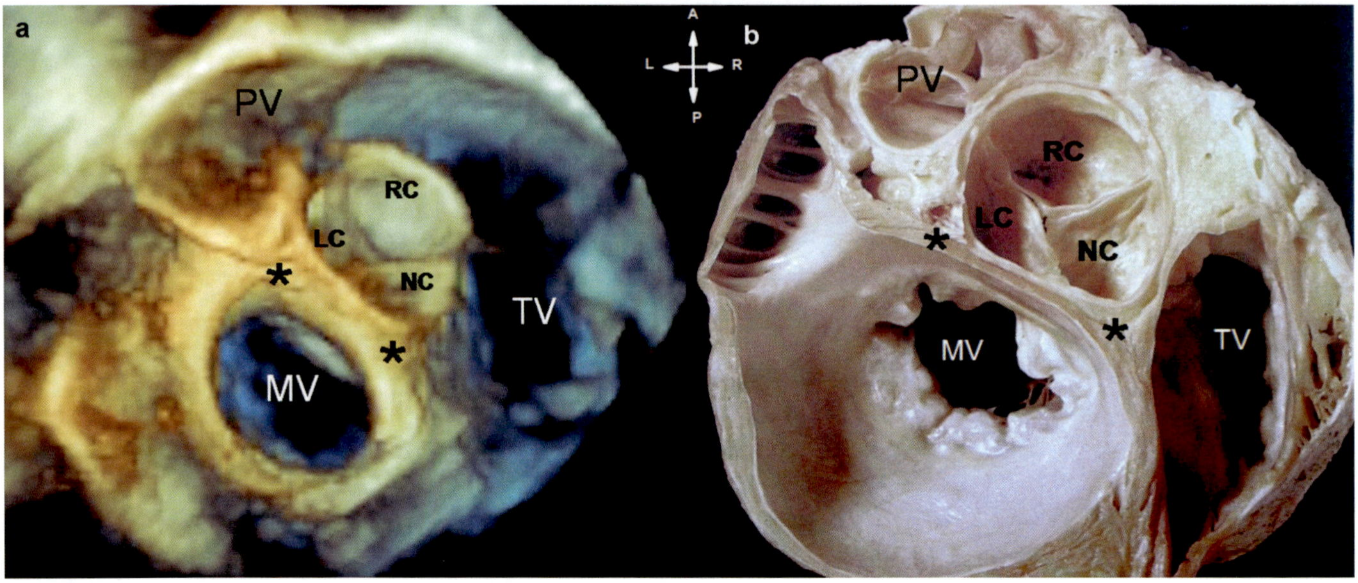

FIGURE 2.1 (a) 3D TEE image in full volume modality of the base of the heart and (b) a corresponding anatomic specimen. The correspondence with the actual anatomy makes this technique a magnificent tool for imaging internal cardiac structures. In this figure, many structures such as the mitral valve (MV), tricuspid valve (TV), pulmonic valve (PV), left coronary (LC), right coronary (RC), and noncoronary aortic (NC) sinuses and leaflets can be recognized. Two *asterisks* mark the position of the left and right fibrous trigones. The aorta is centrally located and is related to both the cardiac chamber and the cardiac valves.

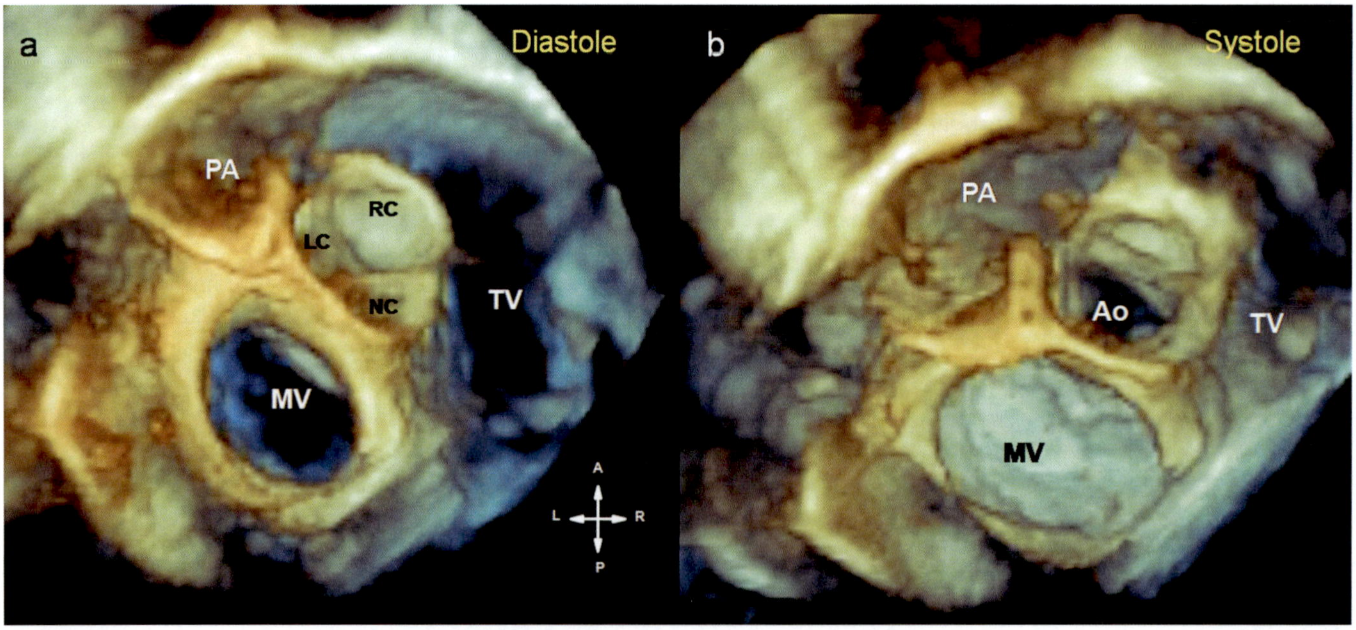

FIGURE 2.2 (**a**) The same heart as in Fig. 2.1 in diastole and (b) in systole. Images obtained with this technique are easily recognizable by nonexperts in echocardiography. Abbreviation as in previous figure. *Ao* aorta, *PA* pulmonary artery.

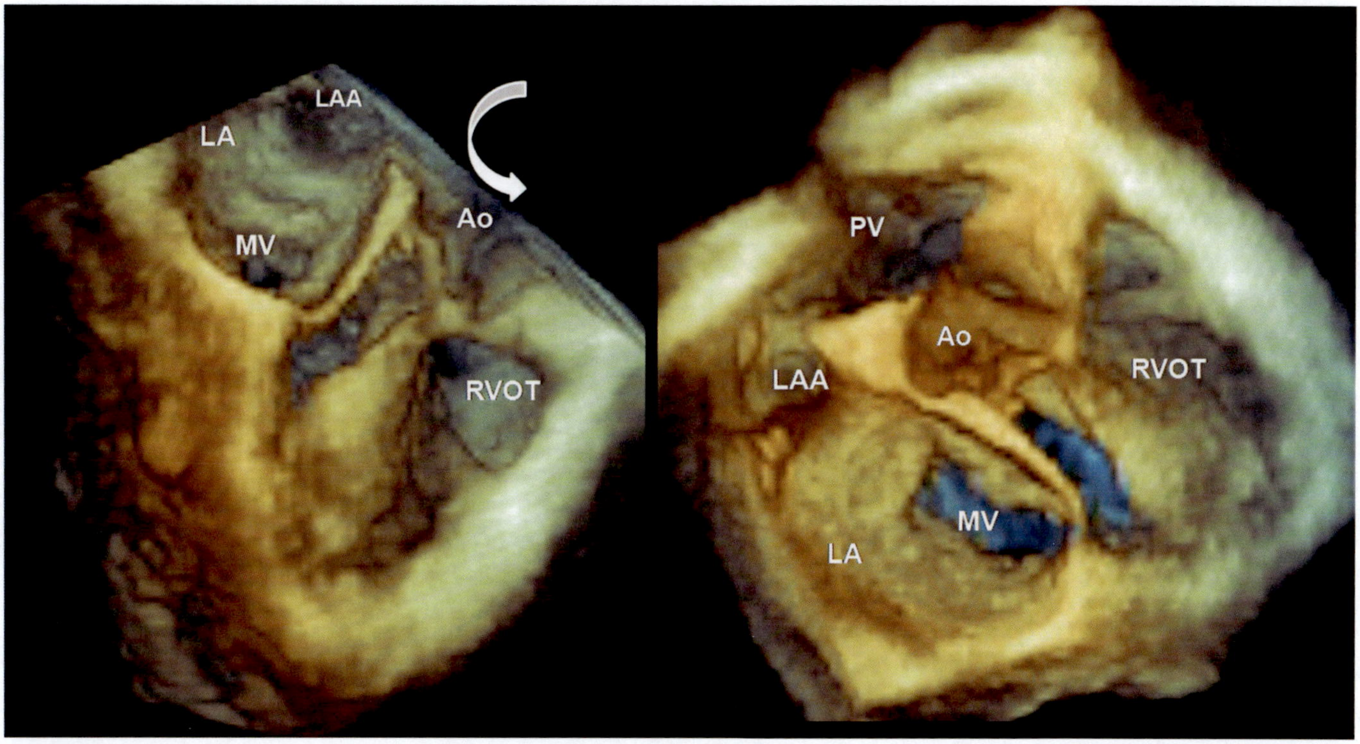

FIGURE 2.3 3D TEE images of the heart in full volume modality displayed in two different perspectives: (a) the orifice and leaflets of the mitral valve are seen only partially because they are hidden by other structures; (b) with a slight angulation and rotation (*curved arrow*) of the volumetric data set, the mitral valve is revealed. *MV* mitral valve; *LA* left atrium; *LAA* left atrial appendage; *Ao* aorta; *RVOT* right ventricular outflow tract; *PV*p ulmonicv alve.

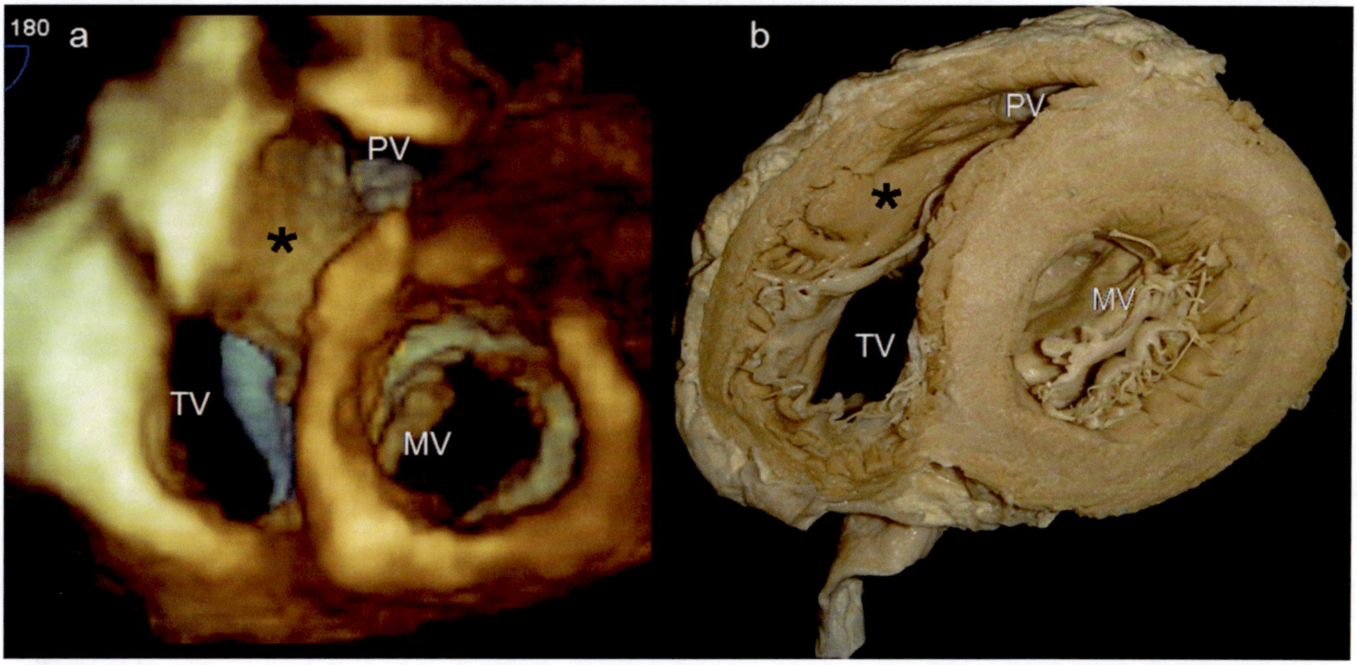

FIGURE 2.4 (a) 3D TEE image in full volume modality after cropping the volume data set through a transverse midventricular plane and (b) the corresponding anatomical specimen. The view from the ventricular perspective shows the ventricular infundibular fold (*asterisk*) separating the tricuspid valve (TV) from the pulmonic valve (PV). This perspective is one shared only with pathologists. *MV* mitral valve.

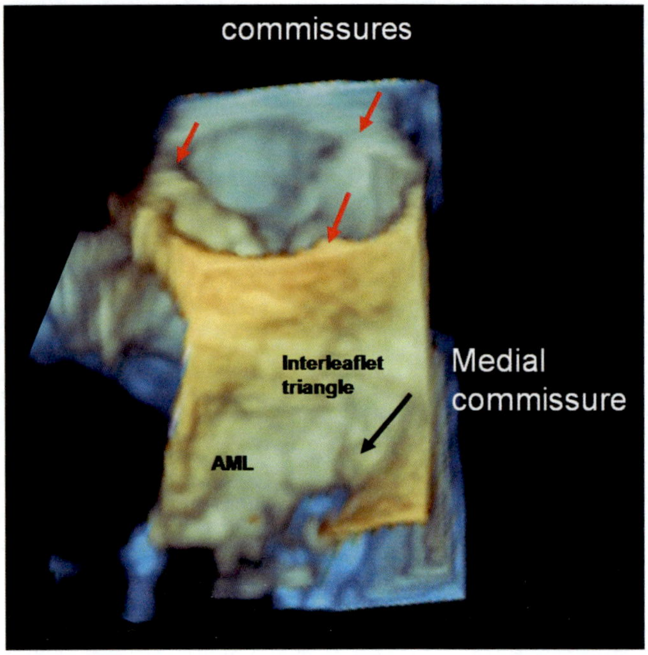

FIGURE 2.5 Real-time 3D TEE image in zoom modality showing fine anatomical details revealed after cropping the volumetric data set. The medial commissure of mitral valve, (*black arrow*) the interleaflet triangle, and the three aortic commissures (*red arrows*) are visualized. *AML* anterior mitral leaflet.

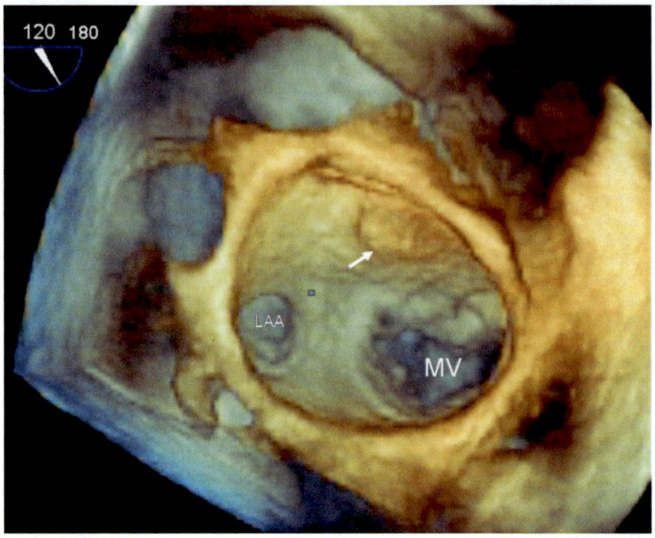

FIGURE 2.6 Real-time 3D TEE image in zoom modality showing the left atrial cavity from the atrial perspective. The mitral valve (MV) and left atrial appendage (LAA) are depicted. An unidentifiable formation abuts against the atrial wall (*arrow*).

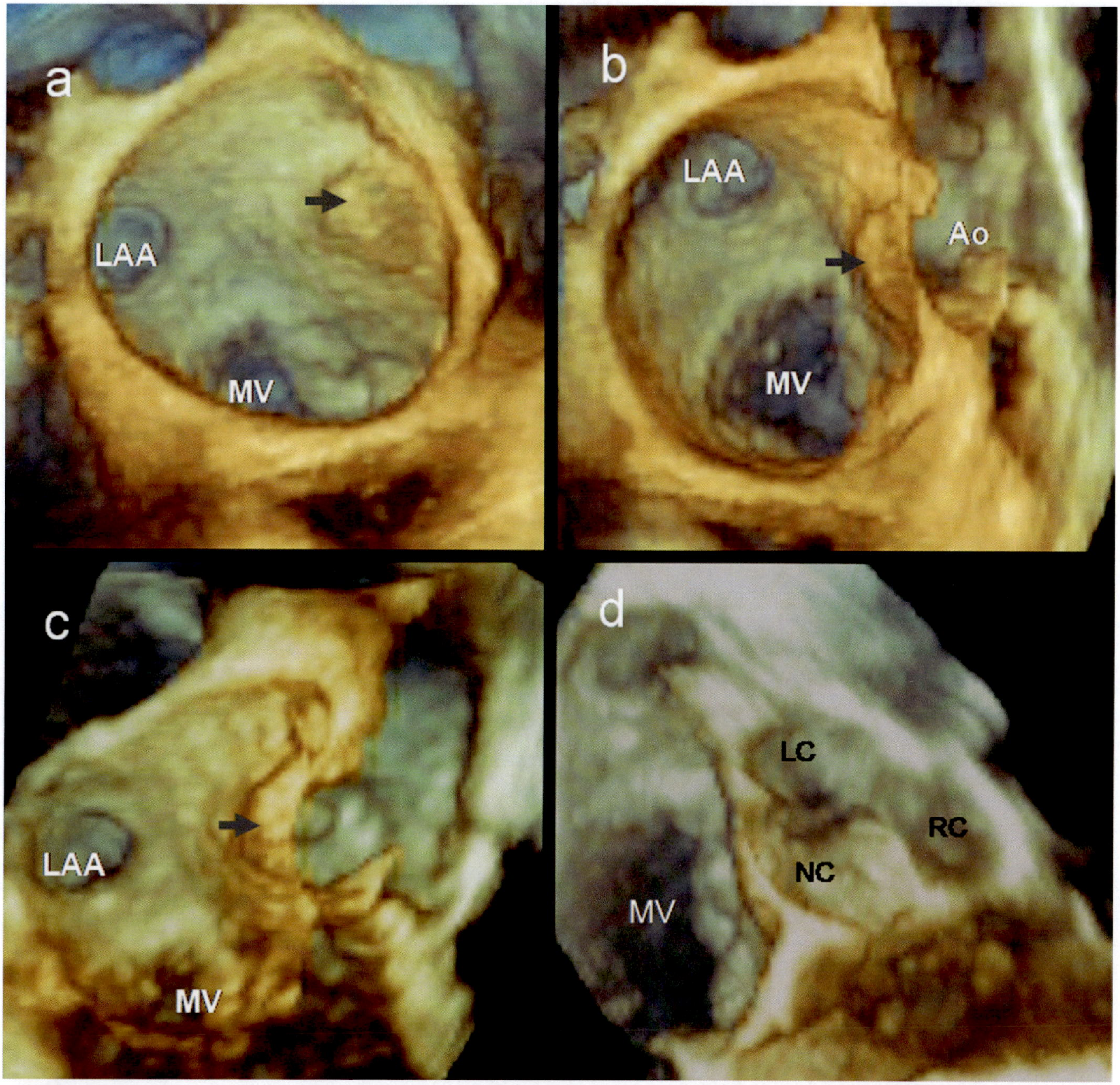

FIGURE 2.7 The figure shows that by rotating the image rightward (b–d), it becomes clear that the curious structure (*arrow*) is a bulge in the atrial wall caused by the noncoronary sinus (NC). *Ao* aorta; *LC* left coronary sinus; *RC* right coronary sinus; *MV* mitral valve; *LAA* left atriala ppendage.

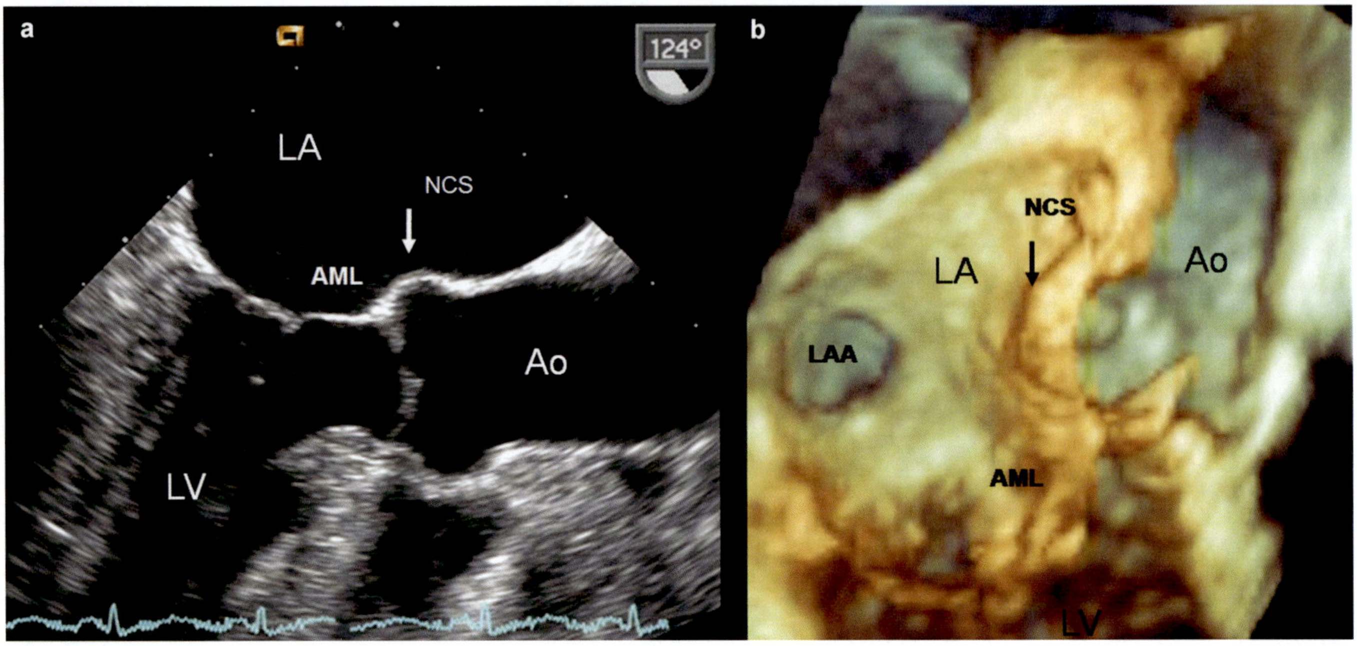

FIGURE 2.8 (a) Conventional 2D TEE and (b) Real time 3D TEE image. With conventional 2D TEE, the noncoronary sinus (NCS) is easily recognizable. *LA* left atrium; *LAA* left atrial appendage; *Ao* aorta; *LV* left ventricle; *AML* anterior mitral leaflet.

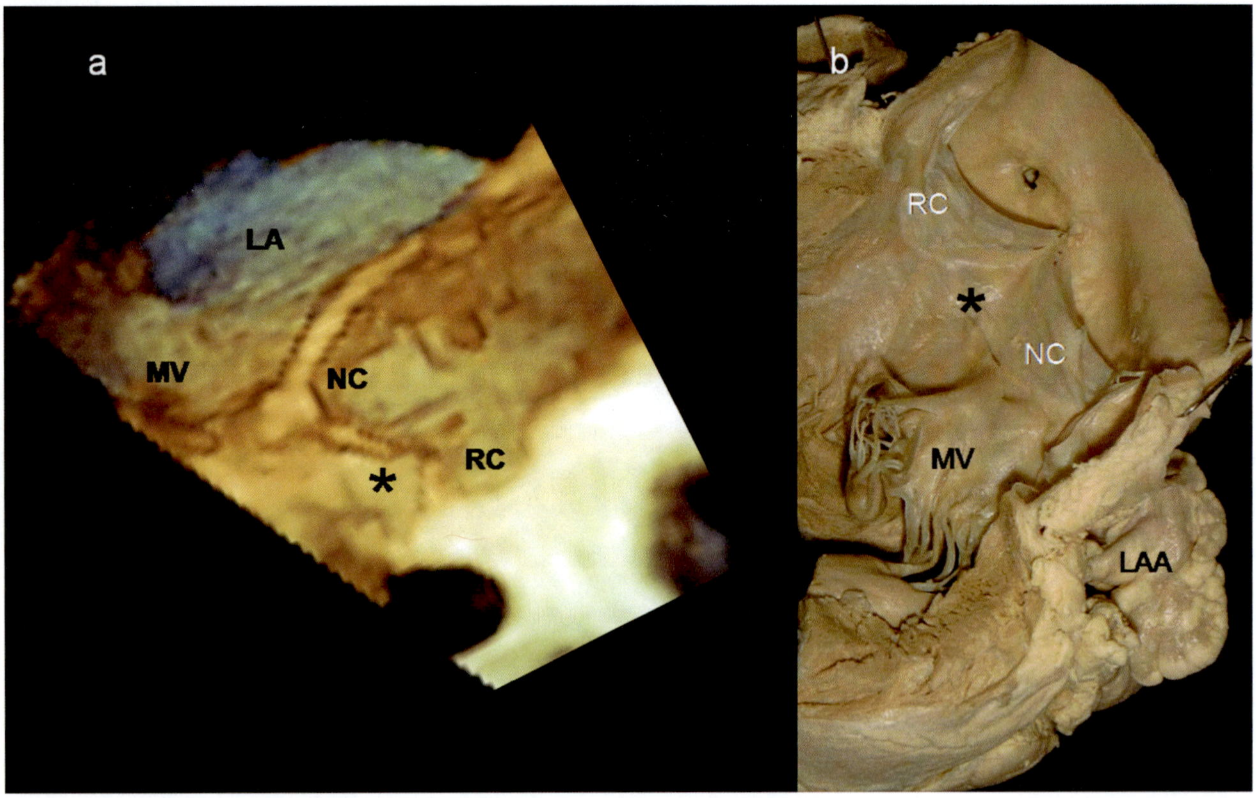

FIGURE 2.9 (a) Real-time 3D TEE image in zoom modality properly cut to show the area (*asterisk*), which is supposed to be the membranous septum and (b) the corresponding anatomical specimen. This small portion of the septum is part of the central fibrous body of the heart along with the right fibrous trigone. The membranous septum is located immediately below the right coronary (RC) and the non-coronary (NC) aortic sinuses. However, the "en face" image does not allow identification of the septum as a distinct structure. *MV* mitral valve; *LA* left atrium; *LAA*l efta triala ppendage.

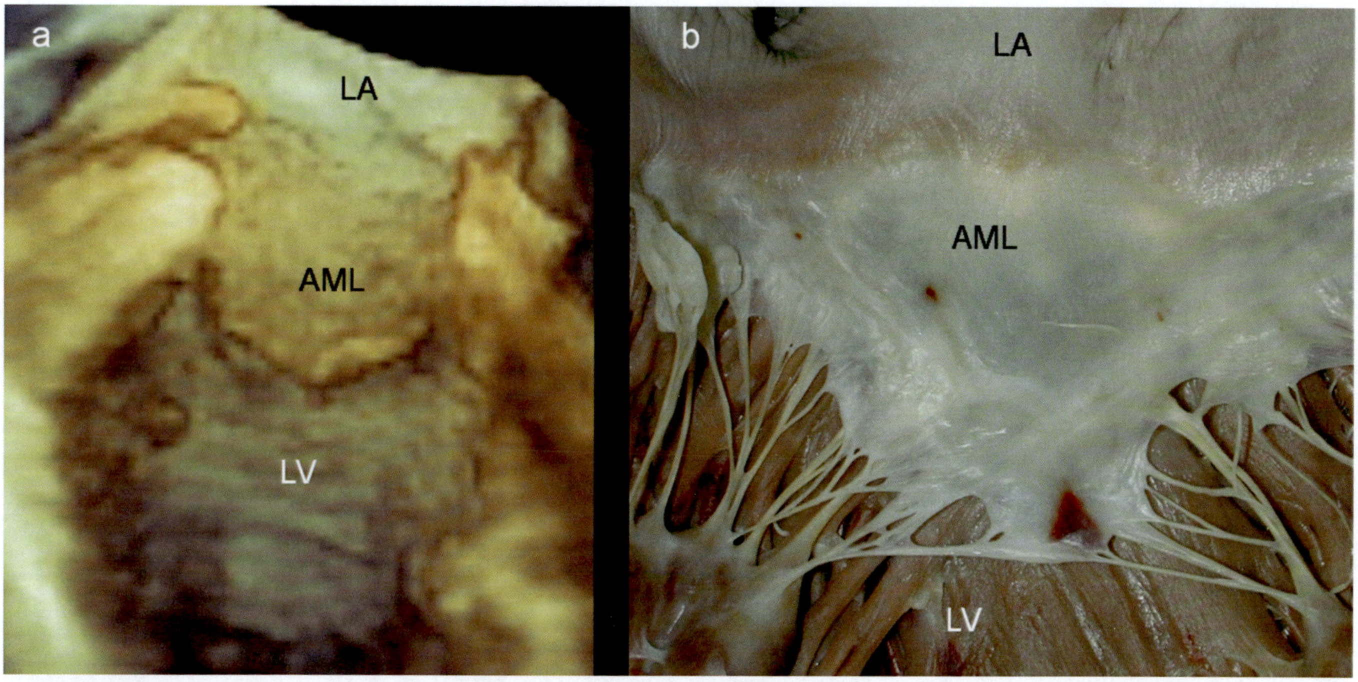

FIGURE 2.10 (a) Real-time 3D TEE image in full volume modality cropped properly to visualize the anterior mitral leaflet (AML) from an "en face" perspective and (b) the corresponding anatomical specimen. This unique viewpoint clearly reveals the roughly triangular shape of the leaflet. *LV* left ventricle; *LA*l efta trium.

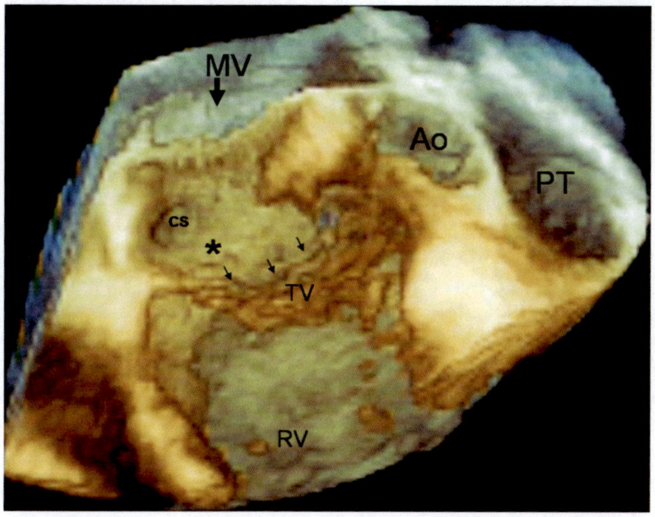

FIGURE 2.11 3D TEE image in full volume showing part of the right atrium and ventricle (RV) after cropping the antero-lateral portion of the heart. The cut visualizes the entry of the coronary sinus (CS) into the right atrium. Once the ostium of the CS and the septal hinge line of the tricuspid valve (*arrows*) are identified, the isthmus in between can be clearly visualized (*asterisk*). This isthmus is the so-called "septal" isthmus that is ablated to interrupt the "slow" pathway in atrio-ventricular nodal reentrant tachycardia. *Ao* aorta; *MV* mitral valve; *PT* pulmonary trunk.

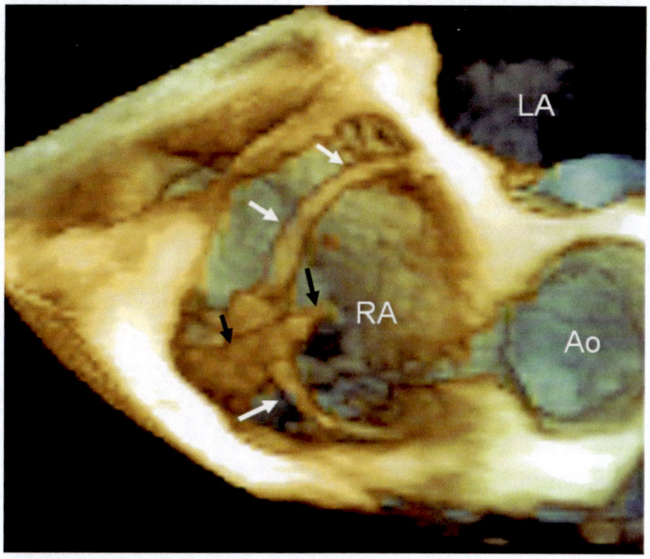

FIGURE 2.12 Real-time 3D TEE image in zoom modality showing two catheters in the right atrium (RA; *black* and *white arrows*). One of them (*white arrows*) can be followed for a long tract into the RA cavity. *LA* left atrium; *Ao* aorta.

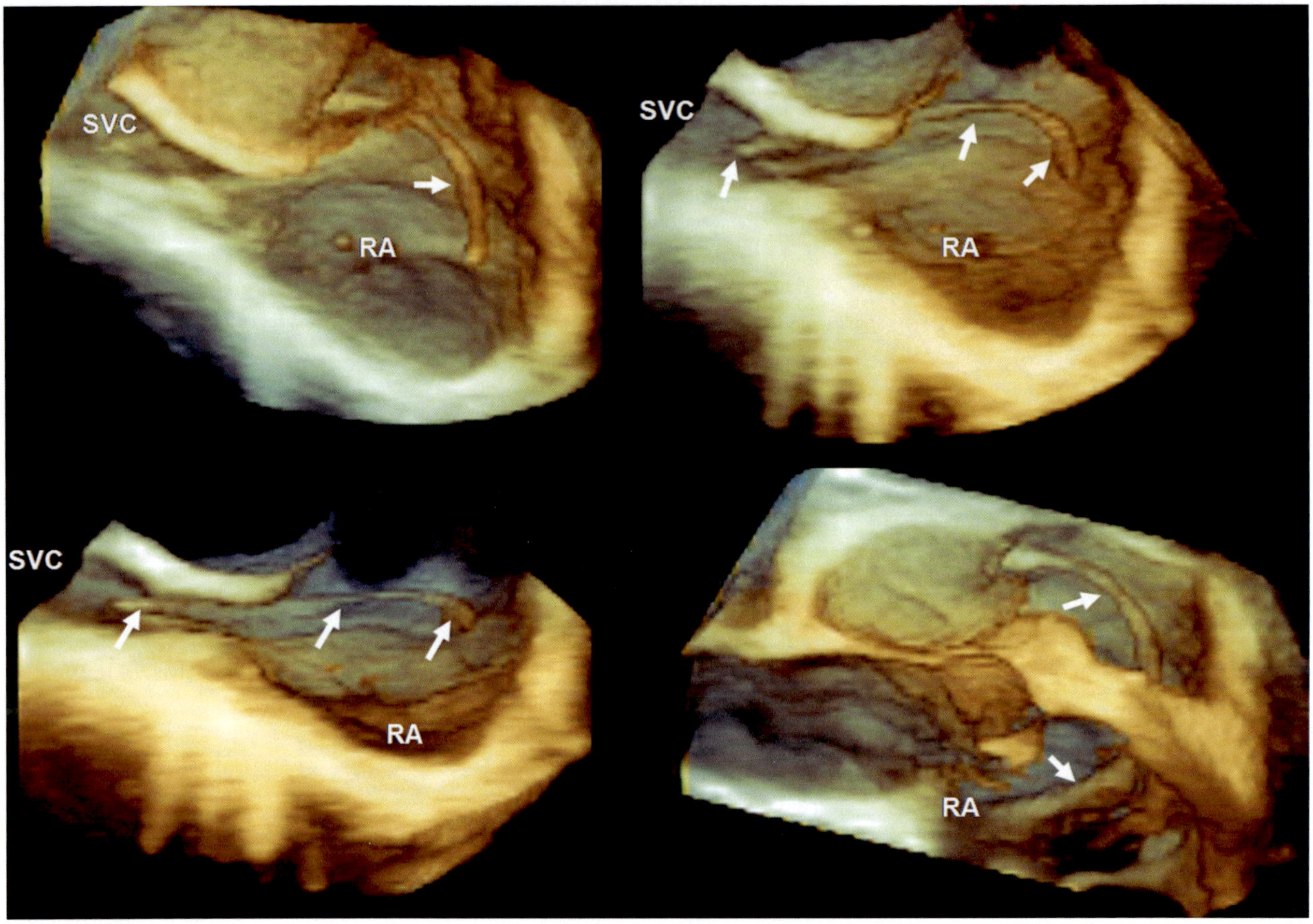

FIGURE 2.13 Real-time 3D TEE image in zoom modality showing how with proper cuts the entire course of the catheter (*arrows*) from the superior vena cava (SVC) into the right atrium (RA) is revealed.

CHAPTER 3

The Mitral Valve

Three-dimensional TEE offers impressive, high quality images of the mitral valve, as seen from both the atrial and ventricular perspectives. These superb views are achieved by an ideal, perpendicular angle of incidence of the ultrasound beam as well as a close proximity of the transducer to the mitral valve. The atrial perspective offers an optimal viewpoint that simulates the exposed view during cardiac surgery, and it is one of the most useful views for evaluating the finest anatomical details of the valve (see Movie 3.1).

MOVIE 3.1 The atrial perspective offers an optimal viewpoint that simulates a "surgical perspective".

Mitral annulus: From an atrial perspective, the mitral annulus (or hingeline) can be recognized as a roughly elliptical line to which leaflets are anchored at the atrioventricular junction in a D-shaped configuration (Fig. 3.1). The longest diameter runs from commissure to commissure at the ends of the zone of coaptation, whereas the shortest runs through the midpoint of the anterior leaflet (AML) to the midpoint of the posterior (mural) leaflet. As seen in Fig. 3.2, real-time 3D TEE allows a reader to view two portions of the annulus, which are of different consistency: the anterior portion (the straight line of the "D" indicated by arrows) and the posterior portion (the curved line of the "D" marked with a black dotted line). When seen from the atrial perspective, the anterior portion forms a robust hinge connecting the annulus with the base of the aorta (known as the mitral-aortic curtain). The posterior portion forms a C-shaped ring connecting the atrial and ventricular myocardium. The fine structure of the mitral-aortic curtain can be seen from the ventricular perspective in real-time 3D TEE by cropping the ventricular myocardium, creating a view that is shared only with pathologists (Fig. 3.3). When imaged from this viewpoint, the anterior portion of the annulus disappears, and a fibrous sheet is seen connecting the anterior leaflet with the inter-leaflet triangle beneath the left coronary and noncoronary aortic leaflets.

The annulus is not lying in a single plane; rather, it has a 3D "saddle-shaped" configuration. Peaks are located in the midpoint of the anterior and posterior segments (shortest diameter), whereas corresponding valleys lie near commissures (longest diameter). Seen from an atrial perspective, the saddle-shaped configuration cannot be appreciated (Fig. 3.4). Figures 3.5 and 3.6 show a cut plane

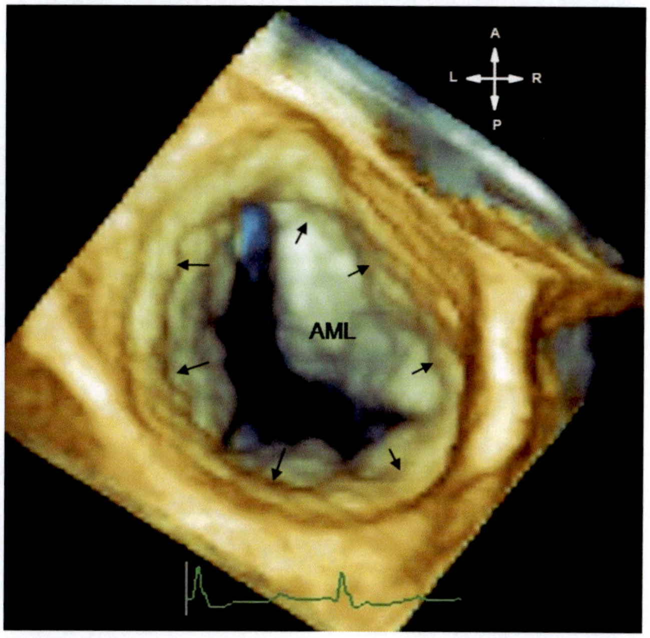

FIGURE 3.1 Real-time 3D TEE visualization of the mitral annulus and mitral leaflets in zoom modality from the atrial perspective. The *black arrows* indicate a roughly elliptical line to which the leaflets are anchored. This line likely corresponds to the mitral annulus. *AML* anterior mitral leaflet.

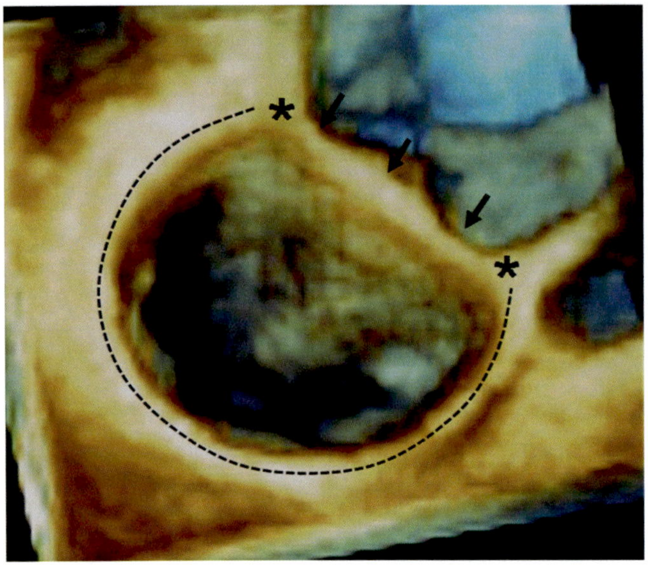

FIGURE 3.2 Real-time 3D TEE visualization of the mitral annulus and mitral leaflets in zoom modality from the atrial perspective. The *arrows* point to the anterior portion of the annulus, while the *dotted line* corresponds to the posterior portion. The anterior portion is a relatively robust hinge of connective tissue ending on two fibrous trigones (*asterisks*). The maximum stress on the mitral valve is at these trigones. The clinical implication is that all annuloplasties must be anchored to the trigones for firm support. The posterior portion is rather heterogeneous, with gaps in fibrous continuity. The posterior portion is therefore weaker than the anterior portion, and more frequently it contributes to annular dilation and calcification.

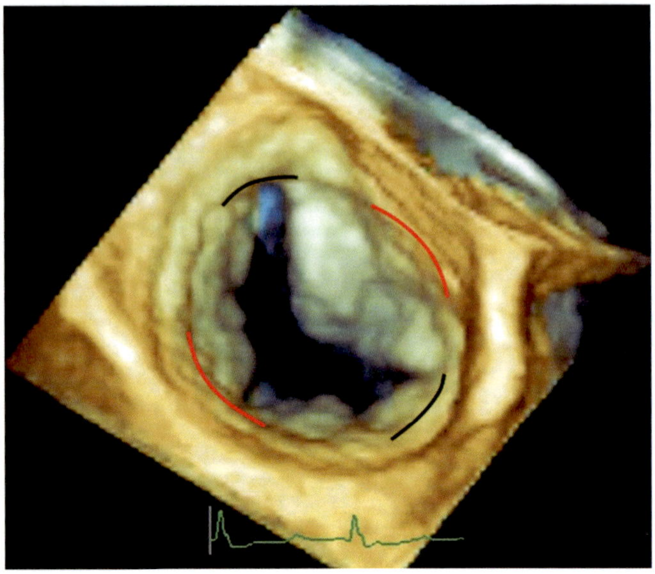

FIGURE 3.4 Real-time 3D TEE of the mitral annulus. *Red lines* mark "peak" segments and *black lines* mark respective "valleys." From the atrial perspective, all four segments seem to be placed in the same plane. The difference in shades of colors does not allow perception of the different heights of the four segments.

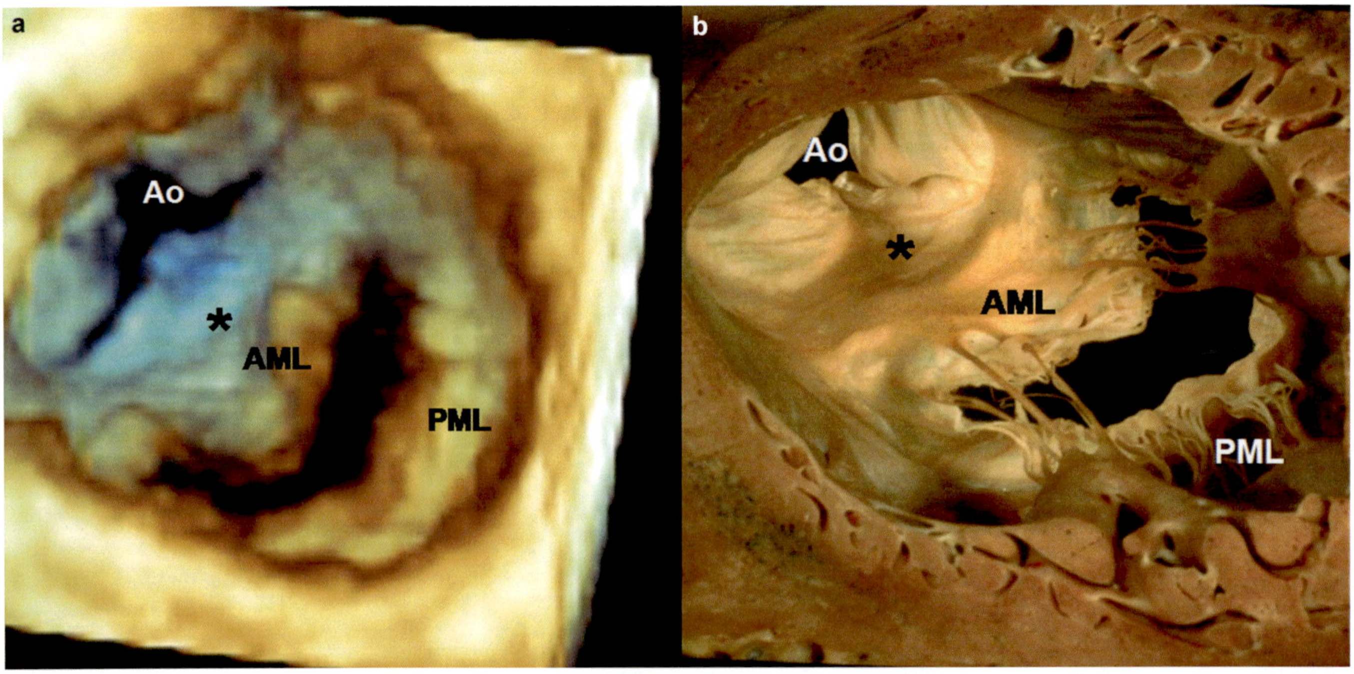

FIGURE 3.3 (a) Real-time 3D TEE of the mitral valve from the ventricular perspective and (b) the corresponding anatomic specimen. The *asterisks* mark the interleaflet triangle. From this perspective, it is clear that there is no well-defined fibrous mitral hinge, but rather a sheet of fibrous tissue that connects the anterior mitral leaflet with the interleaflet triangle. From this perspective, the mitral and aortic valves can be seen sharing a part of the annulus and, hence, can be considered as a single anatomic and functional unit, like a roof on the left ventricle with an entry and an exit. *AML* anterior mitral leaflets; *PML* posterior mitral leaflet; *Ao* aorta.

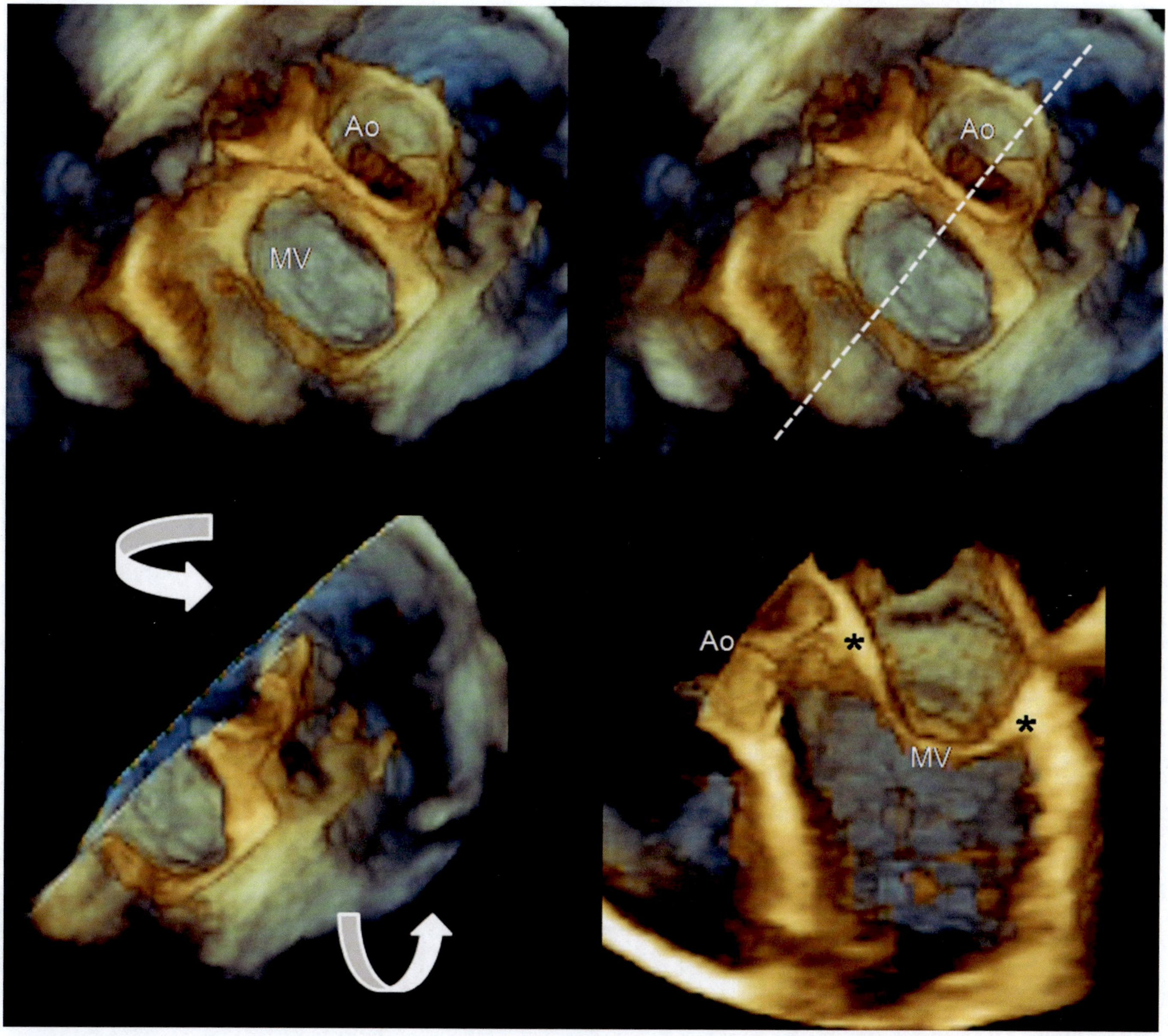

FIGURE 3.5 (a) 3D TEE of a mitral valve from atrial perspective. (b) The image shows the cut plane passing through the "peaks" of the annulus (dotted line), while (c) shows the remaining lateral half after the digital removal of the medial half. The two *curved arrows* mimic the right-to-left rotation and the down-to-up inclination, to obtain needed image (d) in which the *asterisks* identify the hinge-points of the anterior and posterior mitral leaflet. Note that the aortic "peak" is located at a higher point than the posterior peak. *Ao* aorta; *MV* mitral valve.

passing through the peaks and valleys. The planes obtained show the different heights of annular segments.

Mitral leaflets: The normal mitral valve has two leaflets, that are conventionally described as anterior and posterior leaflets separated by two commissures. Commissures and leaflets can be imaged superbly by real-time 3D TEE from both the atrial and ventricular perspectives (Fig. 3.7).

Using real-time 3D TEE imaging, the "anterior" leaflet is seen as truly antero-medial, lying very close to the aortic valve, while the "posterior" leaflet is more accurately postero-lateral. The anterior leaflet has a triangular-shaped free edge and occupies one-third of the annular circumference. However, being deeper than the posterior leaflet, the overall areas of the mitral valve closed by each leaflet are equivalent (Fig. 3.8). Figure 3.9 shows the mitral valve in closed position. The line of coaptation (arrows) is curved, governed by the different shapes of the two leaflets.

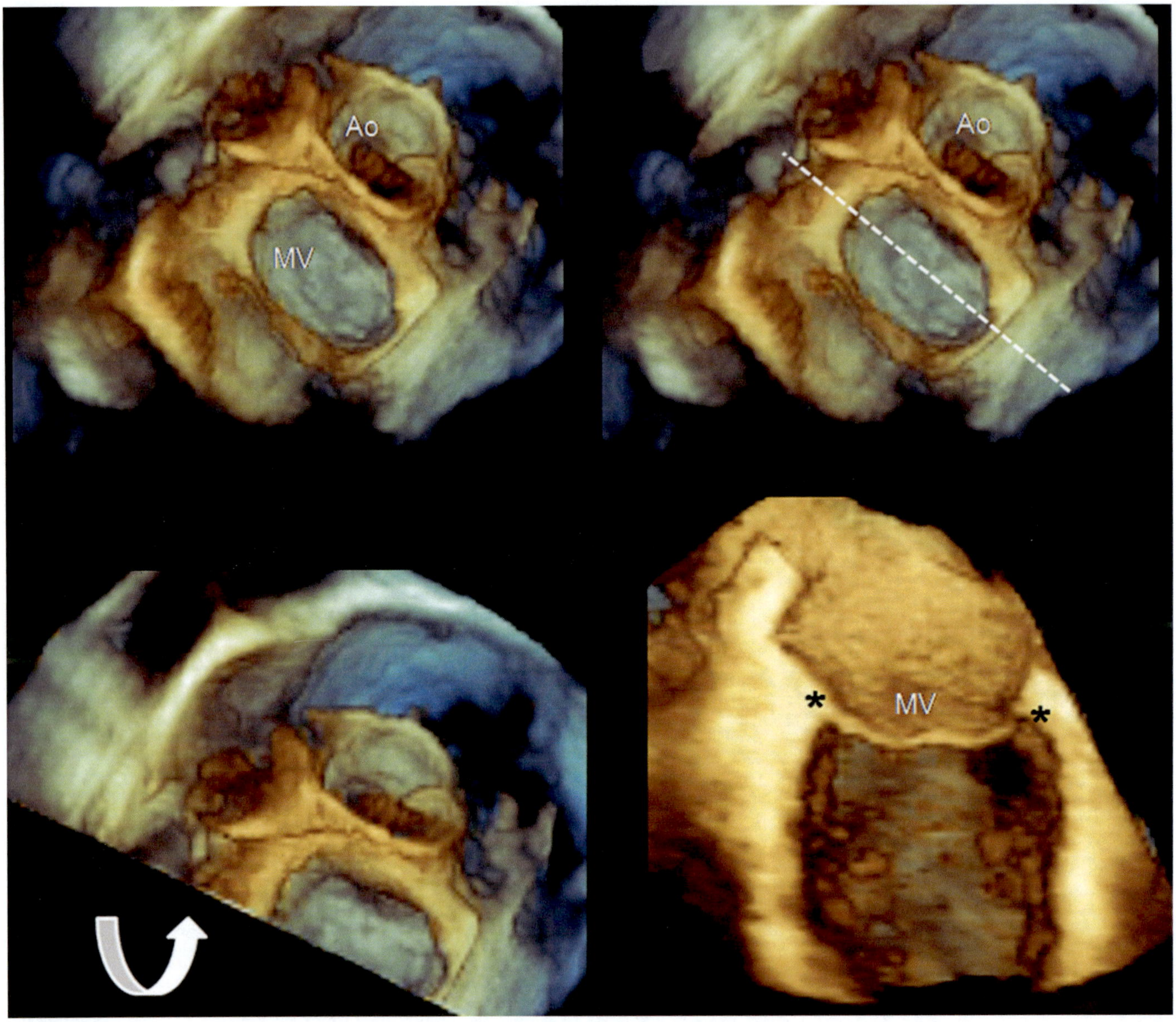

FIGURE 3.6 A four panel 3D TEE image showing the cut plane passing through the "valleys" of the annulus (*dotted line*). In (d) the *asterisks* identify the hinge-points of the mitral leaflets. In this case the hinge-points are located at the same height. Figure (d) is the equivalent to the 2-chamber view obtained with 2D TEE. *Ao* aorta; *MV*m itral valve.

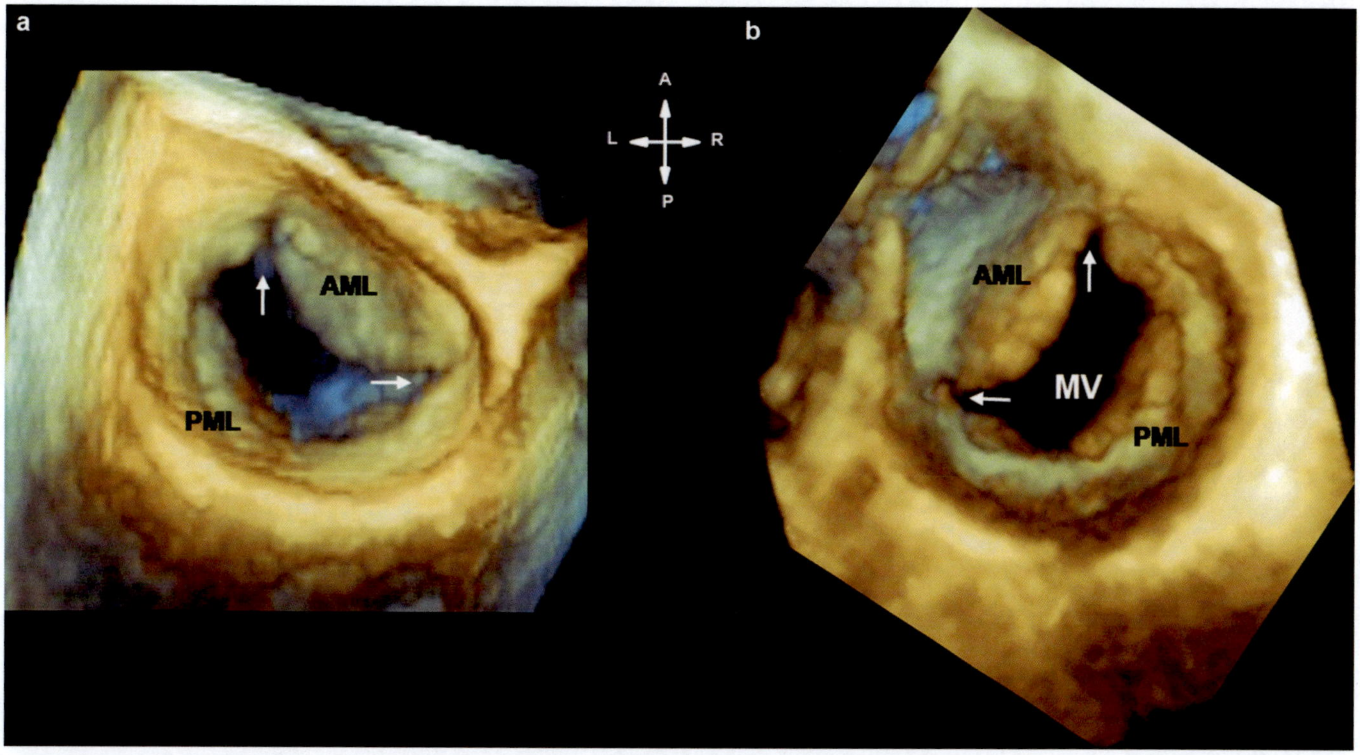

FIGURE 3.7 Real-time 3D TEE from (a) the atrial perspective and (b) the ventricular perspective. The arrows point to the two commissures. As the images demonstrate, the commissures do not reach the annulus, but rather end 3–5 mm before the insertion point. Thus, from a strictly anatomic point of view, the mitral leaflets are hinged along the entire annular circumference and can be considered a single veil. MV mitral valve; AML anterior mitral leaflet; PML posterior mitral leaflet.

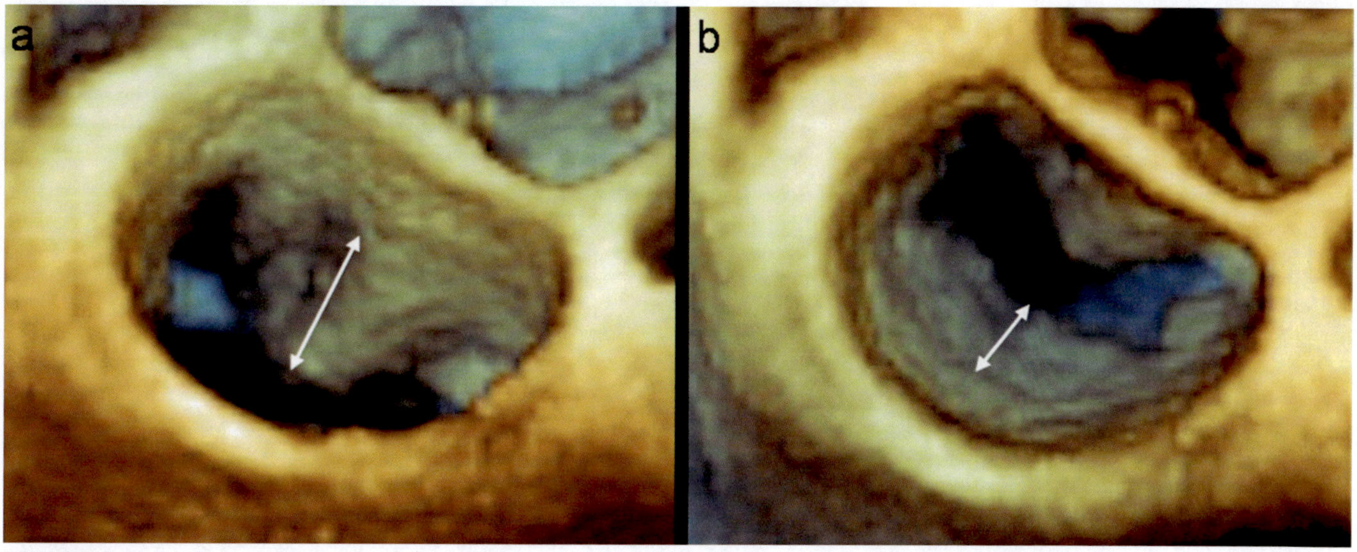

FIGURE 3.8 Real-time 3D TEE of the mitral annulus and mitral leaflets from the atrial perspective in mid-diastole. Two slightly different angulations are shown that optimize the visualization of (a) the anterior leaflet and (b) the posterior leaflet. One of the main advantages of 3D TEE is the ability to rotate or angulate an image while maintaining the relationships between various structures. In this case, the same image was angulated to visualize the depth of anterior (panel a) and posterior (panel b) leaflets (*arrows*).

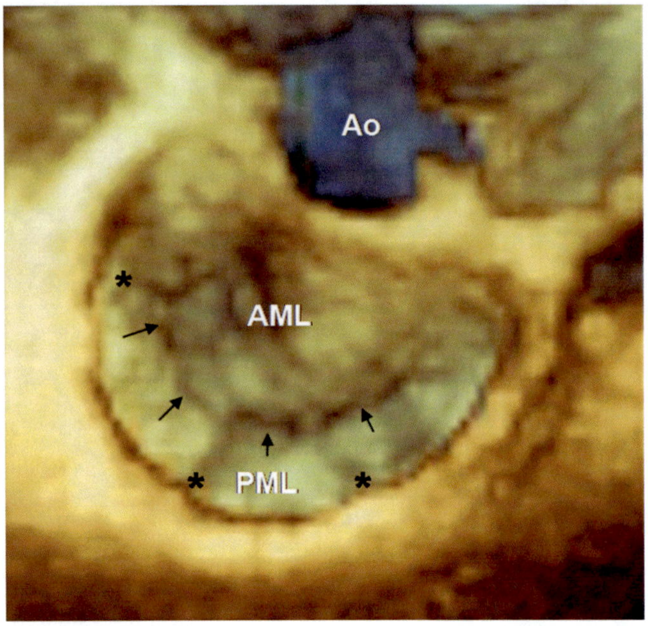

FIGURE 3.9 The mitral valve in the closed position. The *black arrows* indicate the line of coaptation of the two leaflets. The *asterisks* mark the line of coaptation between the scallops. *PML* posterior mitral leaflet; *AML* anterior mitral leaflet; *Ao*a orta.

Small indentations, known as clefts, typically divide the posterior leaflets into three scallops (Fig. 3.10). However, in many instances, particularly when the valve tissue is redundant, there can be four or more scallops. By properly cropping the volume data set, sections comparable to that of 2D TEE can be obtained (Figs. 3.11–3.13), making real-time 3D TEE an intuitively educational tool.

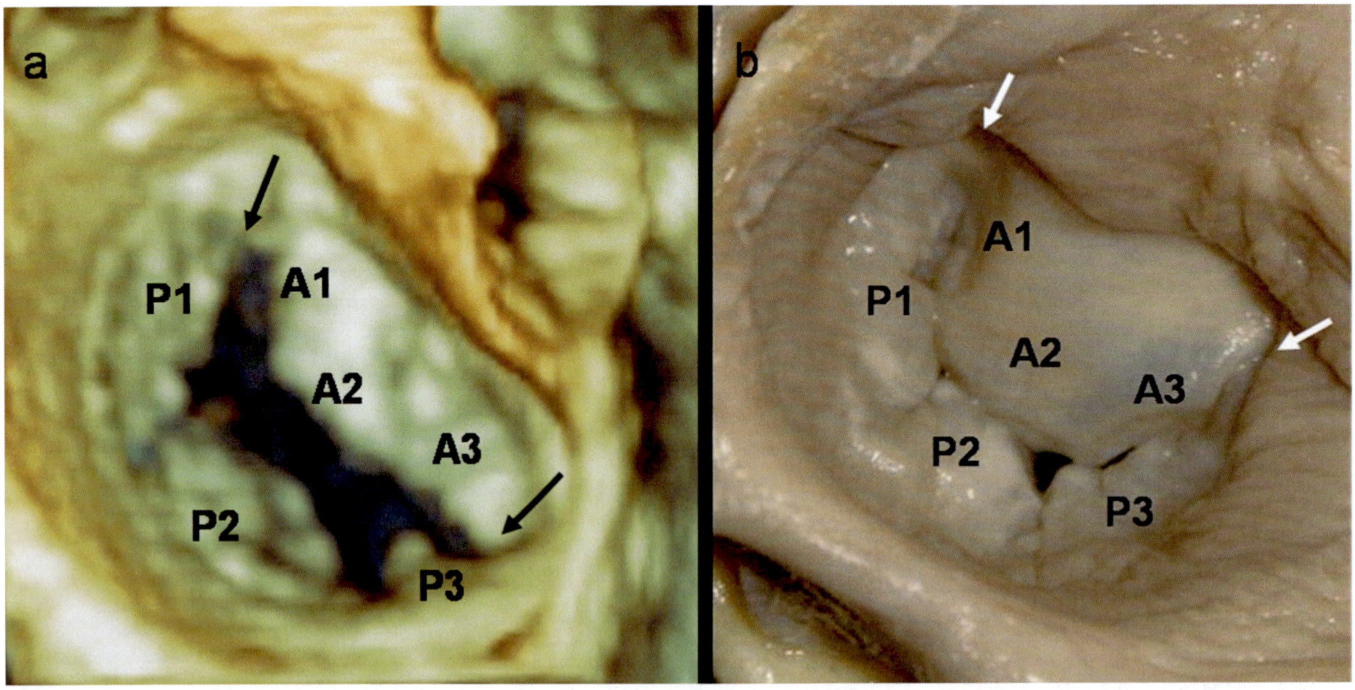

FIGURE 3.10 (a) Real-time 3D TEE image of the mitral valve in mid-diastole and (b) the corresponding anatomical specimen from the atrial perspective. The scallops of the posterior leaflet are clearly visualized. Following Carpentier's classification, these scallops are labeled from lateral to medial as P1, P2, P3 ("P" indicating the posterior leaflet), arbitrarily dividing the leaflet into thirds. The corresponding areas of the anterior leaflet are termed A1, A2, A3, although no anatomic indentations can be observed. The *arrows* point to the two commissures at thee ndo ft hel ineo fc oaptation.

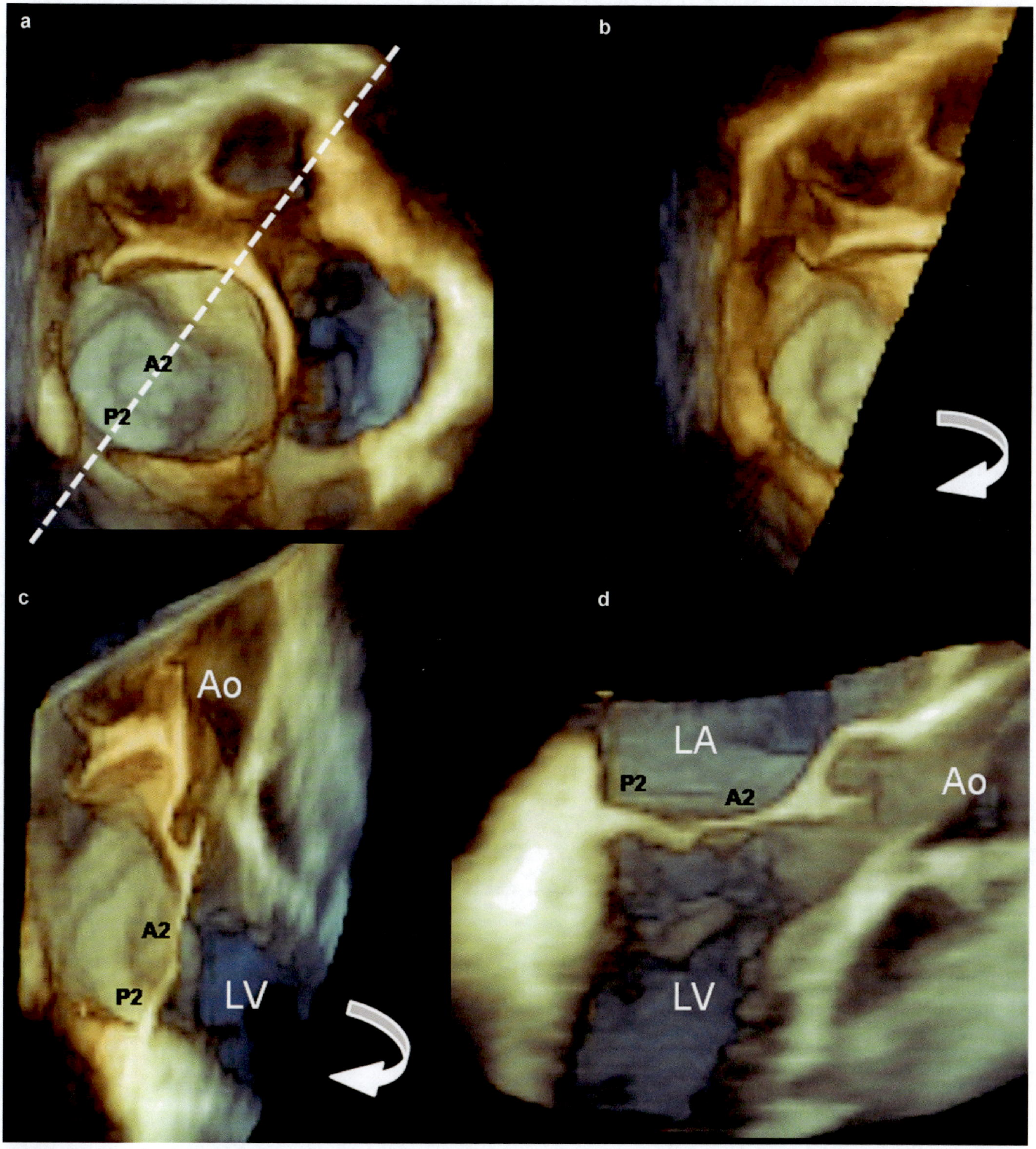

FIGURE 3.11 A four panel 3D TEE image in full volume modality. (a) By using a cutting plane (*dotted line*) passing through the middle part of the A2-P2, the heart is divided in two halves. (b) The posterior oblique half of the heart is then "electronically" removed. (c) The anterior-oblique half of the heart is rotated (*arrows*) to obtain a longitudinal view. (d) Shows a long-axis plane which approximates 2D TEE long axis view, confirming that with this section the middle part of A2 and P2 are visualized. *Ao* aorta; *LA* left atrium; *RA* right atrium; *LV* left ventricle; *RV*r ightv entricle.

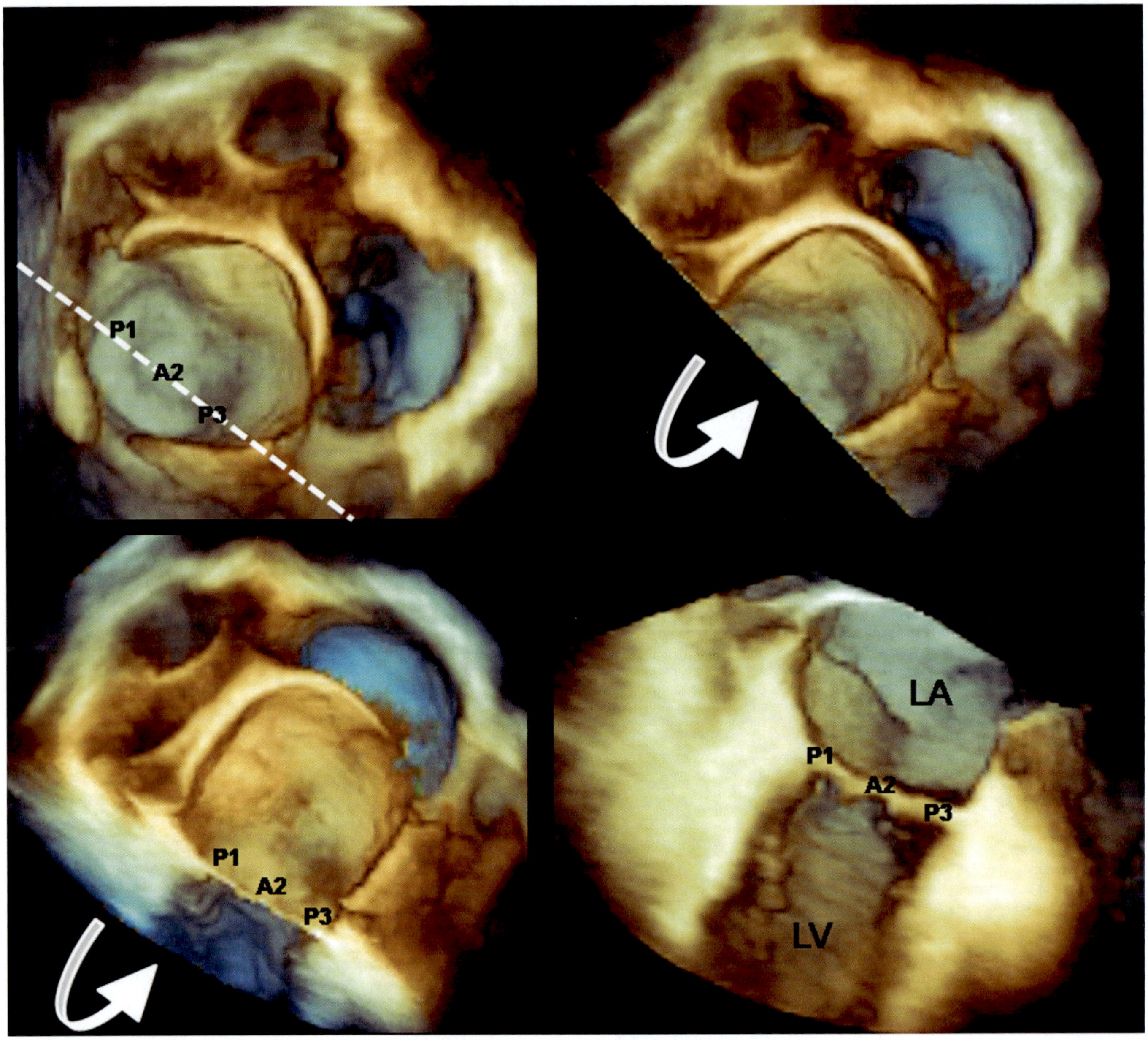

FIGURE 3.12 A four panel 3D TEE image in full volume modality. (a) P1, A2, and P3 can be seen. A cutting plane passing through the coapting line (*dotted line*) divides the volume data set in two halves. (b) The smaller postero-lateral piece is digitally removed. By rotating the antero-medial piece as noted in (b) and (c), a section (d) that approximates the 2-chamber view of the 2D TEE is obtained. This section confirms that the cutting plane passes through P1, A2, and P3. *LA*l efta trium; *LV* left ventricle; *RV* right ventricle.

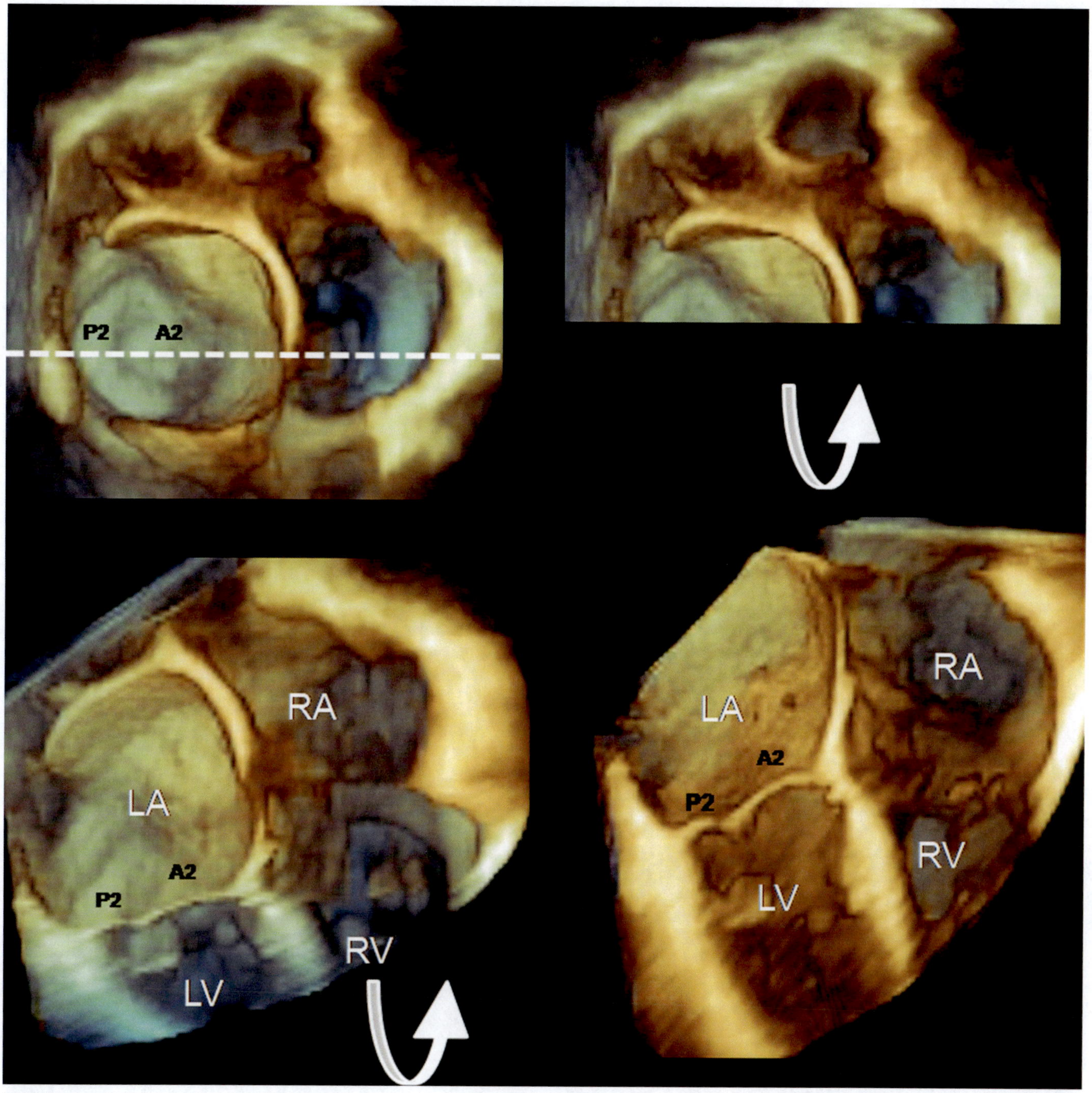

FIGURE 3.13 In this four panel 3D TEE image, the cutting plane passes perpendicularly to the atrial septum (*dotted line*) to obtain a 4-chamber section in (d). In this section, A2 and P2 are imaged. When compared to the long-axis plane (Fig. 3.11d), A2 and P2 are cut obliquely. *LA* left atrium; *RA* right atrium; *LV* left ventricle; *RV* right ventricle.

3.1 3D TEE EXAMPLES OF MITRAL VALVE DISEASE

Real-time 3D TEE will most likely become the imaging modality of choice for evaluating anatomical abnormalities underlying mitral valve disease. Examples are illustrated below.

3.1.1 Mitral Valve Prolapse/Flail

A systematic 2D TEE examination includes 4-chamber, 2-chamber, and long-axis views from the mid-esophageal position, as well as short-axis and long-axis views from the transgastric position. Depending on operator expertise, countless "off axis" views may also be obtained. In this manner, a comprehensive evaluation with 2D TEE can potentially show nearly every pathologic aspect of mitral valve regurgitation caused by a prolapsed or flail valve. However, the identification of mitral scallops in a given plane may vary according to individual anatomy. A large middle scallop (P2) of the posterior leaflet can occasionally be seen in a 2-chamber view, while a large medial scallop (P3) of the posterior leaflet can be sometimes imaged in the long-axis view. Moreover, misidentification of the "culprit" lesion can occur when echocardiographic planes foreshorten the ventricle. A unique advantage of real-time 3D TEE is that it provides a comprehensive picture of the entire mitral valve in one shot, simulating the surgical view of the valve. Furthermore, flail or prolapsed leaflets imaged from this perspective can be seen in motion. This is a rare and valuable view that cannot be seen even in a surgical setting, as intraoperative hearts are empty and motionless (see Movie 3.2). Figure 3.14 shows a mitral valve in diastole and in systole with a flail in the central region of posterior leaflets (P2) (Movies 3.3 and 3.4). Figure 3.15 shows a comparison with actual anatomy at the time of surgical repair. Figure 3.16 shows a ruptured chordae tendineae in a medial portion of anterior leaflet (A3). Figure 3.17 shows a ruptured chordae tendineae in the central portion of anterior leaflet (A2). See also Movie 3.5.

MOVIE 3.2 A unique advantage of real-time 3D TEE is that it provides a comprehensive picture of the entire mitral valve in one shot, simulating the surgical view of the valve. Furthermore, flail or prolapsed leaflets imaged from this perspective can be seen in movement (indeed, the movie shows P2 flail due to ruptured chordae tendineae). This is a rare and valuable view that cannot be seen even in a surgical setting, as intraoperative hearts are empty and motionless.

MOVIE 3.3 Mitral valve in diastole and in systole with a flail in the central region of posterior leaflet (P2) from atrial perspective.

MOVIE 3.4 Mitral valve in diastole and in systole with a flail in the central region of posterior leaflet from ventricular perspective.

MOVIE 3.5 A ruptured chordae tendineae in a central part of anterior leaflet (A2).

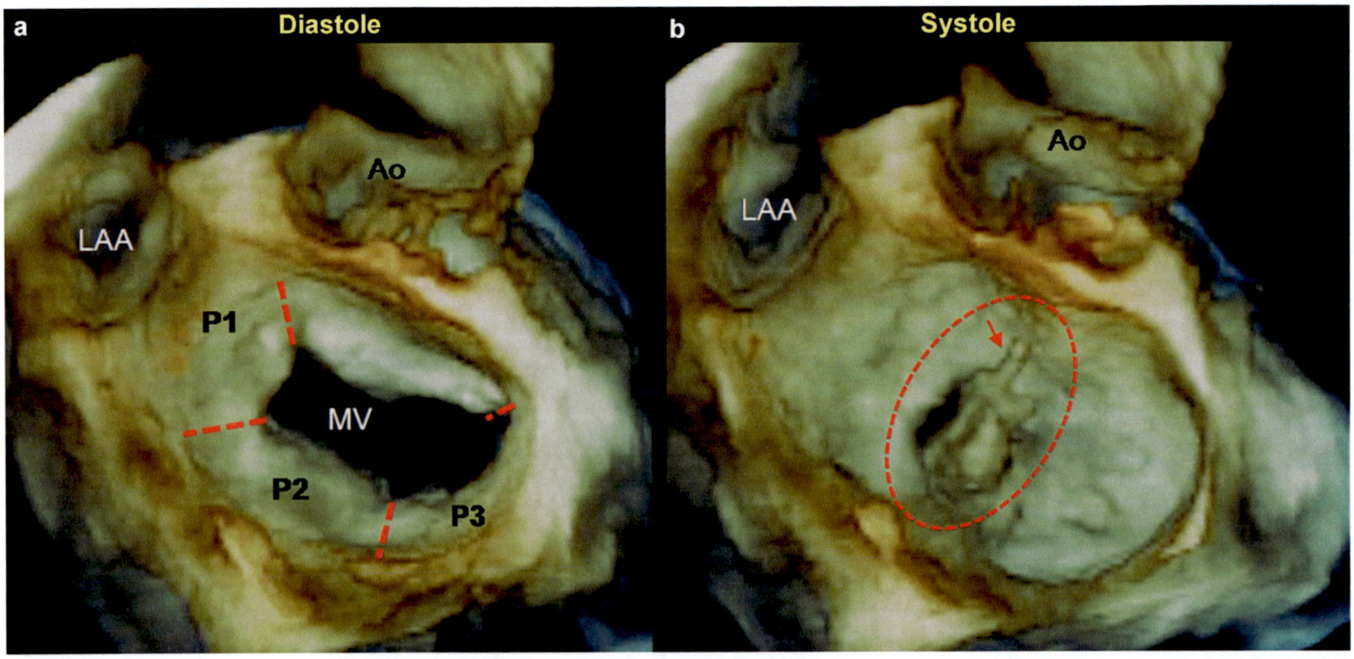

FIGURE 3.14 Real-time 3D TEE image of the mitral valve from the atrial perspective. (a) In the diastolic image, *dotted red lines* roughly divide the posterior leaflet into three scallops. (b) A clear flail of P2 (*dotted red circle*) can be imaged in systole. The fine string-like structure at the margin of P2 is a ruptured cord (*arrow*). *LAA* left atrial appendage; *Ao* aorta; *MV* mitral valve.

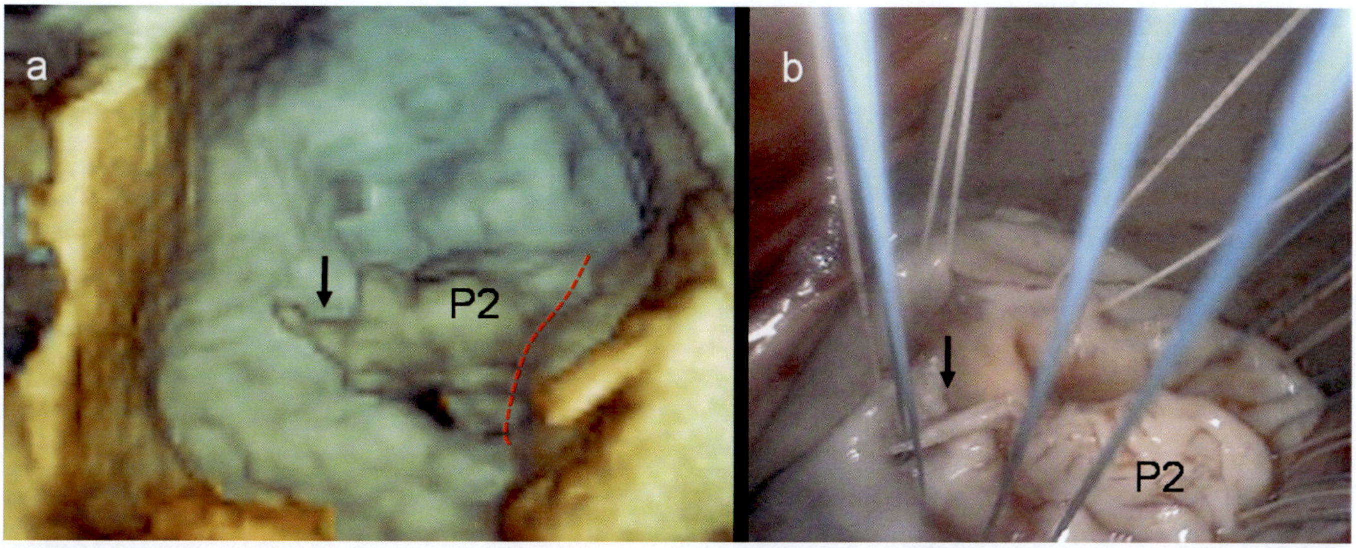

FIGURE 3.15 (a) Real-time 3D TEE of the mitral valve and (b) the corresponding surgical anatomy. The *arrow* points to a ruptured chord. The red dotted line indicates the line of possible surgical resection.

The classic subdivision of the posterior leaflet into three scallops – lateral, middle, and medial – does not always adhere to its anatomical nomenclature. Occasionally, more than three scallops can be seen, while in other cases, the two major indentations that divide the posterior leaflet into three scallops are quite imperceptible. Figure 3.18 shows a large flail segment involving the posterior leaflet. Many scallops can be recognized on the 3D RT TEE image (Movie 3.6). This complex anatomical architecture was later confirmed at surgery.

Not uncommonly, the posterior leaflet of a myxomatous mitral valve has more than three scallops. Figure 3.19 (a) shows the mitral valve of an 84-year-old man with moderate mitral regurgitation caused by myxomatous leaflets. A real-time 3D TEE image from the atrial perspective (a) shows several scallops of the posterior leaflet. (b) A pathologic specimen from a 54-year-old man who died from an aortic dissection showing a myxomatous mitral valve with similar pathological features.

These examples demonstrate the ability of 3D RT TEE to define precisely the pathologic morphology of prolapsed/flail mitral valve tissue. In the future, the use of 3D RT TEE should decrease the necessity of a detailed description of mitral morpho-pathology, since images of the valve in motion can be shown to the surgeon.

MOVIE 3.6 Shows a large flail segment involving the posterior leaflet. Many scallops can be recognized on the 3D RT TEE image. This complex anatomical architecture was confirmed at surgery.

3.1.2 Functional Mitral Regurgitation

It is well established that functional mitral regurgitation (both ischemic and nonischemic) is caused by regional or global geometric ventricular remodeling, without primary valve leaflet pathology. Typically, in ischemic mitral regurgitation, a posterior/inferior scar tethers to the medial part of the valve. This leads to an asymmetrical deformation of the valve apparatus with a regurgitant orifice located primarily on the anterior and posterior medial scallops (A3 and P3, respectively). In nonischemic mitral regurgitation, such as in dilatated cardiomyopathy, the increase in ventricular volume and the global remodeling toward a

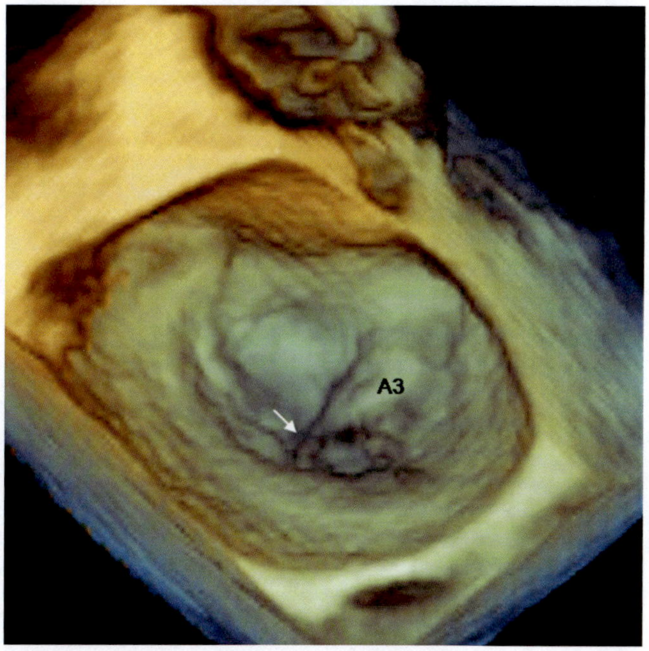

FIGURE 3.16 Real-time 3D TEE image of the mitral valve in zoom modality from the atrial perspective. A ruptured chorda tendinea (*arrow*) in the medial portion of the anterior leaflet (A3) is imaged.

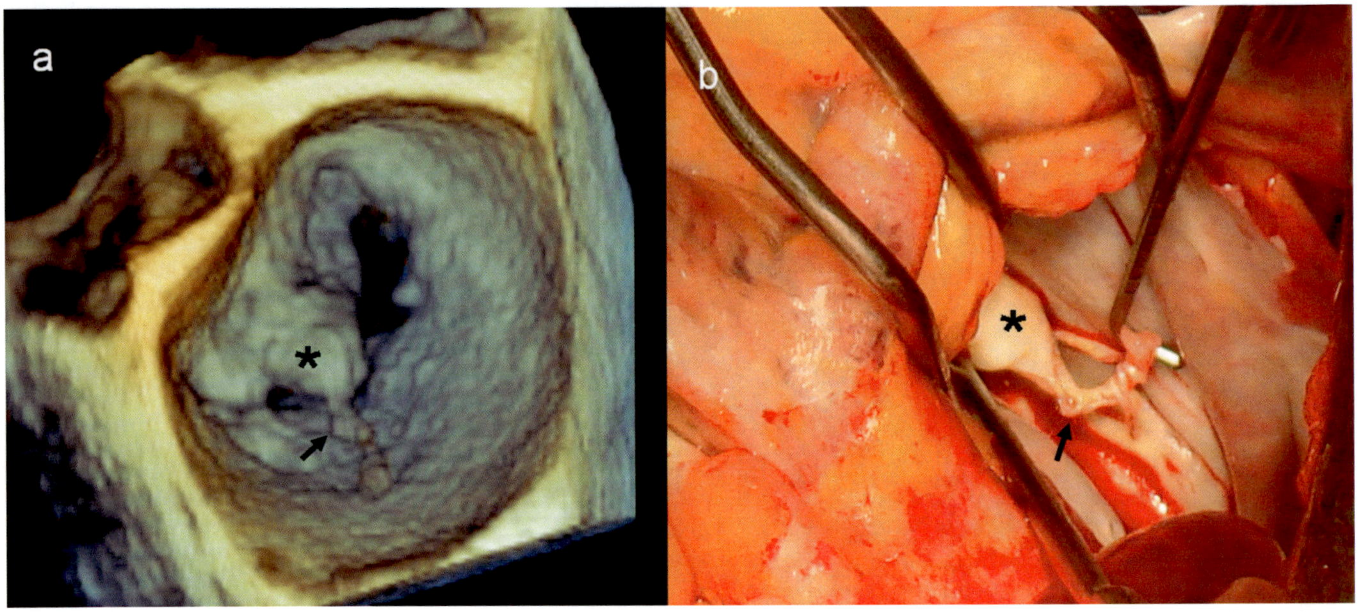

FIGURE 3.17 (a) Real-time 3D TEE image of the mitral valve in zoom modality from the atrial perspective. A ruptured chordae tendineae (*arrow*) is shown in the central portion of the anterior leaflet (*asterisk*); (b) the corresponding surgical anatomy.

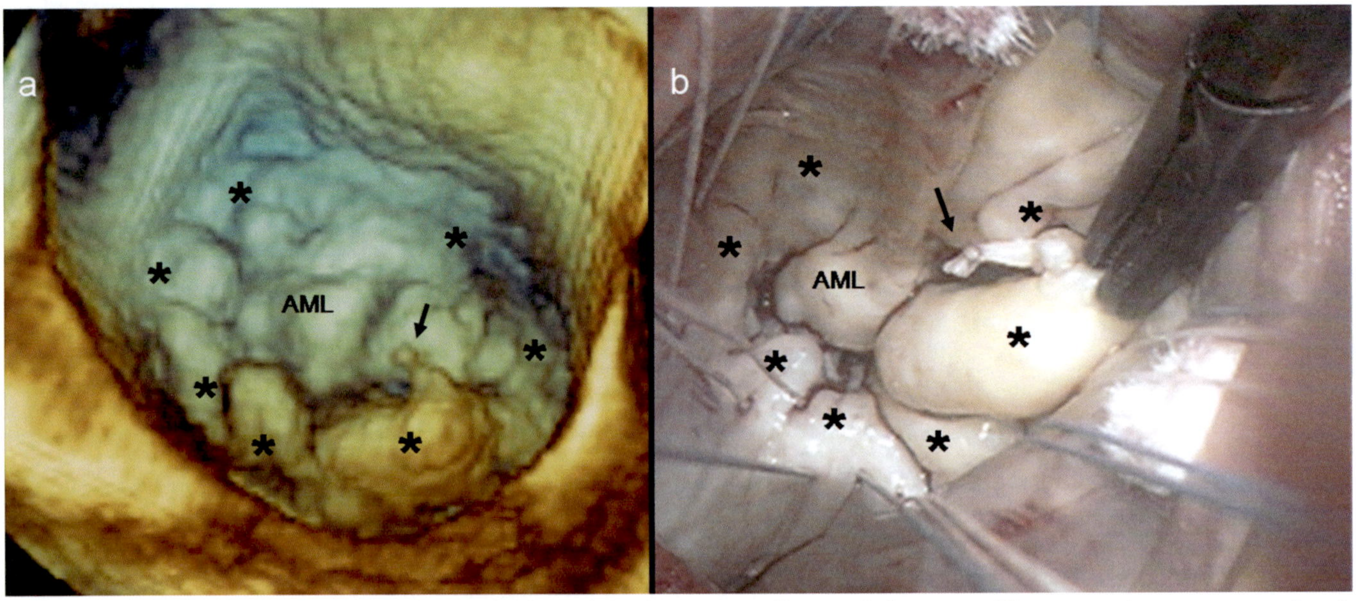

FIGURE 3.18 (a) Real-time 3D TEE of the mitral valve and (b) the corresponding surgical anatomy. The *arrow* points to a ruptured cord. The *asterisks* indicate several scallops forming the posterior leaflets. *AML* anterior mitral leaflet.

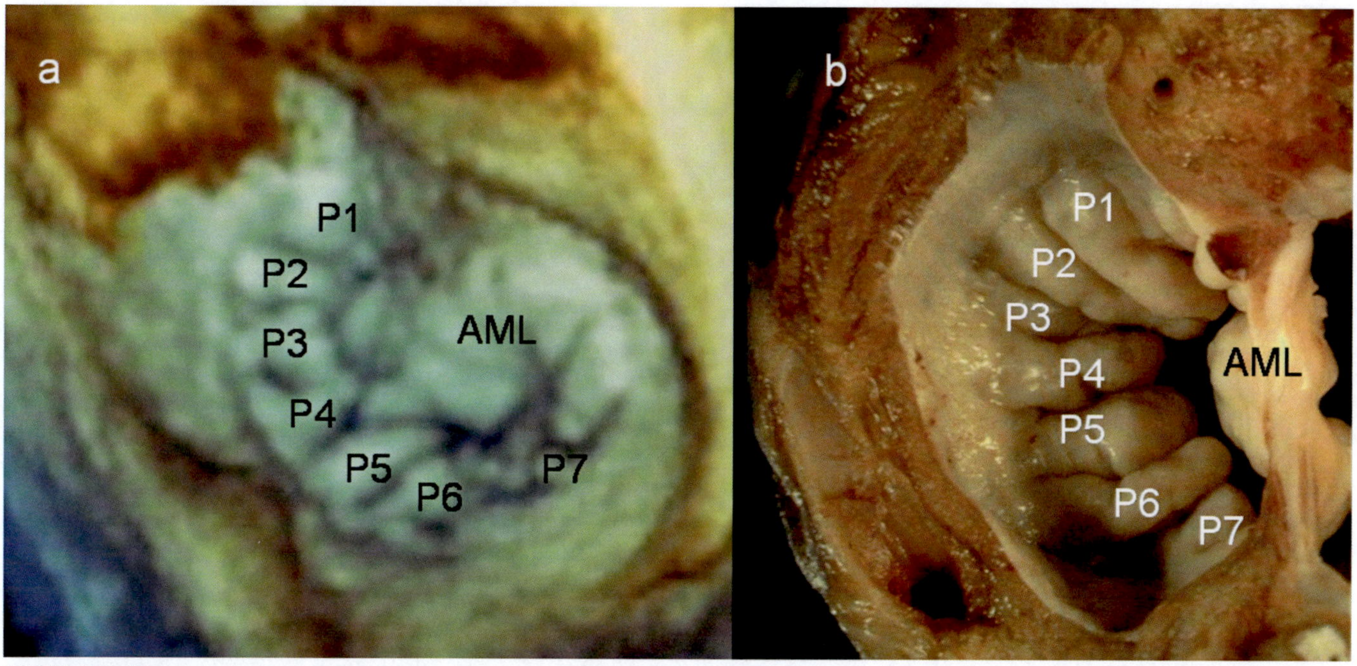

FIGURE 3.19 (a) Real-time 3D TEE of a myxomatous mitral valve with several scallops and (b) an anatomical specimen showing similar pathological features. *P1–P7* scallops of posterior mitral leaflet; *AML* anterior mitral leaflet.

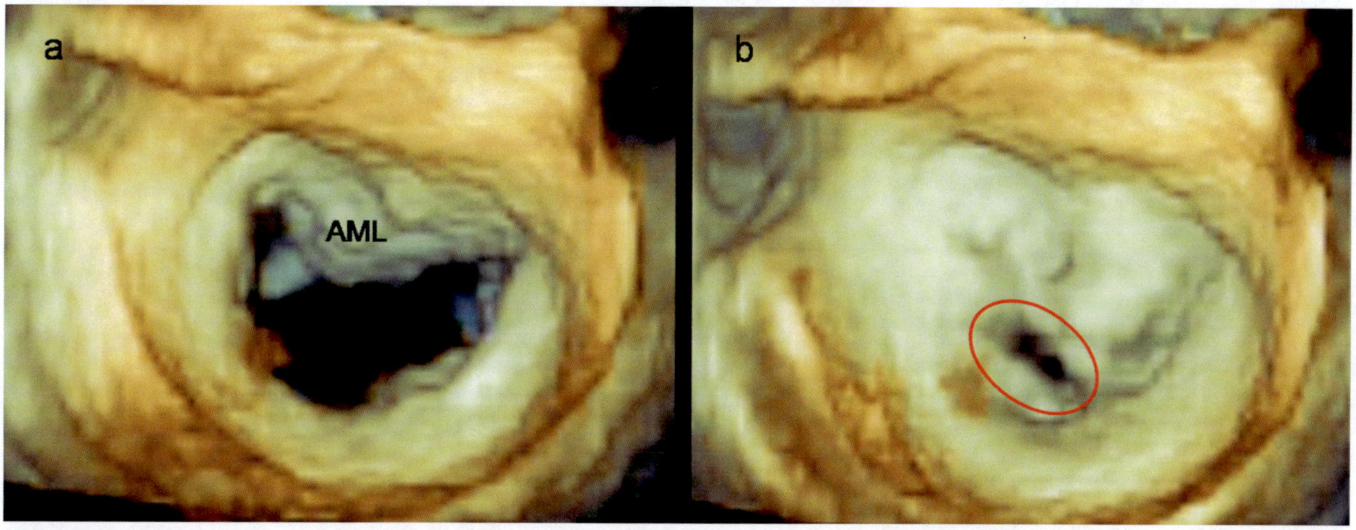

FIGURE 3.20 (a) Ischemic mitral valve in diastole and (b) in systole. A central ellipsoidal regurgitant orifice, mainly due to tethering of P2, is clearly imaged (*red circle*). *AML* anterior mitral leaflet.

globular ventricular shape lead to mitral valve annular dilation and apical displacement of leaflet coaptation. In such settings, mitral regurgitation is mainly due to a "symmetric" loss of coaptation, usually along the entire coaptation line. Mechanisms of regurgitation are even more complex when a localized wall motion abnormality is associated with left ventricular dilatation and globular-shaped remodeling.

A unique ability of real-time 3D TEE is to reveal the site, shape, and magnitude of regurgitant orifices from the atrial perspective. It must be noted that regurgitant orifices can be "mis-imaged" by an inappropriate use of the gain or other control settings on the machine. With a low gain, artifactural holes along the commissural line can appear, whereas with a high gain setting actual regurgitant holes can be diminished or can disappear from view entirely. Therefore, proper setting of gain is critical in evaluating the presence and location of regurgitant orifices. There are no guidelines for establishing the proper gain setting. However, it can generally be

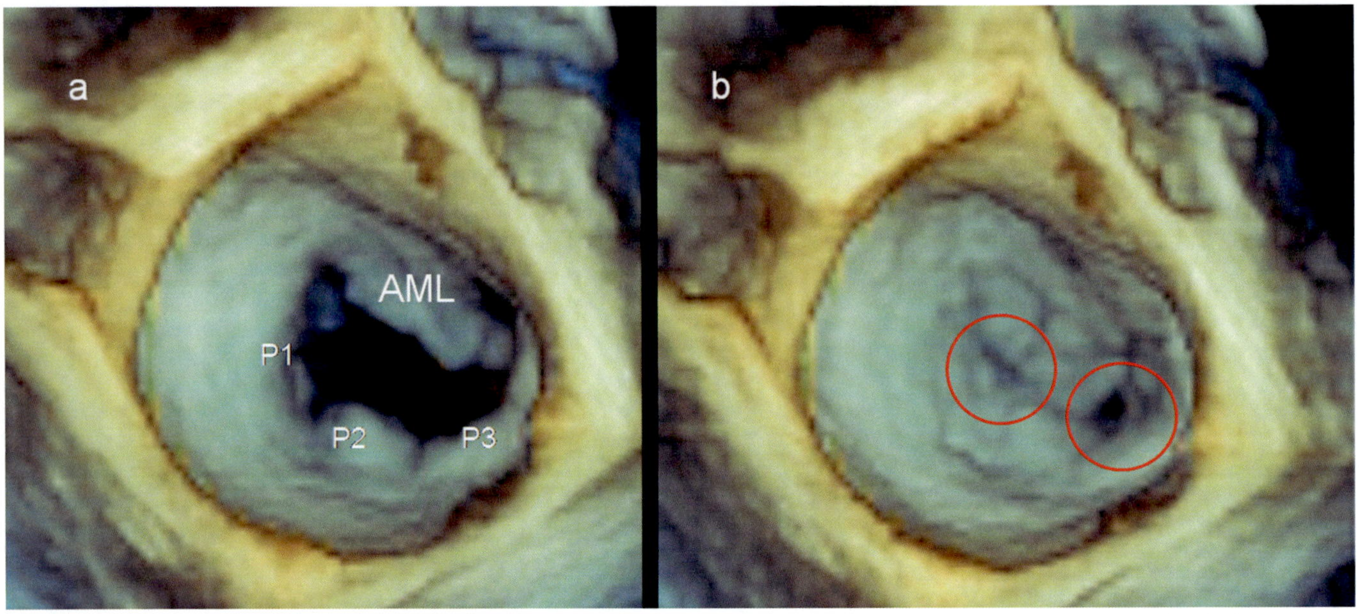

FIGURE 3.21 Ischemic mitral valve (a) in diastole and (b) in systole. Two regurgitant orifices are imaged (*red circles*). The larger one is located medially, corresponding to the P3/A3 area. *AML* anterior mitral leaflet; *P1–P3* scallops of posterior mitral leaflet.

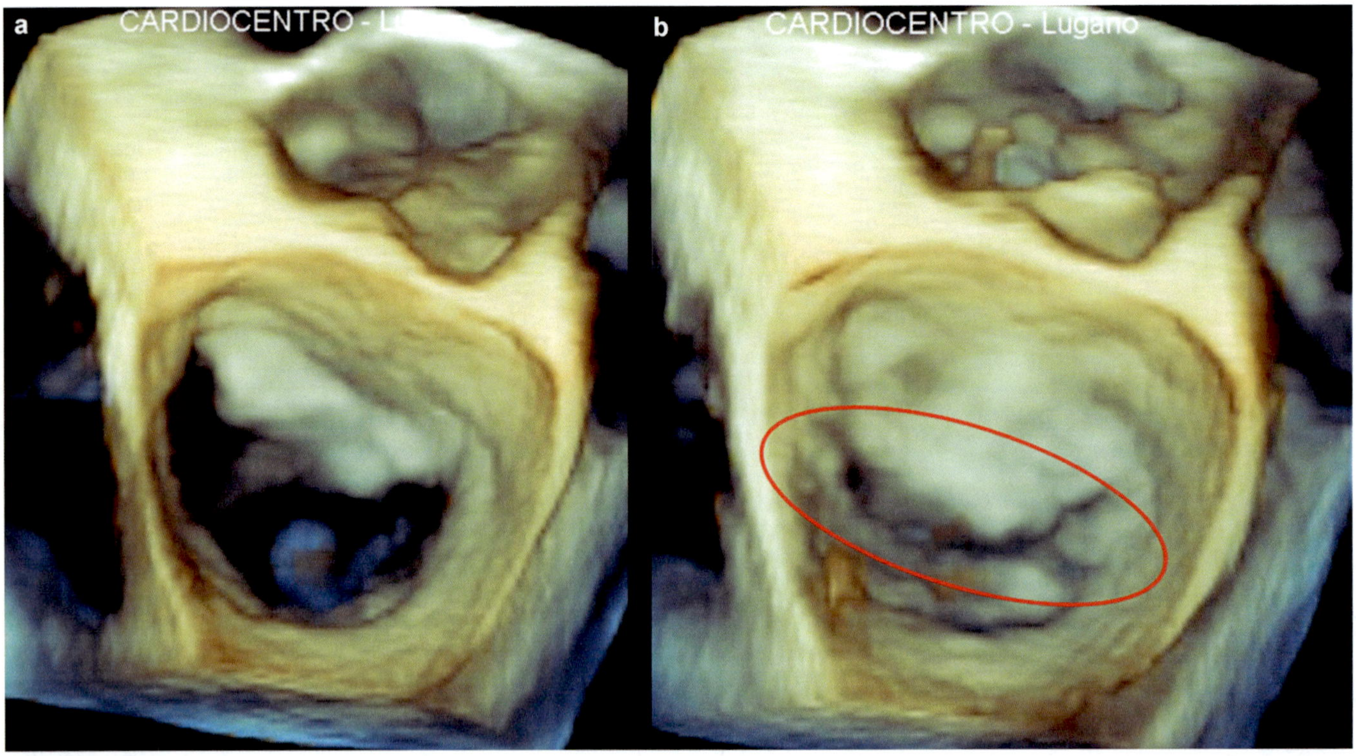

FIGURE 3.22 Ischemic mitral regurgitation associated with globular remodeling (a) in diastole and (b) in systole. In this example, the regurgitant orificei nvolvest heen tirec oaptationl ine.

stated that at a gain setting just below the disappearance of noises (following the usual practice for color Doppler), the presence of orifices is unlikely to be due to image artifacts.

Depending on the complex and mixed mechanisms of functional mitral regurgitation, real-time 3D TEE may show variable shapes of regurgitant orifices, from single to multiple holes. These are typically caused by a failure of the coapting line to form a semilunar-shaped line of complete leaflet closure. Figures 3.20–3.22 demonstrate these pathological features. Movies 3.7 and 3.8 show an ischemic mitral regurgitation with an asymmetric regurgitant orifice located near the medial commissure.

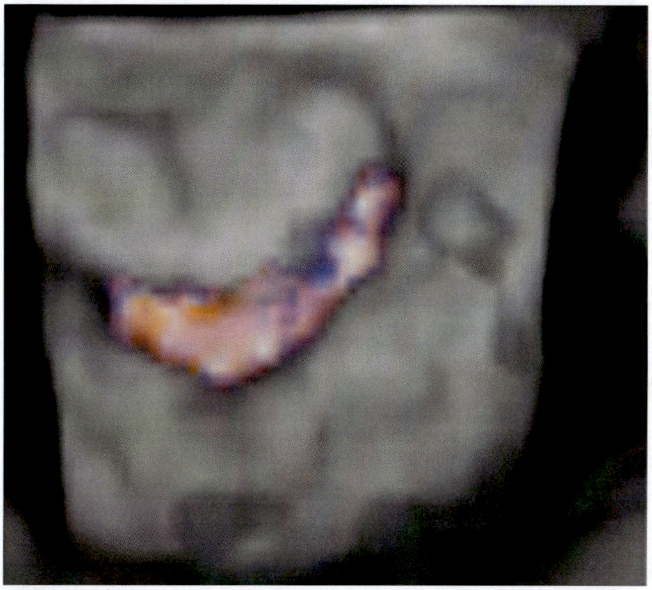

FIGURE 3.23 3D TEE full volume color Doppler image of "vena contracta" from ventricular perspective" (the patient is the same as inFi g.3. 22).

MOVIE 3.7 Ischemic mitral regurgitation with an asymmetric regurgitant orifice located near the medial commissure.

MOVIE 3.8 Same patient of the movie 3.7. Color Doppler full volume modality confirms the localization of regurgitant jet near the medial commissure.

MOVIE 3.9 Two anatomical regurgitant orifices from atrial perspective.

MOVIE 3.10 Same patient of movie 3.9. The two anatomical orifices correspond to two regurgitant jets.

Awareness of this asymmetry might help to avoid underestimation when the proximal isovelocity surface area (PISA) method is used to quantitatively assess the magnitude of mitral regurgitation (Fig. 3.23). Two or more anatomical regurgitant orifices usually correspond to two or more regurgitant jets (Figs. 3.24 and 3.25 and Movies 3.9 and 3.10).

3.1.3 Mitral Stenosis

As in the case of mitral regurgitation, real-time 3D TEE is likely to become the most useful technique for evaluating pathological features of mitral stenosis. Typically, stenotic mitral valves resulting from rheumatic heart disease have funnel-shaped configurations. Therefore, a reliable measurement of such a valve area by planimetry requires imaging the residual mitral orifice in a manner that depicts the valve as the "smallest in the space" and the "greatest in time." One of the limitations of conventional 2D TEE is that these measurements can be achieved only through a transgastric view, without verification that the chosen

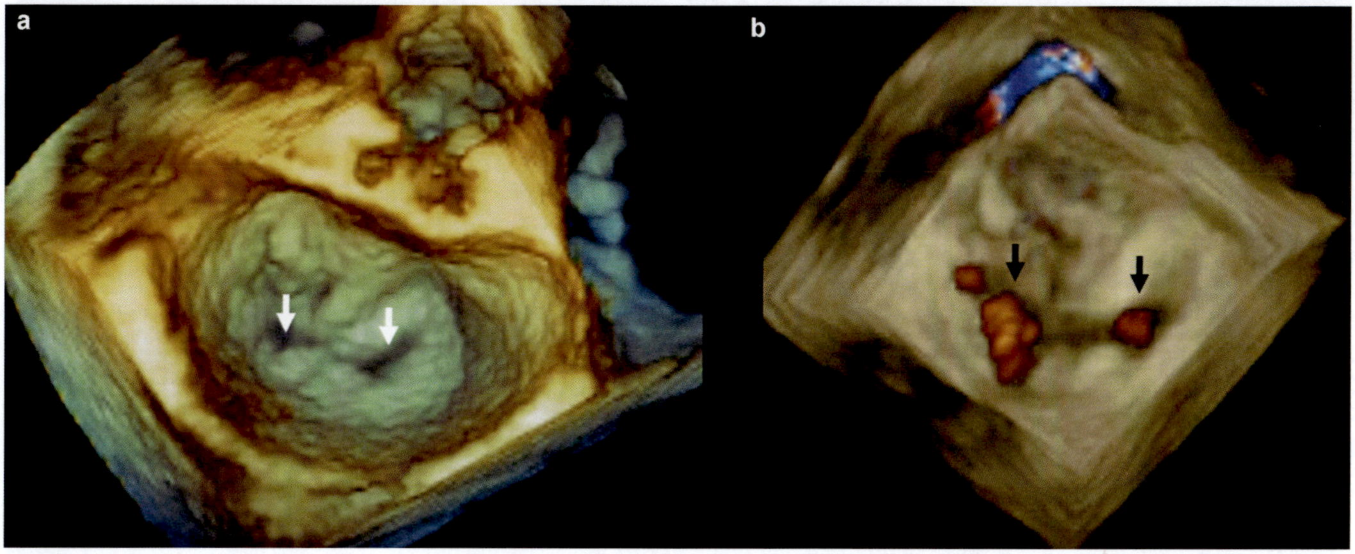

FIGURE 3.24 (a) 3D TEE in zoom modality from the atrial perspective showing an ischemic mitral regurgitation with two regurgitant orifices (*white arrows*) and (b) in full volume color Doppler showing two corresponding regurgitant jets (*black arrows*).

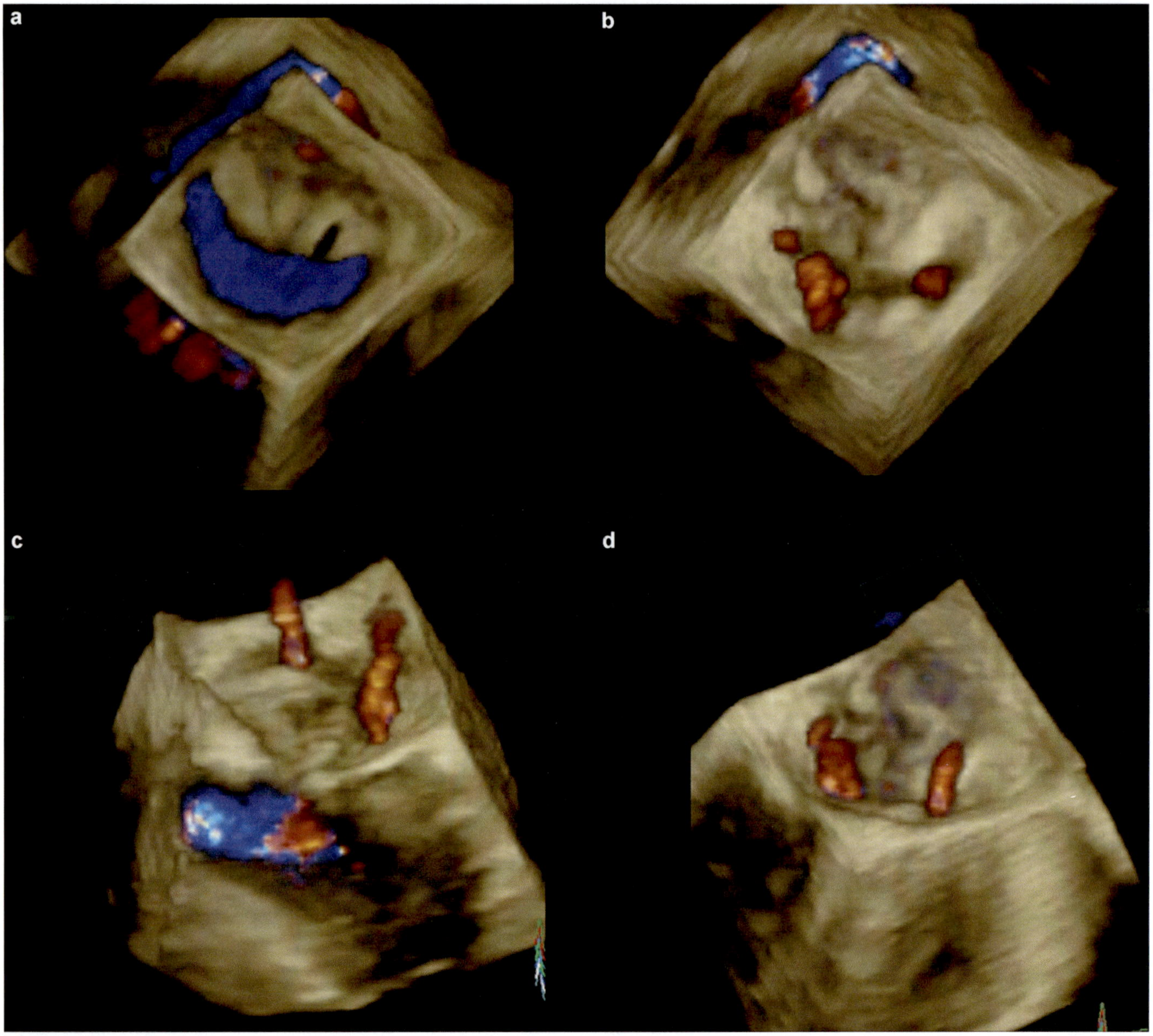

FIGURE 3.25 Same patient as in Fig. 3.24 showing two regurgitant jets from (b) the atrial perspective, (c) the antero-lateral perspective, and (d) the postero-medial perspective. (a) Shows the flowt hrough the mitral valve in middiastole.

plane corresponds to the smallest valve area. With real-time 3D TEE, the narrowest valve orifice is always imaged, both from above and below the mitral valve (the atrial and ventricular perspectives, respectively). Measurements can be properly made by cropping the volume data set at the level of the image plane that corresponds to the smallest area. The fact that the narrowest valve area is always displayed improves accuracy and reduces interobserver variability. Figure 3.26 shows an example of mild stenosis and Fig. 3.27 an example of severe mitral stenosis, with a pathological specimen showing similar morphological features (Movie 3.11).

Figures 3.28 and 3.29 show a calcified valve with mitral stenosis and corresponding surgical specimens from the atrial and ventricular perspectives, respectively. Using real-time 3D TEE, several pathological details of

MOVIE 3.11 An example of mild rheumatic mitral stenosis.

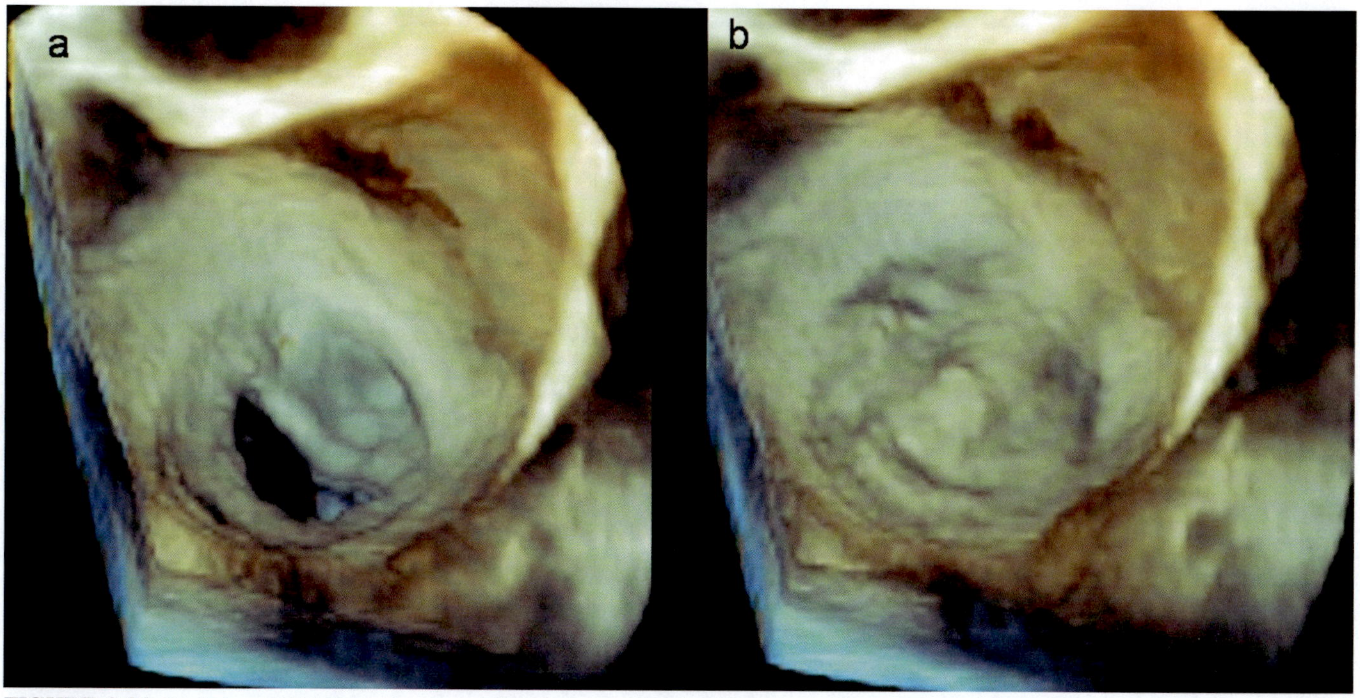

FIGURE 3.26 Real-time 3D TEE in zoom modality showing a mild mitral stenosis from the atrial perspective (a) in diastole and (b) in systole.

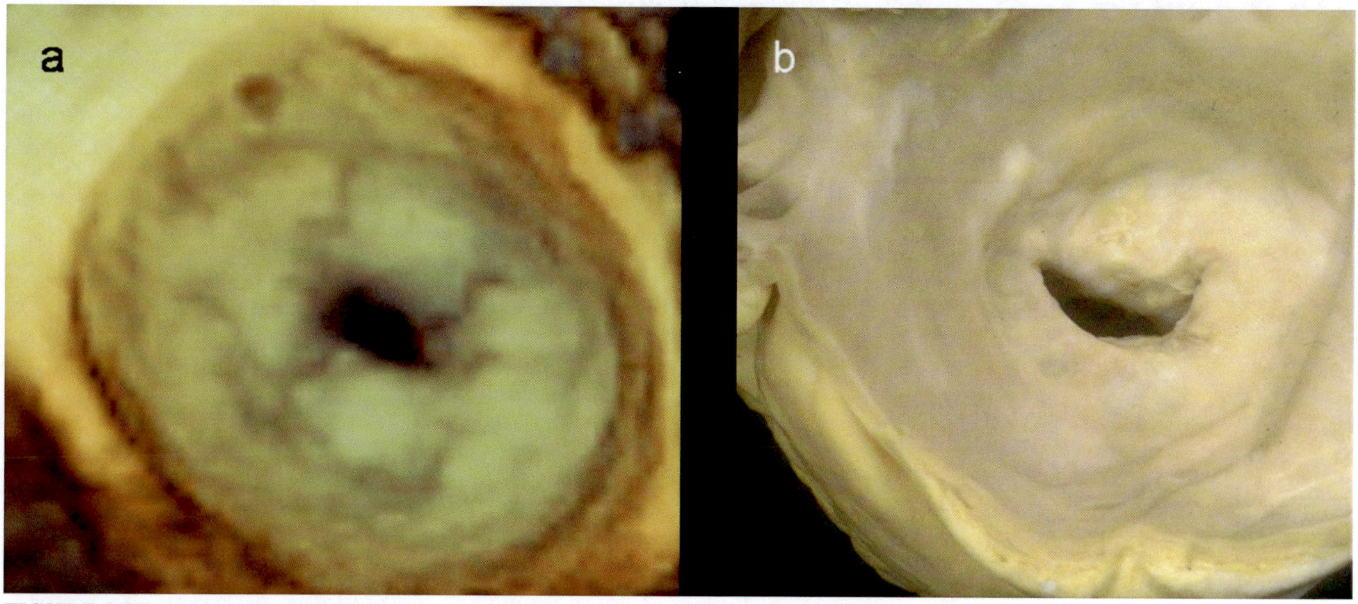

FIGURE 3.27 (a) Real-time 3D TEE in zoom modality showing a severe mitral stenosis from the atrial perspective in diastole. (b) A pathologicals pecimenw iths imilara bnormalities.

the stenotic mitral valve can be appreciated including the extent of commissural fusion. Real-time 3D TEE shows clearly whether the fusion is more pronounced in a single commissure (asymmetrical fusion) (Fig. 3.31) or conversely, whether both commissures are equally affected (symmetrical fusion) (Fig. 3.27). These data may be relevant in the clinical decision regarding balloon mitral valvuloplasty.

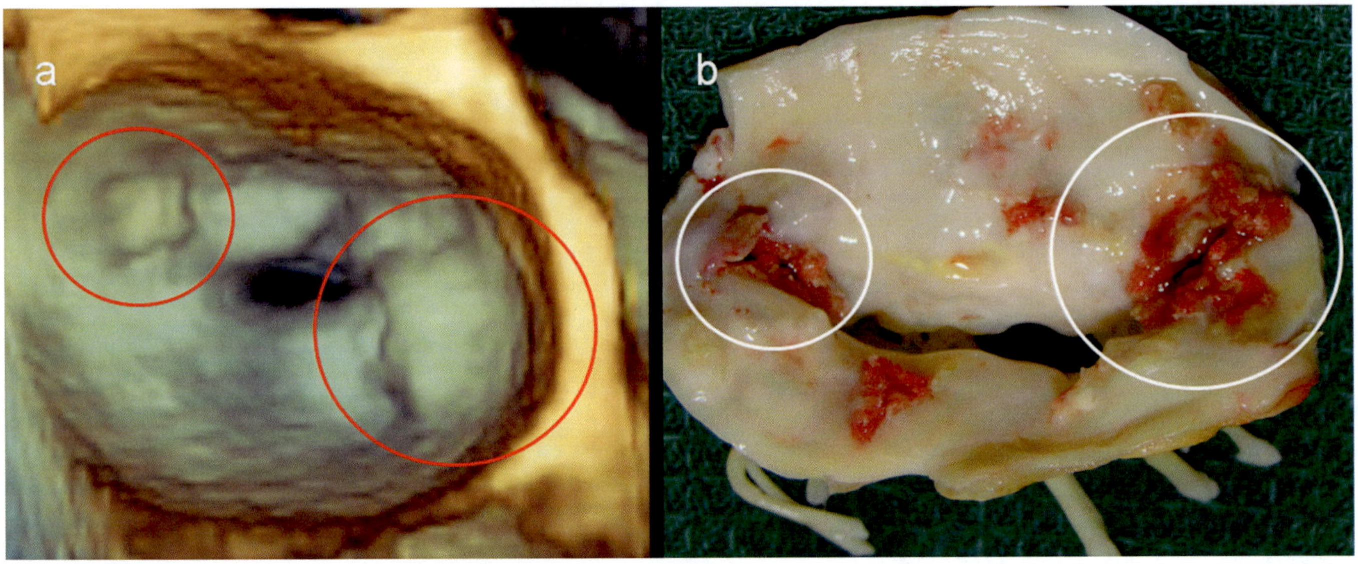

FIGURE 3.28 (a) Real-time 3D TEE in zoom modality showing a calcified valve with mitral stenosis in diastole from the atrial perspective and (b) the corresponding surgical specimen. *Red* and *white circles* encircle the commissural calcifications. In 3D echocardiography, shades of gray or colors provide a perception of depth rather than of texture. Consequently, calcification can be difficult to recognize.

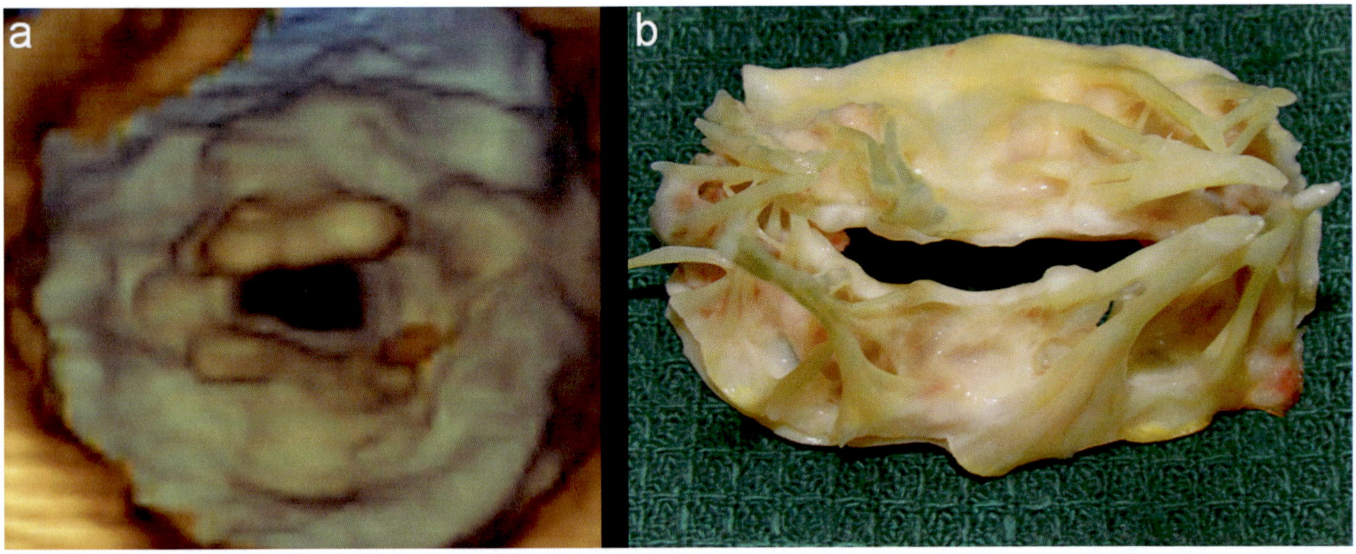

FIGURE 3.29 (a) Real-time 3D TEE in zoom modality from the ventricular perspective. (b) A surgical specimen from the same perspective.

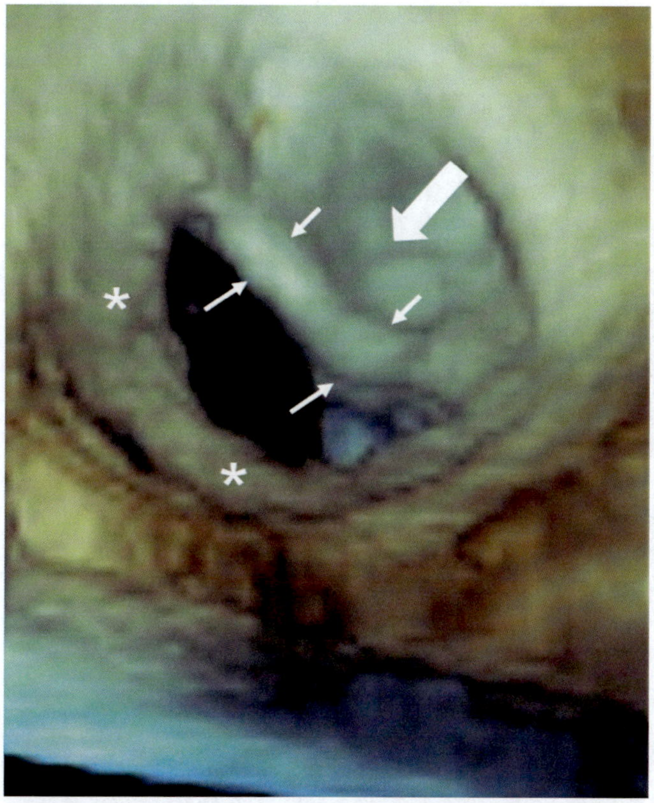

FIGURE 3.30 The same case shown in Fig. 3.24. Several pathological details can be described. The free margin of the anterior leaflet (*small arrows*) appears thicker than the body. In diastole, the body of the anterior leaflets abuts the left ventricle (*large arrow*). The *asterisks* identify the fusion between scallops forming a single rigid posterior leaflet. The fusion of commissures among scallops is one of the earliest pathological abnormalities of rheumatic mitral stenosis.

3.1.4 Calcification of the Mitral Annulus

Calcification of the mitral annulus is a frequent sequela of aging, ranging from a focal deposit, usually located on the posterior annulus, to extensive deposits both on the posterior and anterior annulus. Other conditions such as hypertension and renal insufficiency can accelerate calcium deposits on the mitral annulus, occasionally leading to a mass-like abnormality consisting primarily of calcium. Associated mitral regurgitation, usually mild, is not uncommon, while ring-shaped calcification may reduce leaflet excursion leading to functional mitral stenosis (i.e., without commissural fusion). This condition is a form of fibro-degenerative mitral stenosis, usually with a small pressure gradient. While the diagnosis of a calcified mitral annulus is easy to make with 2D images since calcifications are brighter than the surrounding structures, the diagnosis is more cumbersome with real-time 3D TEE. Shades of gray or colors mainly provide perception of depth rather than of texture. Thus, focal calcifications are rarely detected, especially when they are encased in the annulus. Extensive calcifications might be recognized in real-time where they interfere with the annulur motion. Occasionally, depending on where calcifications extrude, real-time 3D TEE images display them clearer than 2D images (Fig. 3.32).

Caseous calcification of the mitral annulus is a rare variant of annulus calcification. The echocardiographic finding of caseous calcification is incidental, mostly unrelated to patient symptoms. This kind of mitral annular calcification contains various degrees of central liquefaction that makes the echocardiographic images quite peculiar. Usually it appears as a large, round, echo-dense homogeneous mass with smooth borders encircling a central area of echolucency, situated in the posterior region of the mitral annulus. Quite often, the diagnosis is made with transthoracic 2D echocardiography. Sometimes the mass is better defined with TEE. Because of the central area of echolucency, this anomaly is easily diagnosed by using 2D TTE or TEE since their tomographic nature makes it possible to differentiate the echo-dense (calcific) peripherical shield and the central area of echolucency. As with the simple annular calcification, the diagnosis of caseous calcification of the mitral annulus with real-time 3D TEE is difficult. When seen from the left atrial perspective, the mass appears as a tumor protruding into the left atrium (Fig. 3.33) and the diagnosis cannot be made. However, by cutting the "tumor" longitudinally, a more familiar anatomical aspect allows for the correct diagnosis (Fig. 3.34).

3.1.5 Mitral Prostheses

Normal and pathological features of prosthetic valves can be superbly visualized by real-time 3D TEE. As with 2D TEE, the atrial side of the prosthesis can be imaged while the ventricular side is hidden by the ultrasonic artifacts caused by the metallic components of the prosthesis. Figure 3.35 shows a bileaflet disc prosthesis in systole and in diastole from the "en face" atrial perspective (Movie 3.12).

Figure 3.36 shows a biological prosthesis in systole and diastole from the atrial and ventricular perspectives (Movies 3.13 and 3.14).

A comprehensive assessment of prosthetic valve thrombi or vegetations (including number, size, and attachment sites) located on the atrial side of the prosthesis can easily be carried out. Figure 3.37 presents the case

MOVIE 3.12 A bileaflet disc prosthesis in systole and in diastole from the "en face" atrial perspective.

MOVIE 3.13 A biological prosthesis in systole and diastole from atrial perspective.

MOVIE 3.14 A biological prosthesis in systole and diastole from ventricular perspective.

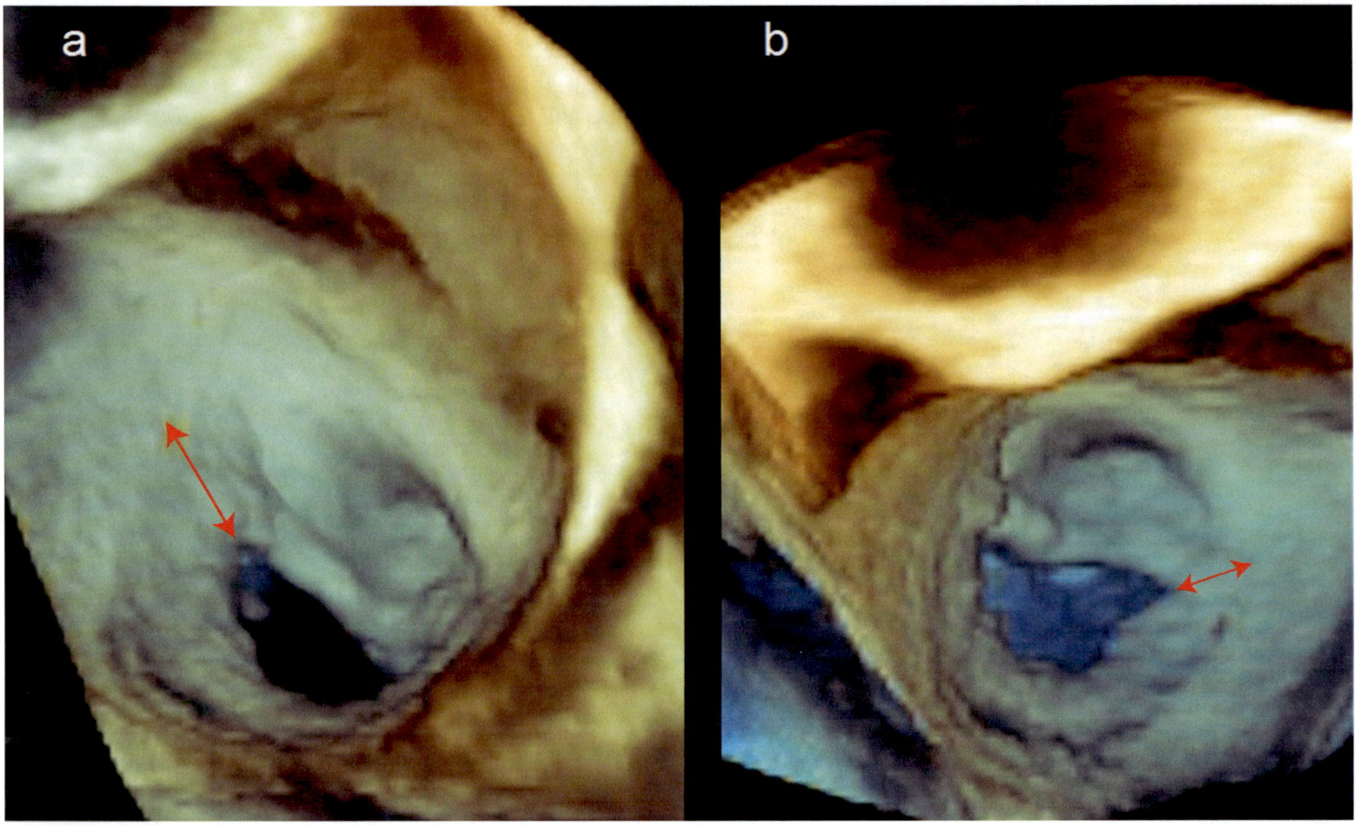

FIGURE 3.31 The same case as illustrated in Fig. 3.24. (a) Depicts the fusion in the antero-lateral commissure (*arrow*). (b) Depicts the fusion in the postero-medial commissure (*arrow*).T hisla tterc ommissure appears less affected.

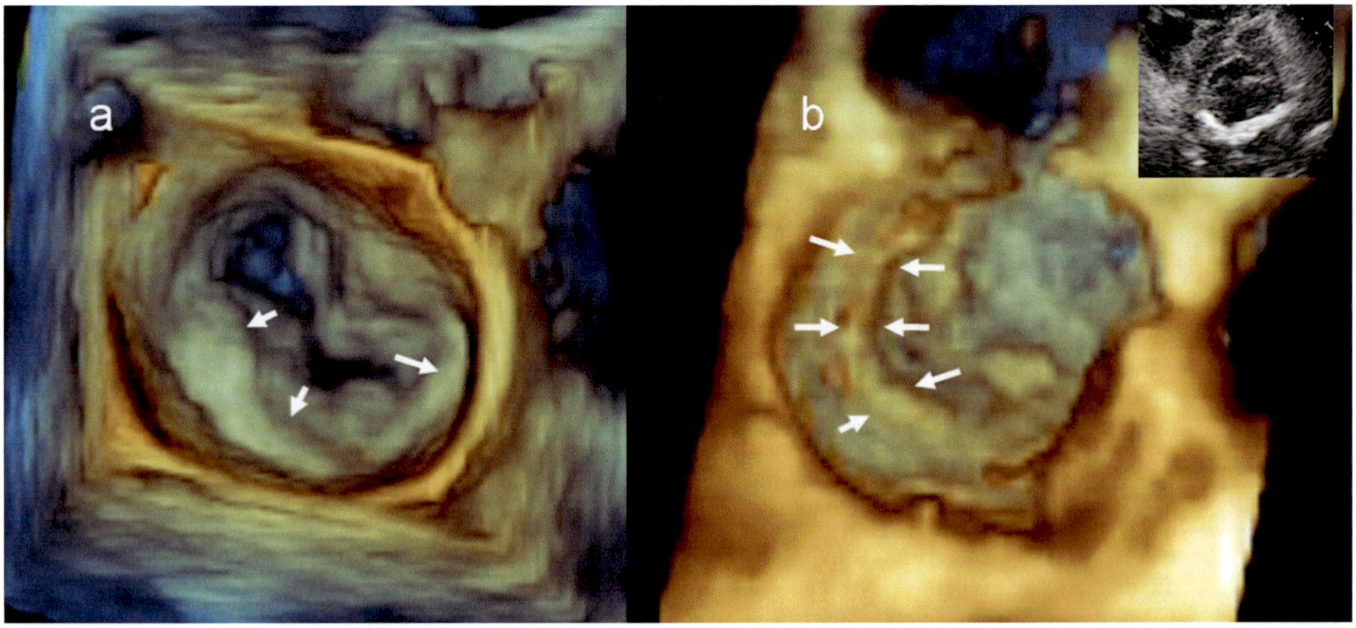

FIGURE 3.32 Real-time 3D TEE image of the mitral apparatus in zoom modality. 2D image in the upper right corner displays extensive calcification of the posterior annulus. (a) With the 3D TEE image from the atrial perspective, the huge calcification is not very clear because in contrast to the 2D image, the texture of the leaflet and the annulus are similar on 3D images. The irregular hinge-line of the posterior leaflet (*arrows*) and the mound-like appearance are the only morphological abnormalities noticeable from this perspective. (b) From the ventricular perspective, calcification is more easily recognizable because the calcification protrudes from the ventricular side of the annulus in the form of a semicircular ridge (*arrows*).

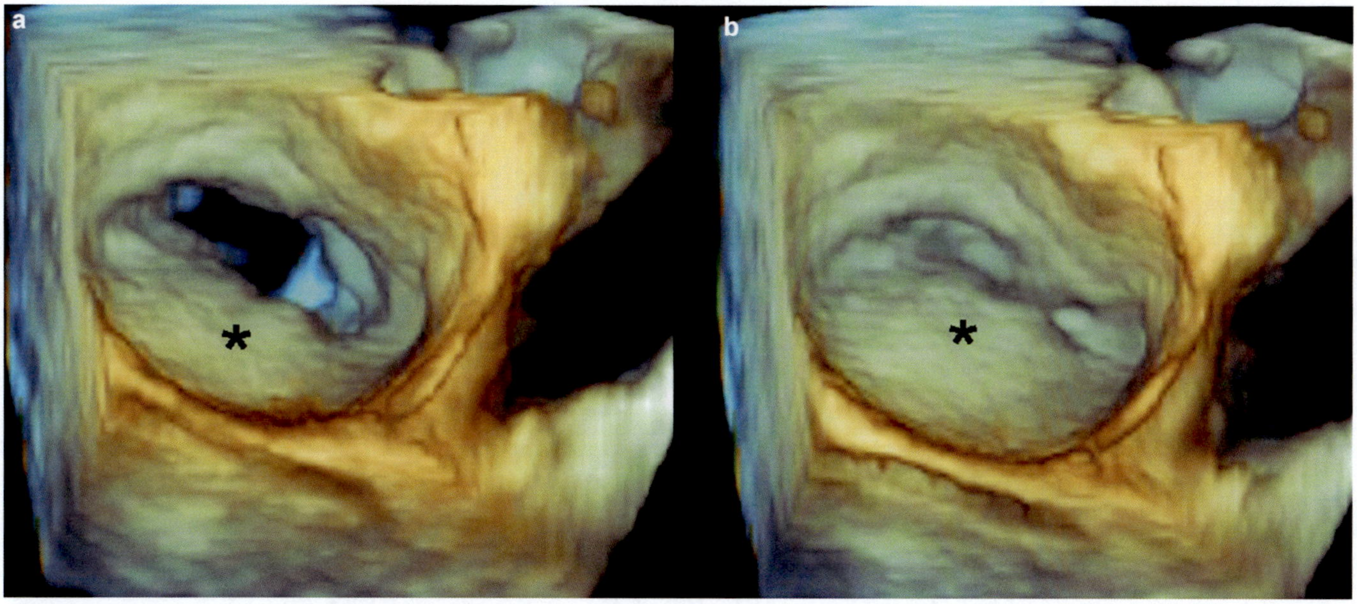

FIGURE 3.33 Real-time 3D TEE image of mitral valve in zoom modality (a) in diastole and (b) in systole. These images show a structure protruding into the left atrium (*asterisk*).

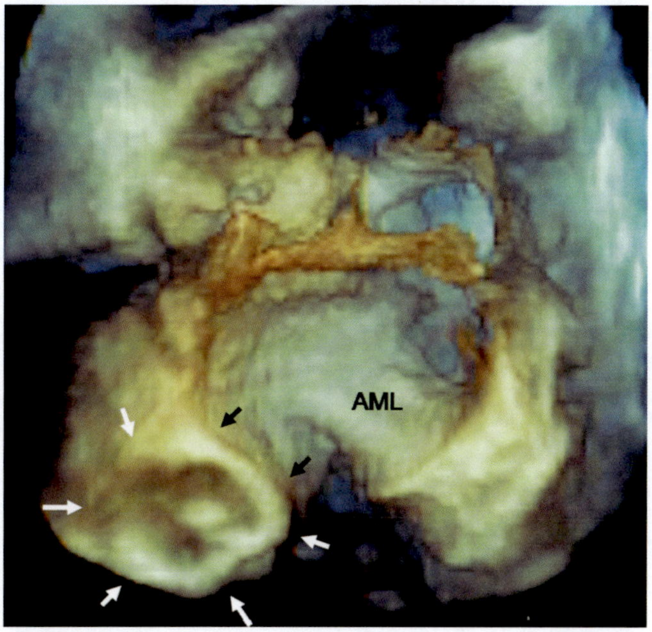

FIGURE 3.34 3D TEE image of the mitral valve in full volume modality after a longitudinal cut through the "tumor." A clear round image with echo-dense homogeneous borders encircling a central area of echolucency appears (*arrows*). *AML*a nteriorm itralv alve.

of a 40-year-old woman with a prosthetic mitral valve who suffered from sensory aphasia, right homonymous hemianopsia, and a mild ataxia of the right upper limb. Real-time 3D TEE clearly displays the prosthetic thrombosis (Movie 3.15).

Three-dimensional TEE may assist in verifying appropriate prosthetic leaflet motion. In Fig. 3.38, a real-time 3D TEE image shows another case of thrombosis. Because of repeat cerebral ischemic events despite anticoagulation therapy, this patient underwent surgical thrombectomy.

With the same accuracy, real-time 3D TEE can evaluate periprosthetic leaks. In Fig. 3.39, two periprosthetic leaks are visualized. Figure 3.40 shows a patient with two paraprosthetic leaks, one anterior (1 o' clock) and one posterior (5 o' clock) clearly visualized by RT 3D TEE, and confirmed subsequently during surgery. In some patients the vena contracta enables recognition of the exact position of the anatomical dehiscence that would otherwise not be detectable (Fig. 3.41) (see also Chap. 10 and Movies 3.16 and 3.17).

3.1.6 Mitral Valve Repair

Real-time 3D TEE will greatly benefit patients who undergo mitral valve repair. It may also help in the long-term follow-up. Figures 3.42 and 3.43 illustrate two cases

MOVIE 3.15 Real-time 3D TEE clearly displays four thrombi localized on the atrial side of the prosthesis.

MOVIE 3.16 An example of a medially located large paraprosthetic leak.

MOVIE 3.17 Color Doppler full volume modality in the same patient identifies severe paraprosthetic regurgitation.

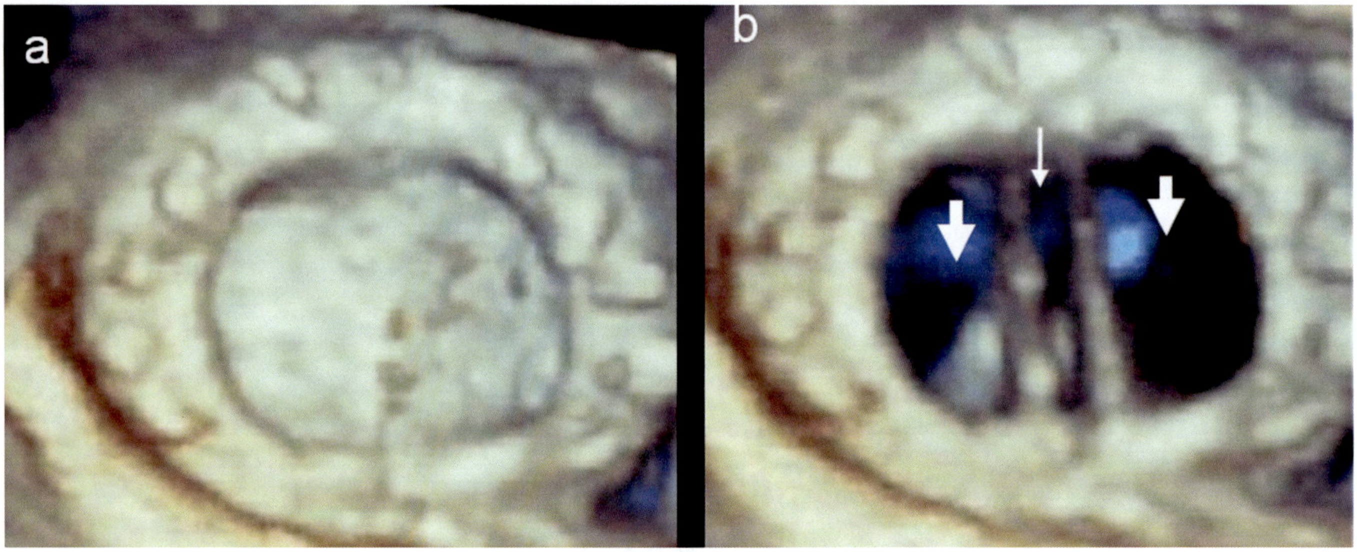

FIGURE 3.35 3D RT TEE of a bileaflet disc prosthesis (a) in systole and (b) in diastole from the "en face" atrial perspective. The two semicircular disks are attached to a rigid ring by small hinges. In diastole the prosthesis consists of three orifices: a small slit-like central orifice between the two opened leaflets (*thin arrow*) and two larger semicircular lateral orifices (*large arrows*). In this example the opening angle of the leaflets relative to the annulus plane is 90°.

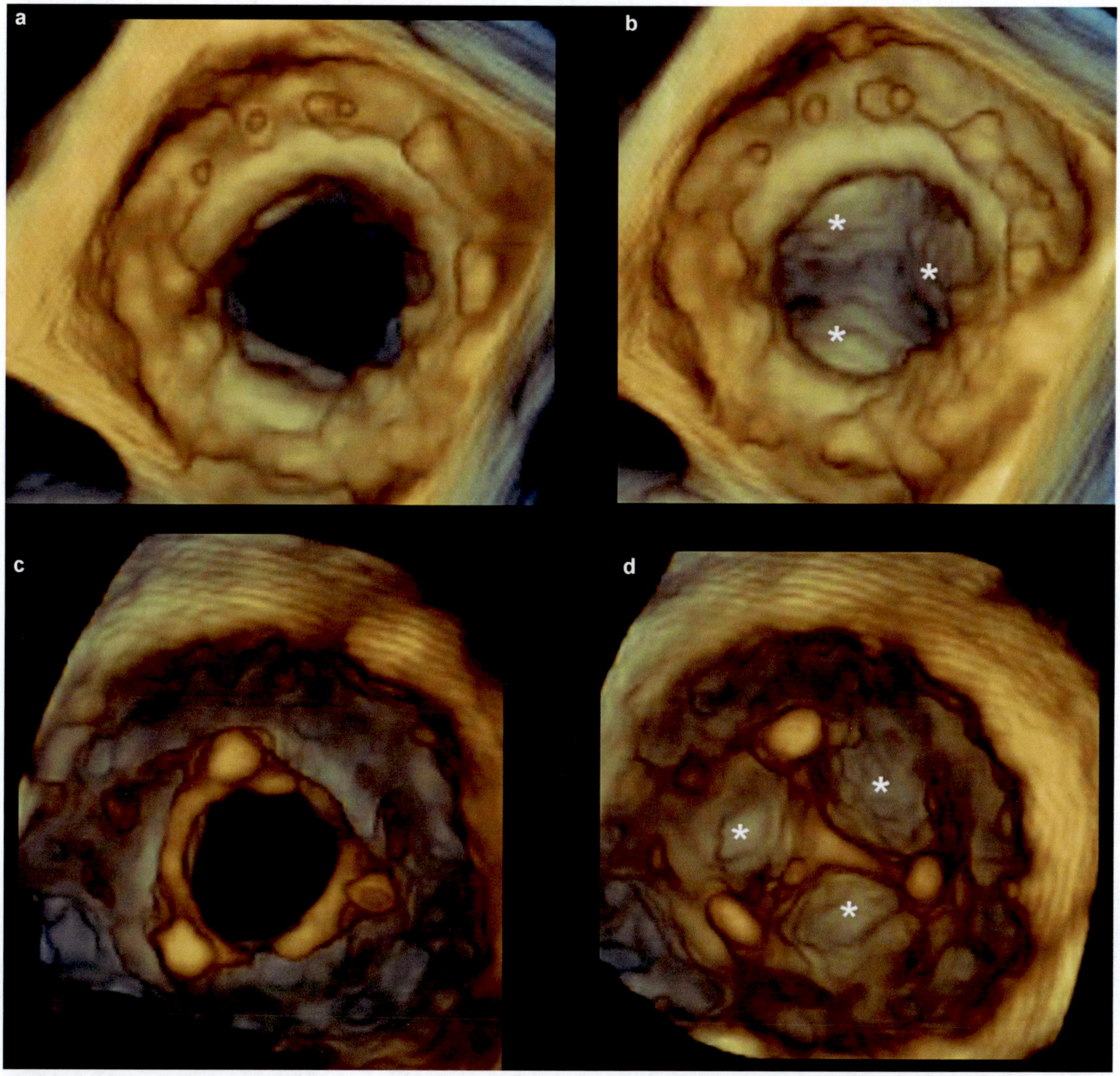

FIGURE 3.36 (a, c) RT 3D TEE image in zoom modality of a biological prosthesis from the atrial perspective (a) in diastole and (b) in systole. The same biological prosthesis from the ventricular perspective (c) in diastole and (d) in systole. *Asterisks* mark the three leaflets in closedposi tion.

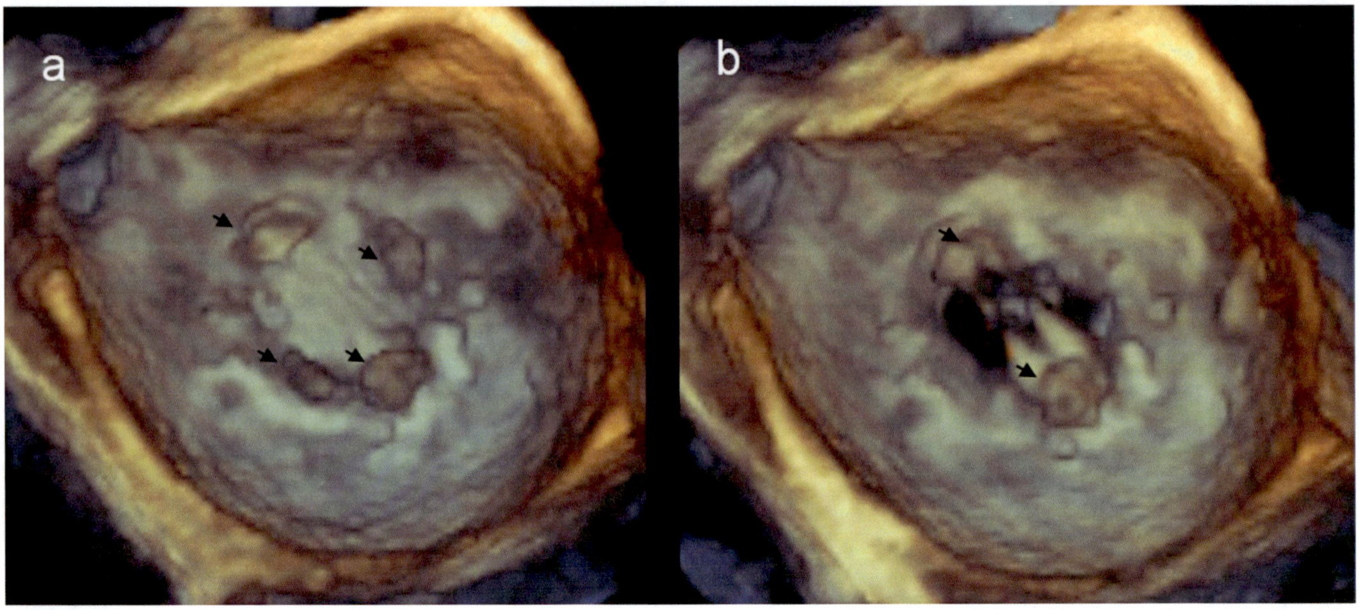

FIGURE 3.37 Real-time 3D TEE of a bileaflet disc prosthesis (a) in systole and (b) in diastole with four thrombi on the atrial side of the prosthesis (*arrows*).

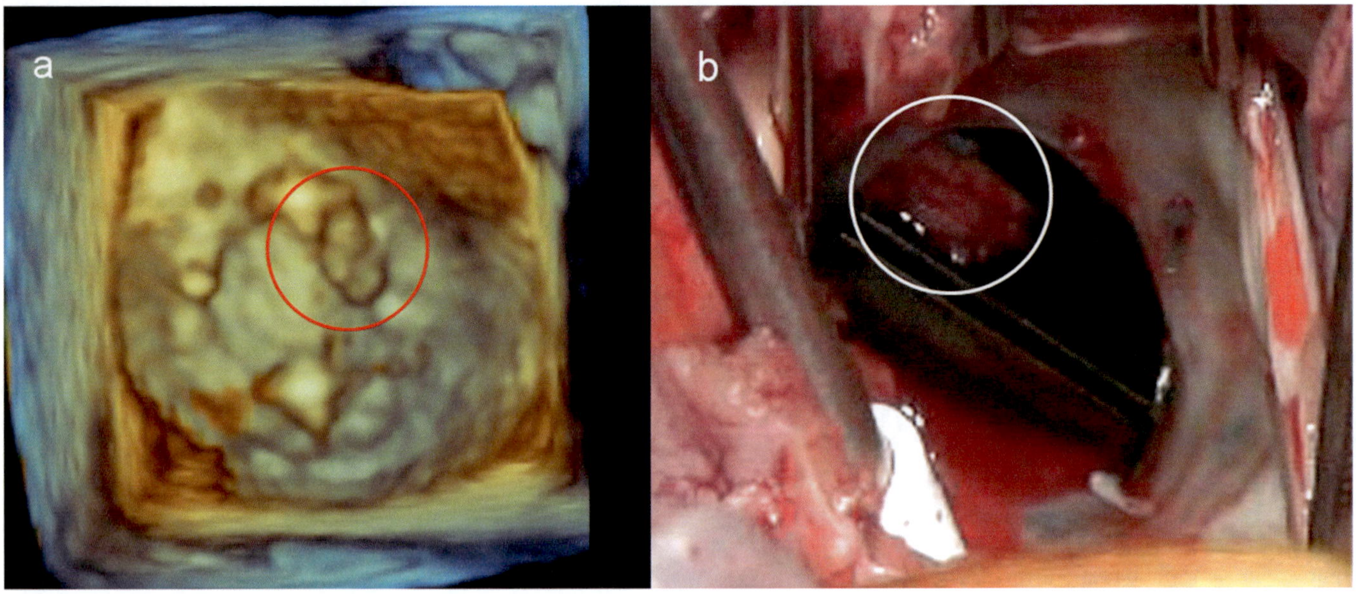

FIGURE 3.38 Real-time 3D TEE image in zoom modality shows (a) a bileaflet disc prosthesis with thrombus (*red circle*). An image taken in the operating room shows (b) the thrombus (*white circle*).

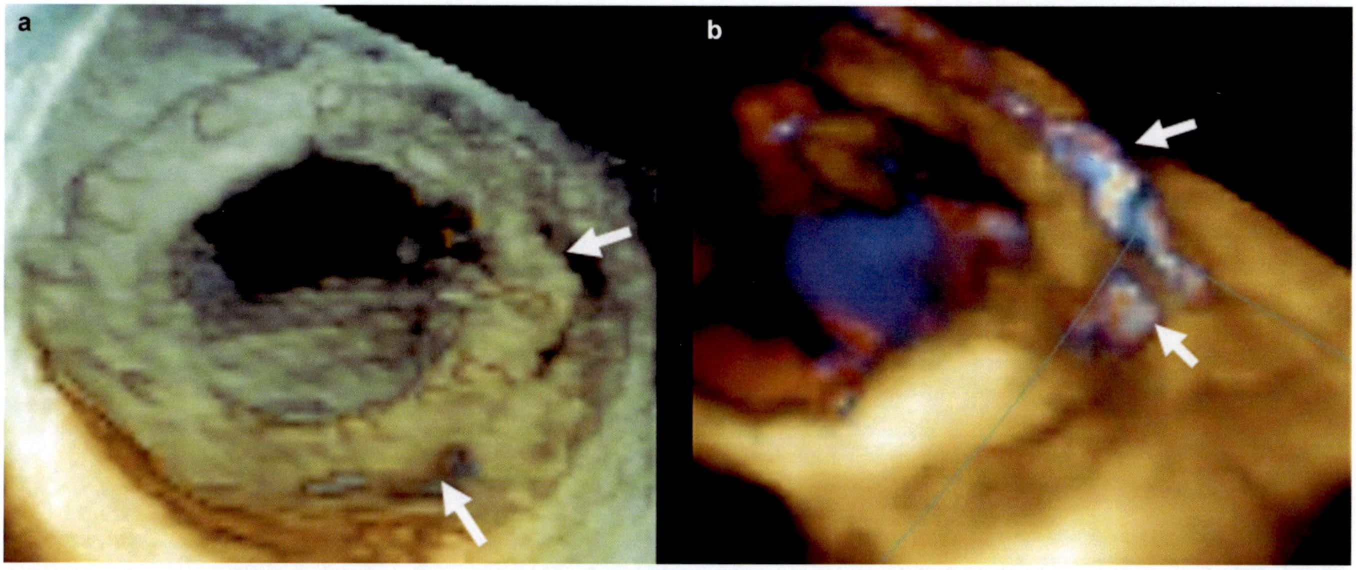

FIGURE 3.39 Real-time 3D TEE image of a bileaflet disc prosthesis showing (a) two periprosthetic leaks. (b) The "vena contracta" of the flow through the leaks (b, *arrows*). The number and size of the leaks were confirmed during surgery.

of successful reconstruction mitral annuloplasty (Movie 3.18) and an Alfieri's stitch respectively.

3.1.6.1 Percutaneous Mitral Valve Repair

Recently, a percutaneous approach has been developed as an alternative to Alfieri's repair. Real-time 3D TEE promises to be the ideal technique for monitoring every step of this complex procedure as shown in the following figures.

Figure 3.44 shows a guide-wire passing into the left atrium through the atrial septum.

Figure 3.45 shows the guide catheter which substitutes for the transseptal apparatus.

Figure 3.46 shows the clip delivery system advancing into the left atrial chamber and centered over the mitral orifice.

Figure 3.47 shows the arms of the clip opening and oriented perpendicularly to the long axis of the leaflet edges.

Figure 3.48 shows the achievement of a double-orifice mitral valve due to leaflet insertion into the closed clip arms.

Finally, Figs. 3.49 and 3.50 show the final result once the clip is released from the clip delivery system and the delivery system and guide catheter are withdrawn (Movie 3.19).

MOVIE 3.18 Example of mitral reconstruction and annuloplasty. The ring is easily identified along its entire circumference. The stitches appear bigger than they are in reality, due to suboptimal z-axisr esolution.

MOVIE 3.19 Final results of percutaneous repair from an atrial perspective. Two adjacent orificesa rec learlyi maged.

3.1.6.2 Imaging Processing

An important advantage of 3D TEE (shared with 3D transthoracic echocardiography) is the ability to measure the object in arbitrary orientations without geometric assumptions. Quantitative analysis of acquired volumetric data uses a software system (QLAB version 6.0 Philips Medical Systems, Andover, MA). By using the MPR modality, which consists of three planes (coronal, sagittal, and transverse) and one 3D volume image, it is possible to measure an anatomically exact distance and area, especially in the "en face" view. A cut plane perpendicular to the "en face" view depicting the tips of the mitral valve leaflets allows the most accurate measurements of the valve area. Accordingly, 3D TEE may become the new standard for mitral valve orifice measurements in patients with mitral stenosis (Figs. 3.51 and 3.52).

Mitral valve quantification (MVQ) is a program specifically designed to quantitatively analyze the mitral valve apparatus. This program requires the operator to correctly align different axes and enter reference points. Diameters and height of the saddle-shaped mitral annulus, leaflet prolapse height, lengths, surface and volume, aortic orifice to mitral plane angle, and the position of papillary muscles can be assessed (Figs. 3.53–3.55).

Similarly, quantification of leaflet tenting, quantitative assessment of annular dilation, remodeling of its saddle-shape configuration, and symmetrical displacement of papillary muscles, be assessed in the dilated cardiomyopathies (Fig. 3.56).

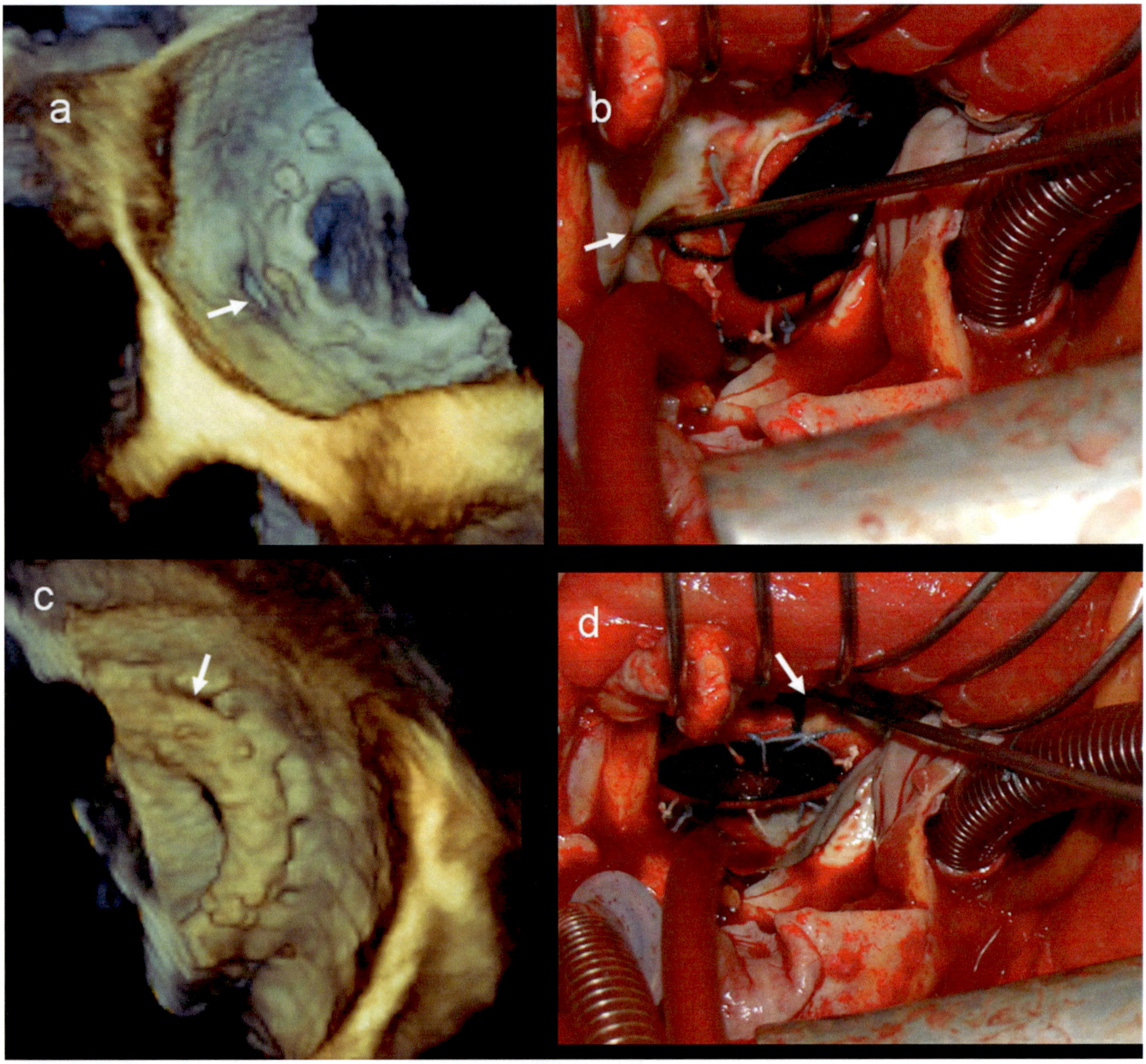

FIGURE 3.40 Real-time 3D TEE image of a bileaflet disc prosthesis showing (a) one periprosthetic leak in the anterior position (*arrow*) and one (c) in the posterior position (*arrow*);(b,d)t hec orresponding surgical views.

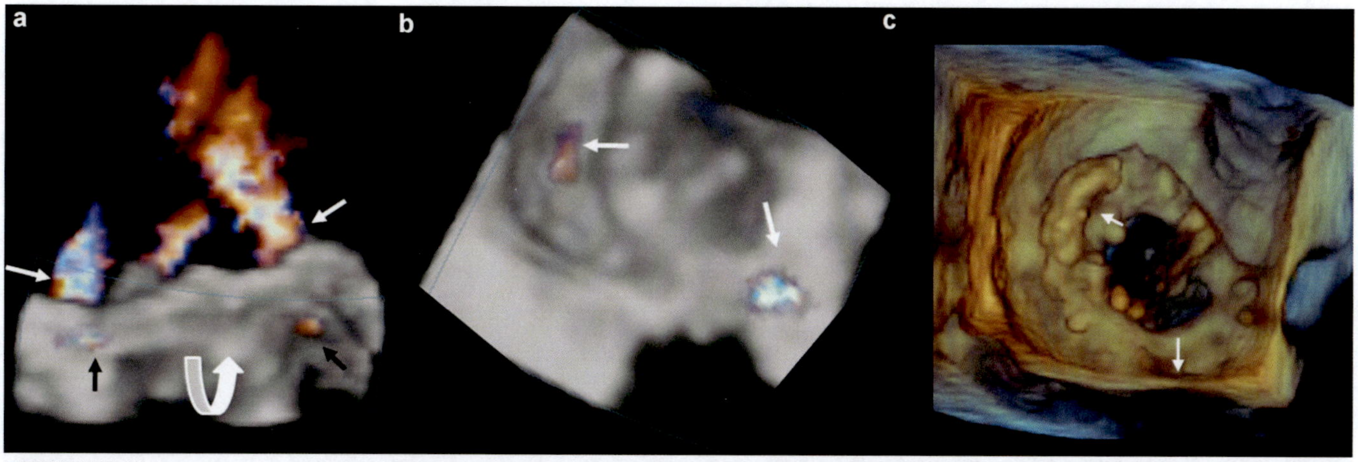

FIGURE 3.41 3D TEE image of a bileaflet disc prosthesis in 3D color full volume modality showing two periprosthetic jets (a, *white arrows*). The image is angulated to visualize the flow convergence region on the ventricular side of the prosthesis (*black arrows*). By rotating the image downside-up (b, *curved arrows*), the flow convergence region of the two jets is fully displayed indicating the exact location of the anatomical leaks. 3D image of the prosthesis (c) in zoom modality. The *arrows* point to the anatomical locations of the two leaks based on the indications of color. Without color Doppler, it would have been difficult to recognize the dehiscences based only on anatomical images.

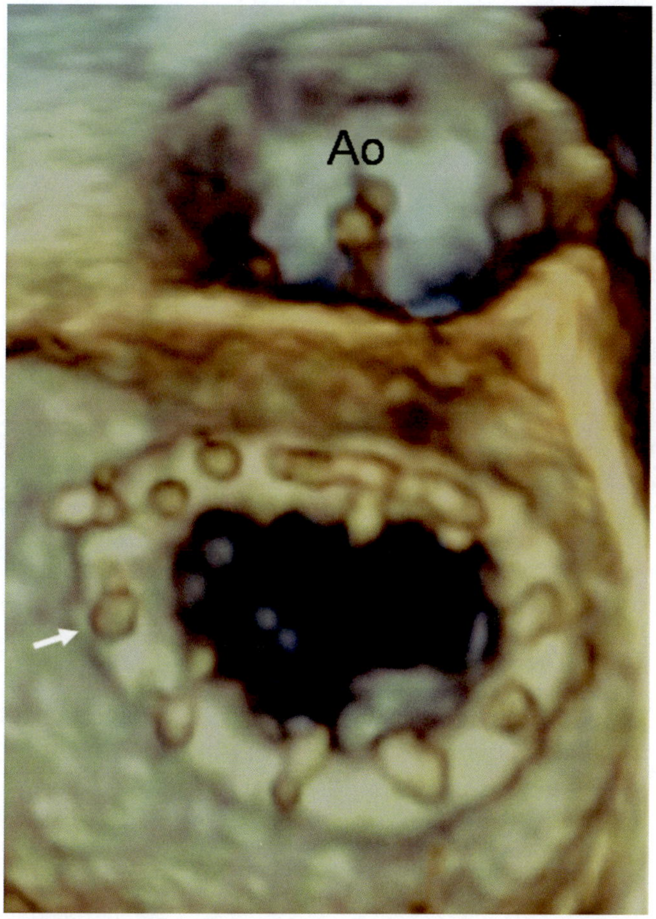

FIGURE 3.42 3D RT TEE image of mitral valve annuloplasty. The ring is easily identified along its entire circumference. The stitches (*arrow* is pointing to one of them) appear bigger than they are in reality, due to suboptimal *z*-axis resolution. *Ao* aorta.

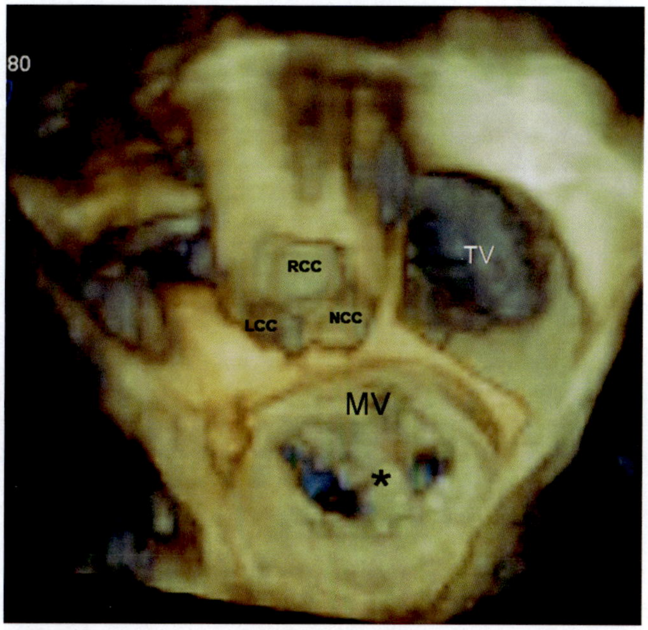

FIGURE 3.43 Real-time 3D TEE image of mitral reconstruction and Alfieri's stitch viewed from the atrial perspective. The *asterisk* points to the site of the stitch. In this patient an asymmetric double orifice was created. *MV* mitral valve; *TV* tricuspid valve; *LCC* left coronary cusp; *RCC* right coronary cusp; *NCC* noncoronary cusp.

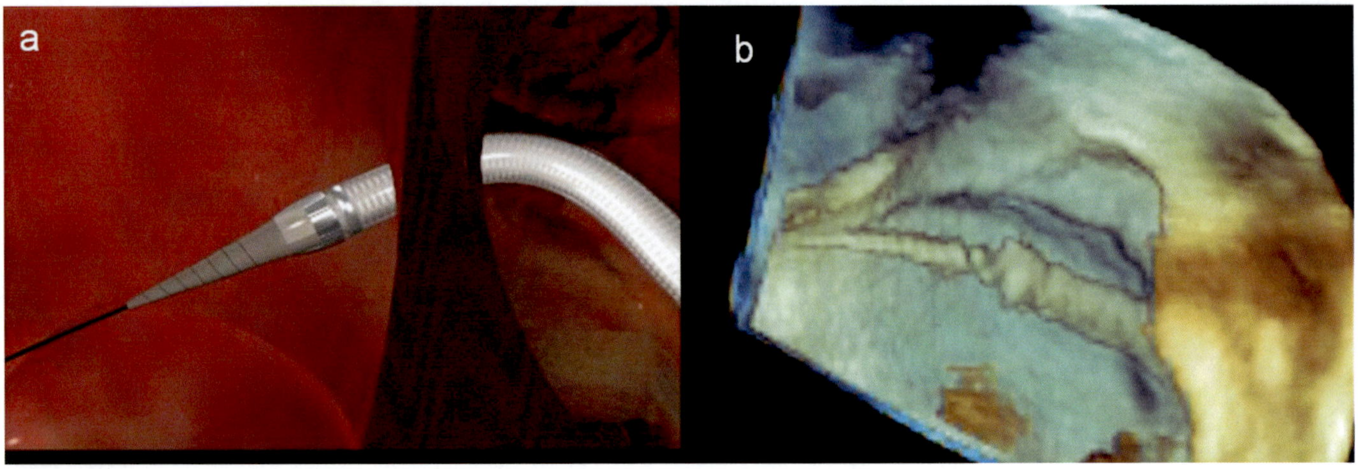

FIGURE 3.44 Real-time 3D TEE image of a guide-wire passing into the left atrium. (a) Shows a demonstration image provided by the supplier. (b) Shows a corresponding real-time 3D image.

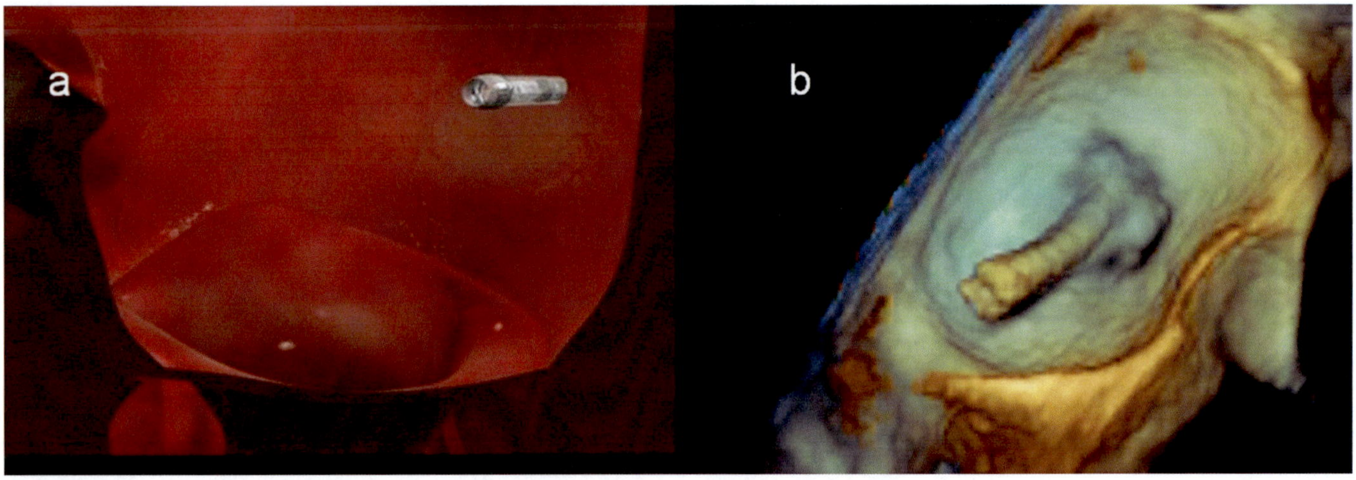

FIGURE 3.45 Real-time 3D TEE image of a guide catheter passing into the left atrium. (a) Shows a demonstration image provided by the supplier. (b) Shows the corresponding real-time 3D image.

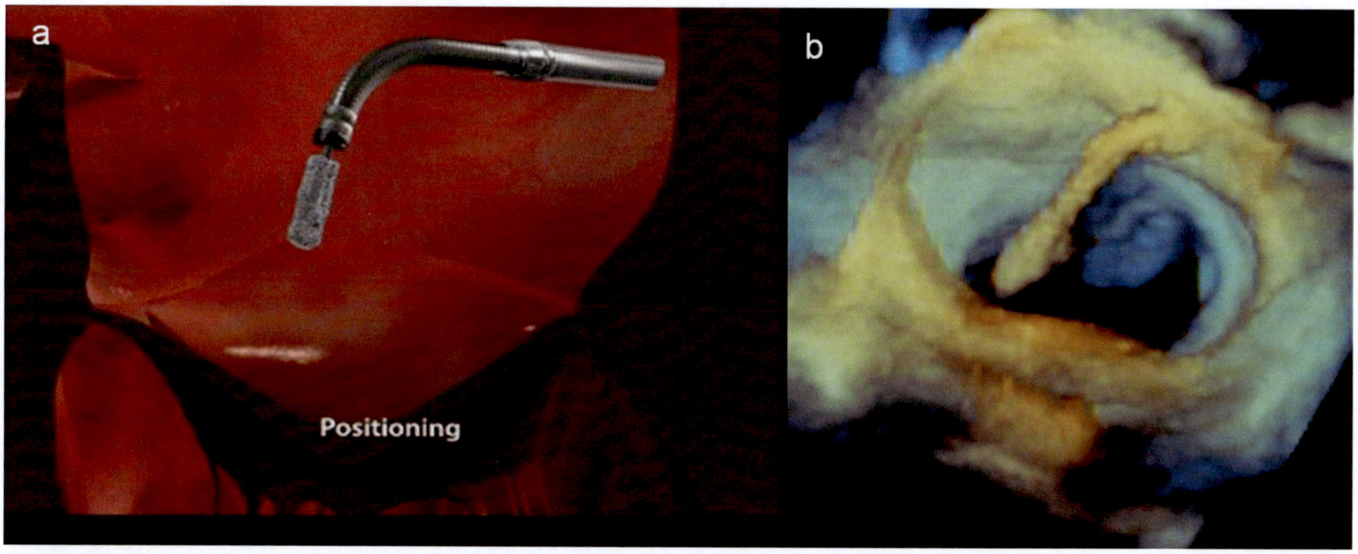

FIGURE 3.46 Real-time 3D TEE image of the clip delivery system positioning over the mitral orifice. (a) Shows a demonstration image provided by the supplier. (b) Shows the corresponding real-time 3D image.

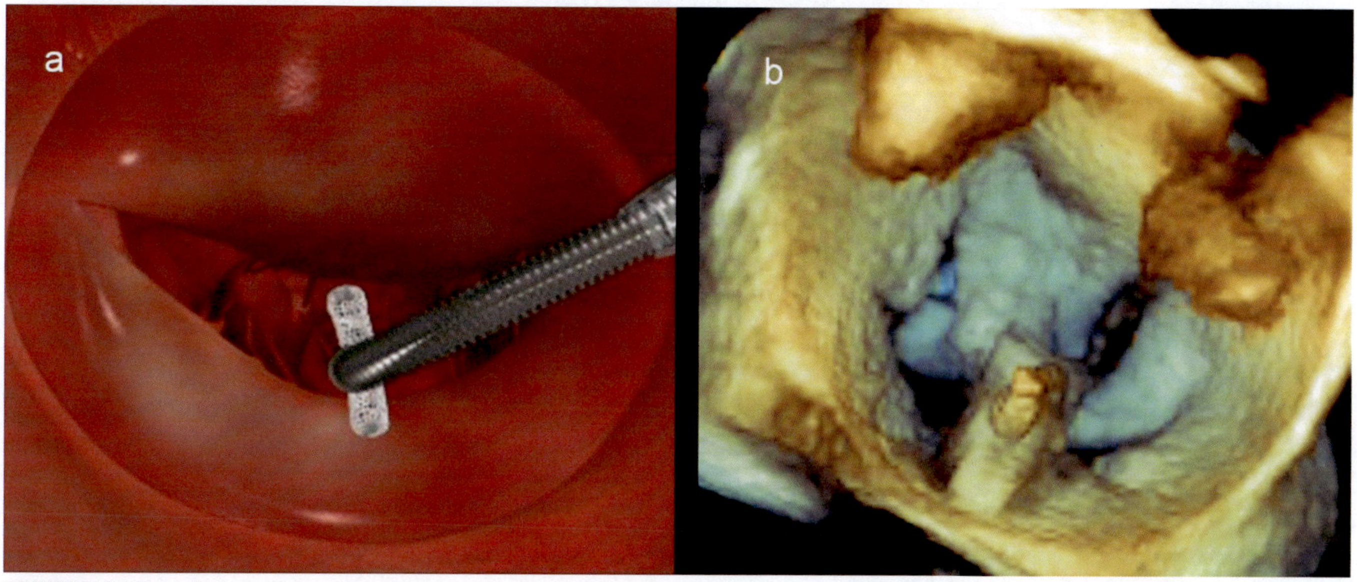

FIGURE 3.47 Real-time 3D TEE image of the clip delivery system oriented perpendicularly to the long axis of the leaflets edge. (a) Shows a demonstration image provided by the supplier. (b) Shows the corresponding real-time 3D image.

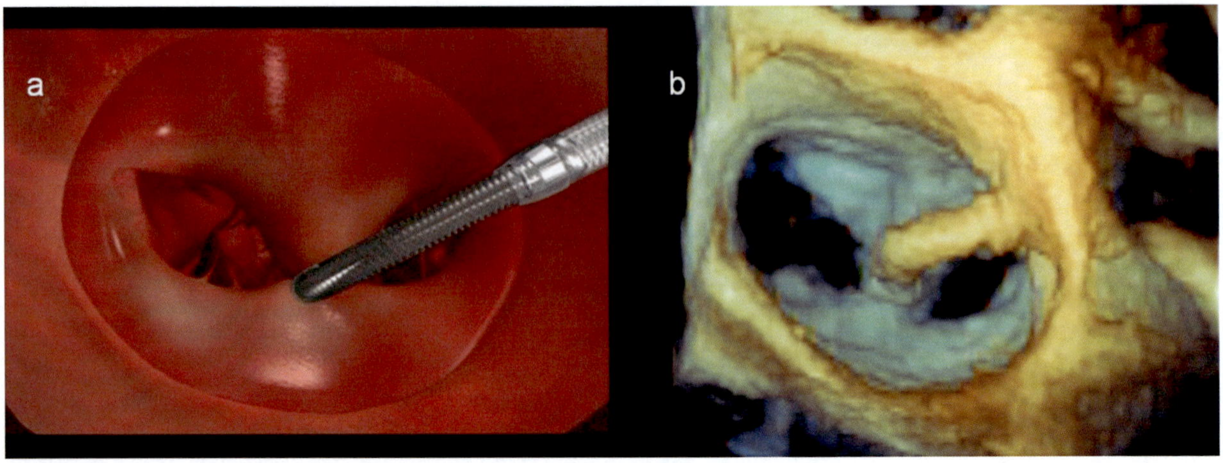

FIGURE 3.48 Real-time 3D TEE image of the clip delivery system anchored to the mitral leaflets. (a) Shows a demonstration image provided by the supplier. (b) Shows the corresponding real-time 3D image.

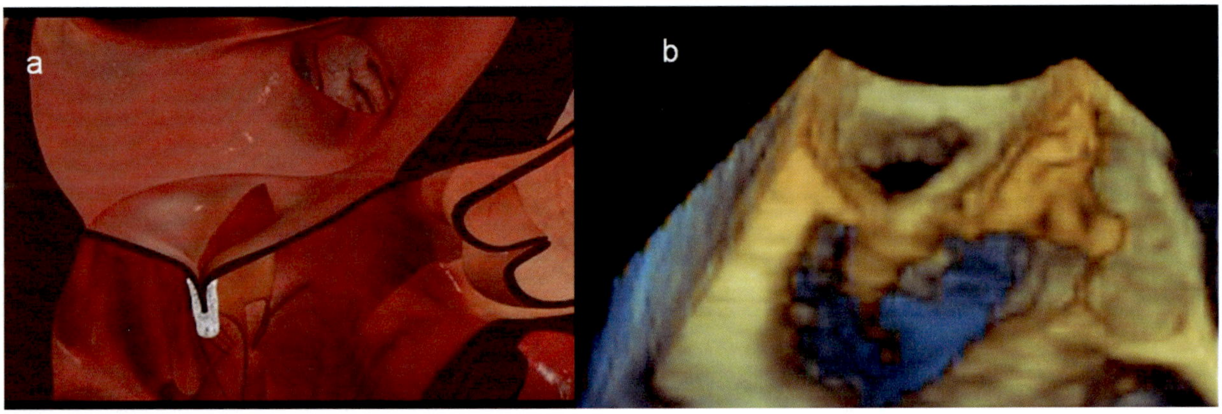

FIGURE 3.49 Real-time 3D TEE image of the final result of percutaneous repair in long axis orientation. (a) Shows a demonstration image provided by the supplier. (b) Shows the corresponding real-time 3D image.

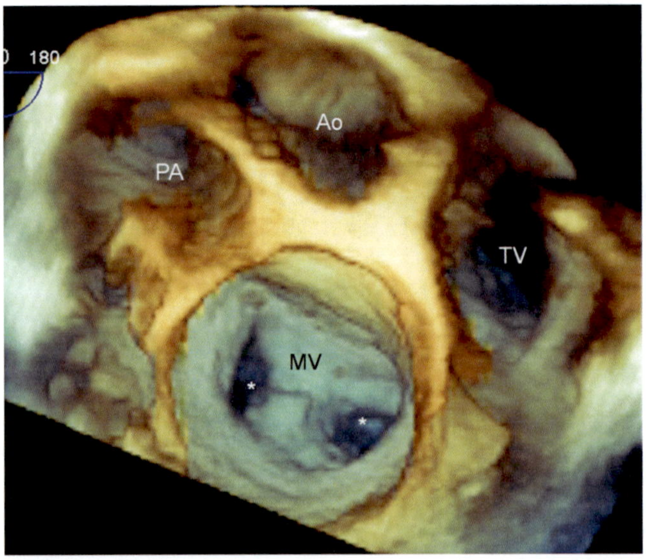

FIGURE 3.50 Real-time 3D TEE image of the final results of percutaneous repair from an atrial perspective. Two adjacent orifices are clearly imaged (*asterisks*). *MV* mitral valve; *PA* pulmonary artery; *TV* tricuspid valve; *Ao*a orta.

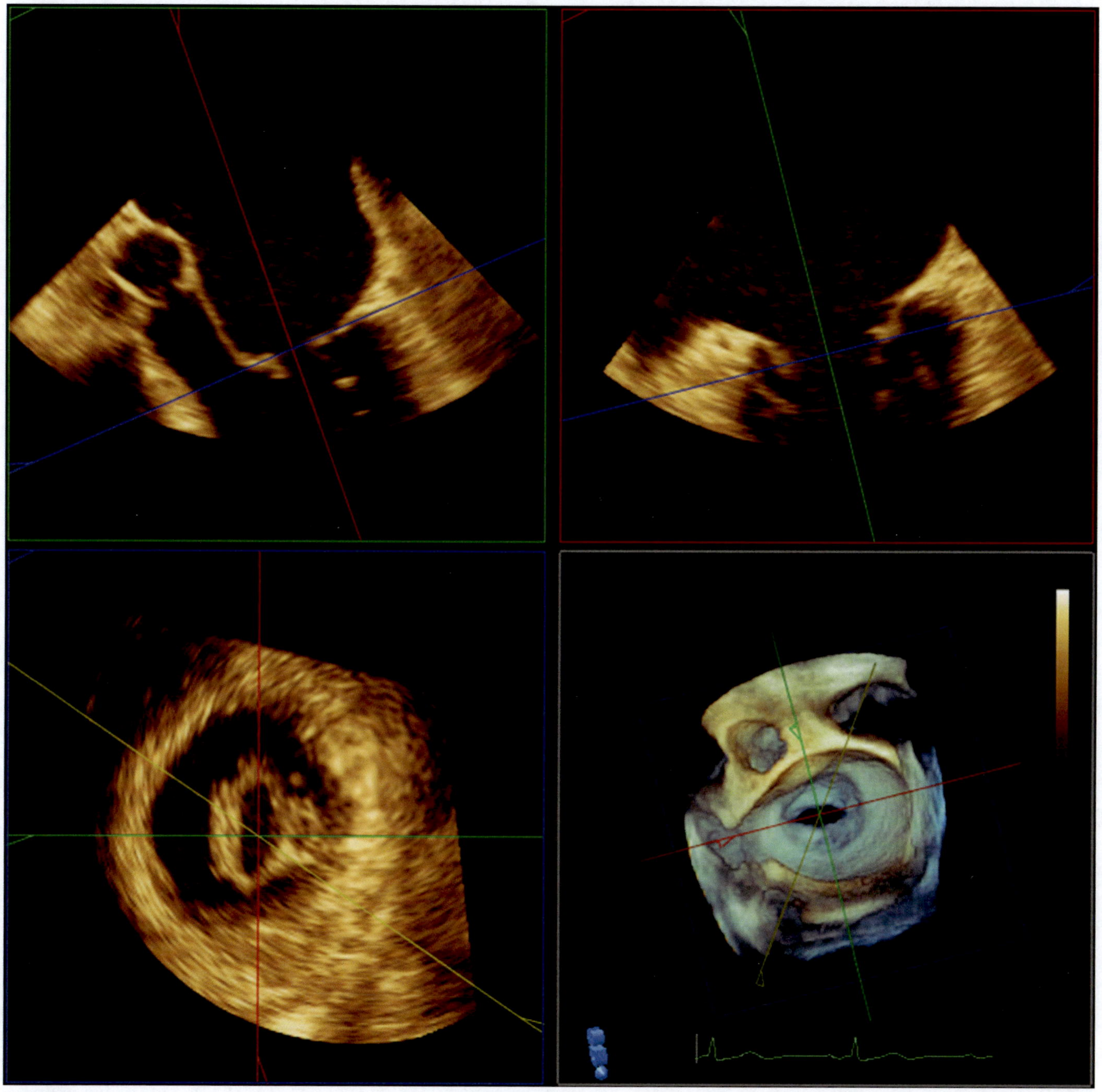

FIGURE 3.51 Moving a cropping platform from the left atrium toward the mitral valve leaflet tips, smallest valve area can be measured accurately.

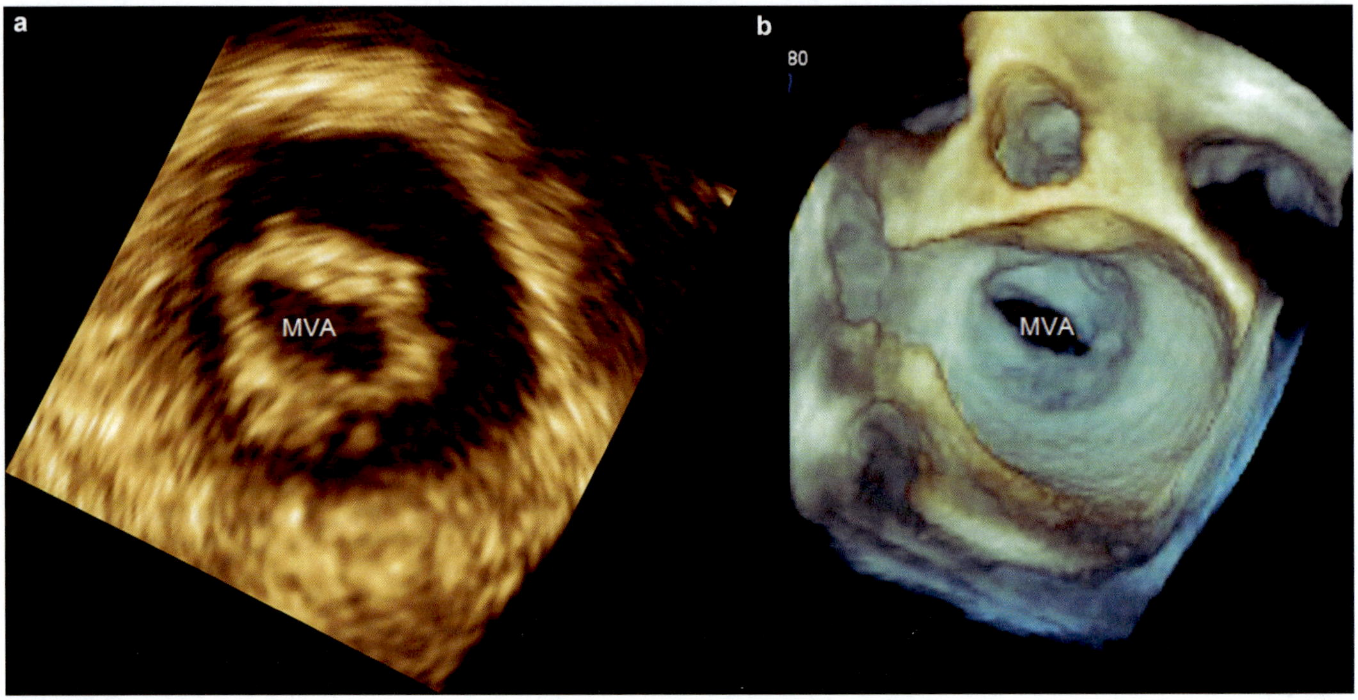

FIGURE 3.52 Thefi gure shows the mitral valve area (MVA) in (a) 2D-derived 3D data set and (b) 3D images.

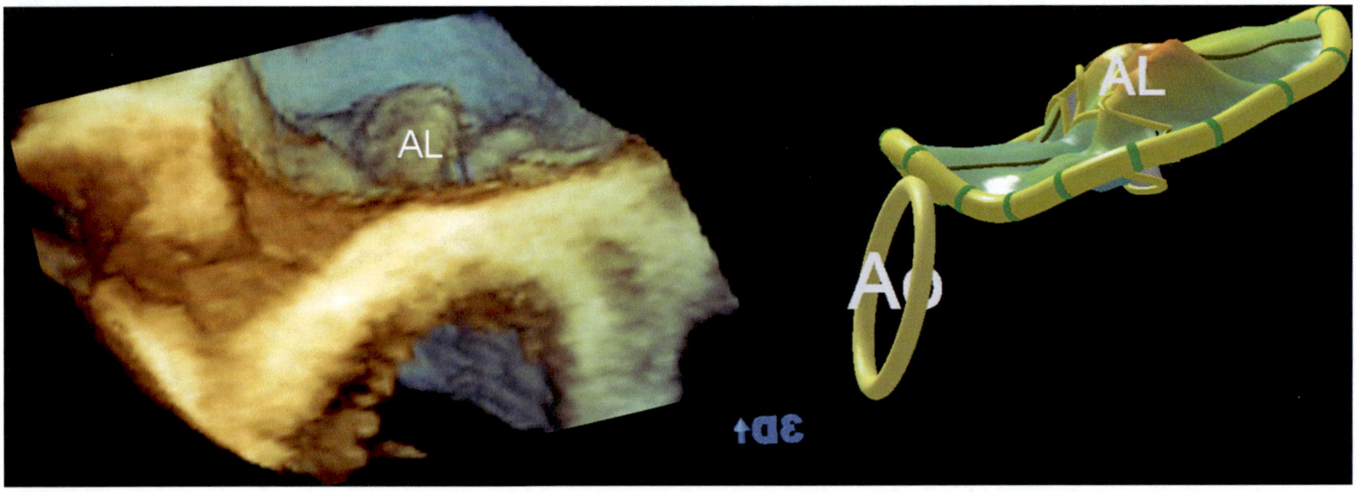

FIGURE 3.53 (a) Prolapse of the anterior mitral leaflet (AL) from lateral view (a) and the corresponding image obtained with quantitative analysis software (b). *Red areas* indicate regions of anterior leaflets (AL) that protrude above the annular plane. *Ao* aortic valve.

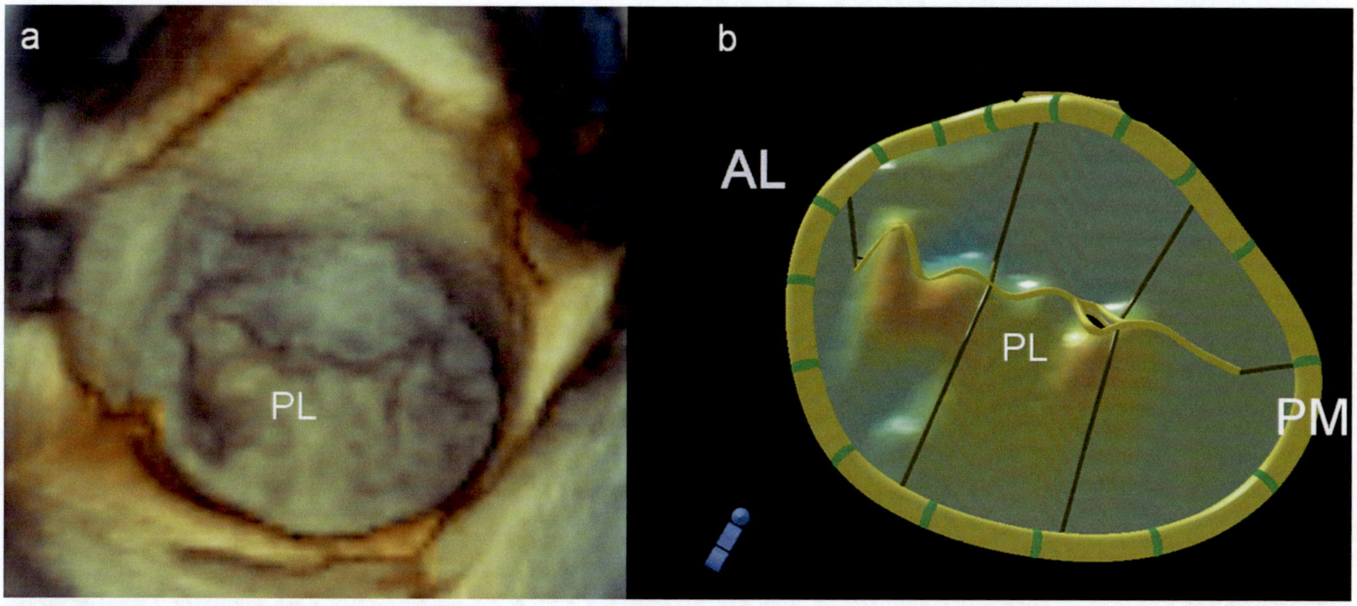

FIGURE 3.54 (a) Severe (multisegmental) prolapse of the posterior mitral leaflet (PL) from the atrial perspective and (b) the corresponding image obtained with quantitative analysis software. *AL* antero-lateral commissure; *PM* postero-medial commissure.

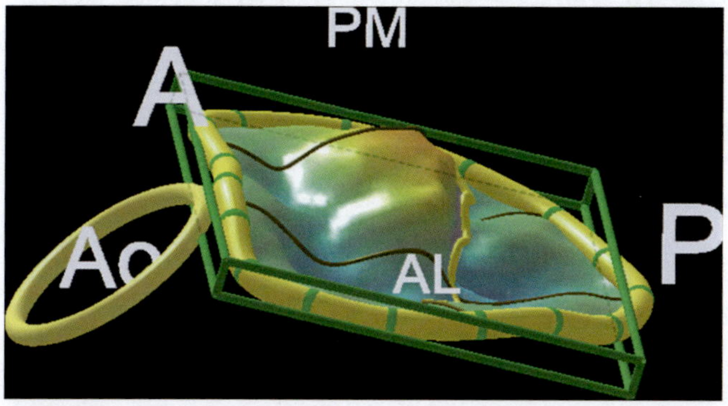

FIGURE 3.55 An image of mitral valve obtained with quantitative analysis software showing the height of the saddle-shaped mitral annulus (*green box*) and the mitro-aortic angle. *PM* postero-medial commissure; *AL* antero-lateral commissure; *A* anterior; *P* posterior; *Ao*a orta.

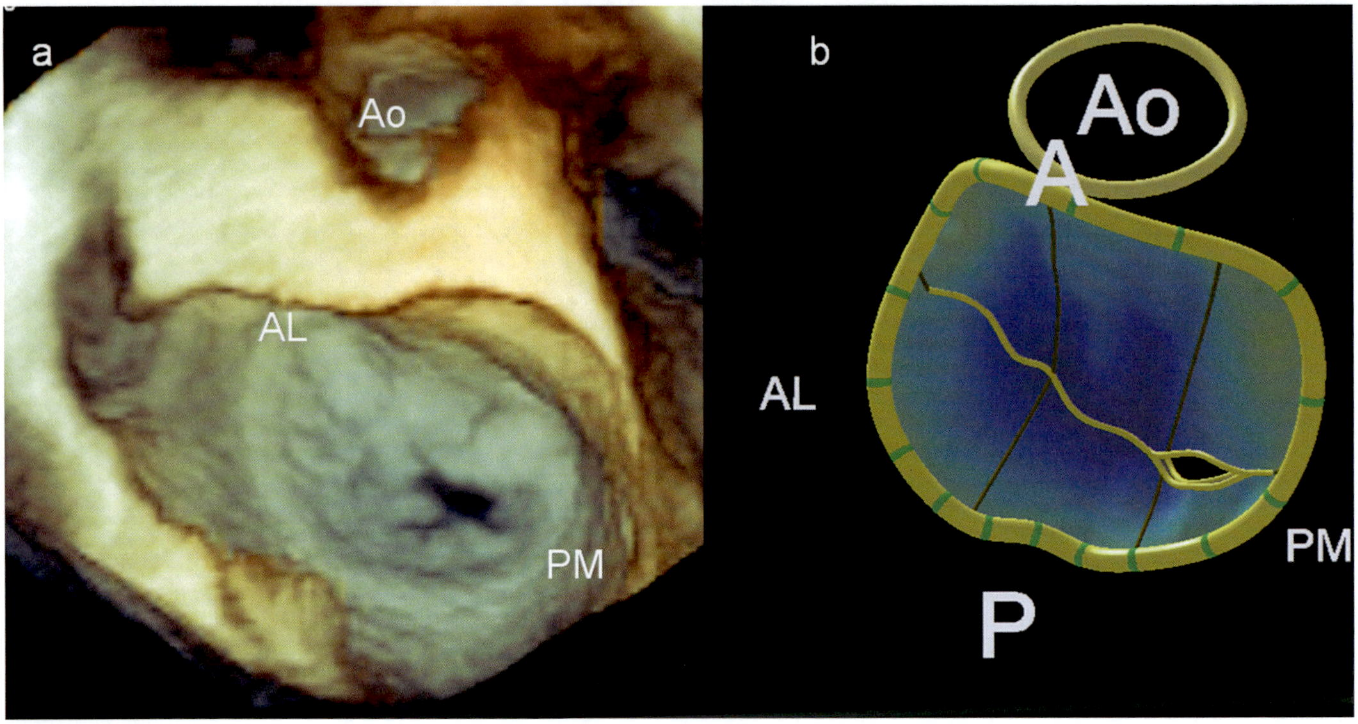

FIGURE 3.56 Mitral valve regurgitation due to the tethering caused by akinesis of the postero-inferior left ventricular wall. A significant regurgitant orifice near the postero-medial commissure (PM) can be appreciated both in (a) real-time 3D TEE and (b) in the valve model obtained with quantitative analysis software. Note that the intense shade of *blue* represents the height of the leaflet tenting. *Ao* aorta; *AL* antero-lateral commissure; *PM* postero-medial commissure; *A* anterior; *P* posterior.

CHAPTER 4

The Aortic Valve and the Aorta

Unlike imaging of the mitral valve, real-time 3D TEE has some limitations in imaging the aortic valve leaflets.[*] There are many reasons for this. First, the aortic valve is anterior to the mitral valve and therefore further from the transducer. Second, the aortic leaflets are thinner than the mitral leaflets. Third, the aortic plane is oblique to the ultrasound beams. Because of these factors, the machine settings are less effective in differentiating aortic leaflets from the background noise. In addition, in a closed position, the body of the leaflets is nearly parallel to the ultrasound beams, resulting in feeble echoes (most are scattering echoes rather than specular echoes). When the gain is adjusted to remove noise, most of the echoes from the leaflet tissue also disappear, leaving mainly "drop-out artifacts." The drop-out artifacts are less evident in systole because when the leaflets are in the open position, they become nearly perpendicular to the ultrasound beams (Figs. 4.1 and 4.2). Overall, it is hardly surprising that aortic leaflets cannot usually be visualized in their entirety with real-time 3D TEE. Despite these difficulties, in some patients we were able to create good images of the aortic leaflets in both diastole and systole. We use these patients for describing the following normal features of the aortic valve and the aortic root (see also Movies 4.1 and 4.2).

MOVIE 4.1 An example of a normal aortic valve with the normal systolic excursion of the aortic leafletsf roma orticp erspective.

[*]The term "cusp" is commonly used when referring to the leaflets of the semilunar valves. It describes the pockets formed by the leaflets owing to their semilunar attachment to the sinuses. Thus, for clarity, we prefer the term "leaflet" to describe the thin flap of tissue, distinguishing them from the sinuses which are part of the arterial wall.

MOVIE 4.2 An example of normal aortic valve with the normal systolic excursion of the aortic leaflets from ventricular perspective.

Aortic root. The aortic root comprises the aortic valve leaflets and their hingelines, the sinuses, the interleaflet triangles, the ventriculo-arterial junction, and the sinutubular junction. The aortic annulus (i.e., the hingelines of the aortic leaflets) has a crown-shaped appearance. Most of these structures can be imaged easily in real-time 3D TEE. Unlike 2D echocardiography, real-time 3D TEE can image all of these features in one image by cropping the aortic root longitudinally (Fig. 4.3).

The normal aortic valve has three semilunar leaflets. The leaflets are seldom perfectly equal in size. Each leaflet has a semicircular hingeline, a body, and a coapting surface. The three leaflets meet centrally along the zones of apposition where adjacent leaflets coapt (Fig. 4.4). The commissures are the highest points of the valvular closure lines. They reach the level of the sinutubular junction, whereas the lower points, the nadirs, cross into ventricular tissue (Figs. 4.5 and 4.6).

The electronic dissection of the volumetric data set reveals some unique details of the aortic sinuses. In Fig. 4.7, the left coronary sinus is imaged together with its corresponding leaflet. Note that the orifice of the left main coronary artery is located in the upper part of the sinus (arrow).

Because of the semilunar attachment of the aortic leaflets, there are three interleaflet triangles that are effective extensions of the left ventricular outflow tract since they are located beneath the level of the leaflets when the valve is in a closed position (Fig. 4.8). Real-time 3D TEE might have difficulty in clearly imaging the interleaflet triangles because the level of resolution does not allow a sufficiently good definition to differentiate these thin areas from adjacent structures. In Fig. 4.8, the arrows point to the position of the interleaflet triangles in between the sinuses.

Figures 4.9–4.11 show each of the interleaflet triangles imaged from different perspectives. The position of the interleaflet triangle between the left and noncoronary aortic sinuses can be recognized since it forms part of the aortic-mitral curtain. In some patients (such as those imaged in the figure), the triangle appears in between the sinuses. The other triangles are featureless, and their position can be recognized only because the surrounding structures are recognizable.

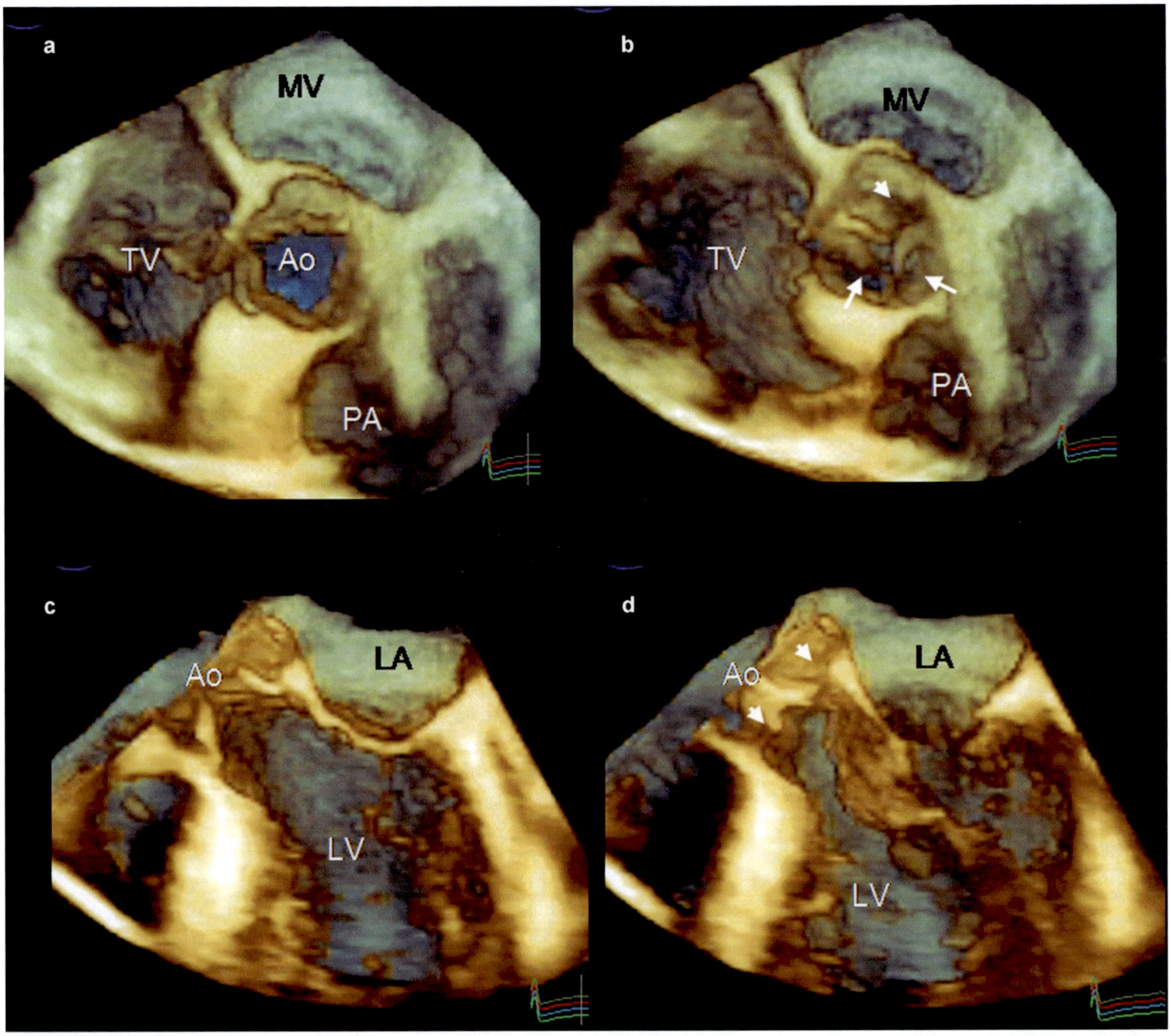

FIGURE 4.1 3D TEE image of the base of the heart in full volume modality: (a) "en face" view of aortic leaflets in systole; (b) "en face" view of aortic leaflets in diastole revealing some "drop-out artifacts" in the body of the leaflets (*arrows*) affecting the quality of the image; (c) long axis view of aortic leaflets in systole; (d) long axis view of aortic leaflets in diastole again revealing the presence of "drop-out artifacts."

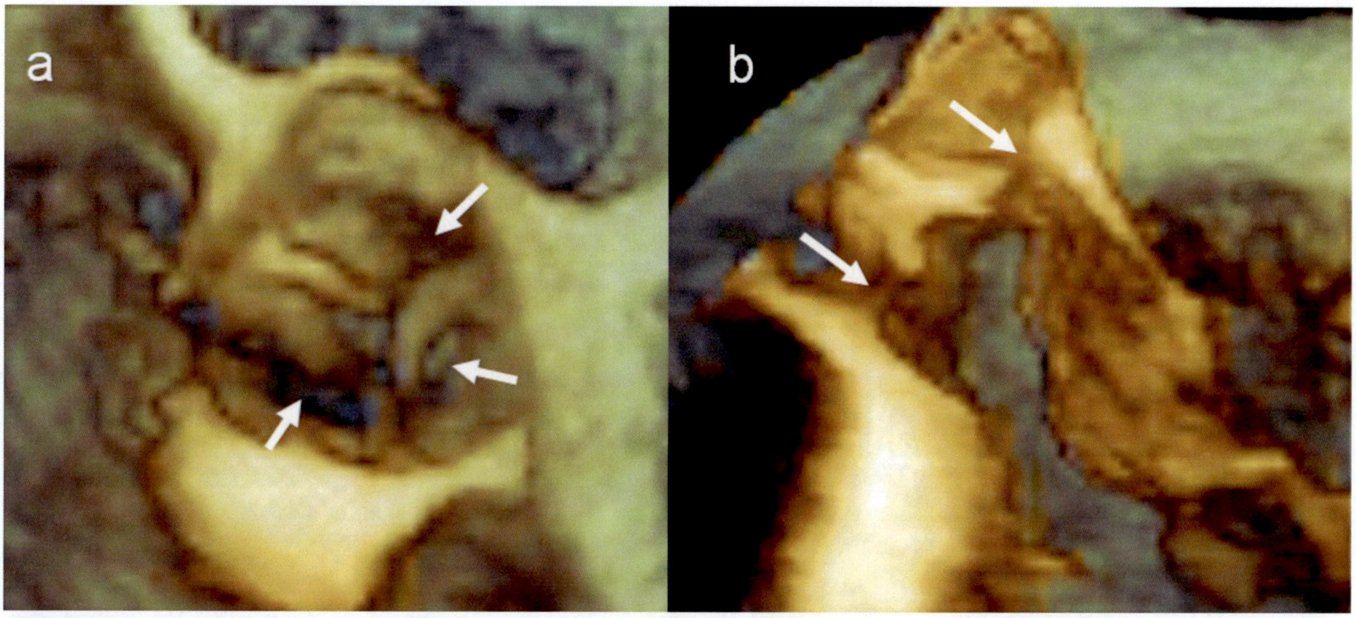

FIGURE 4.2 Magnified image of Fig. 4.1 showing the drop-out artifacts (*arrows*) in both (a) "en face" and (b) long axis views.

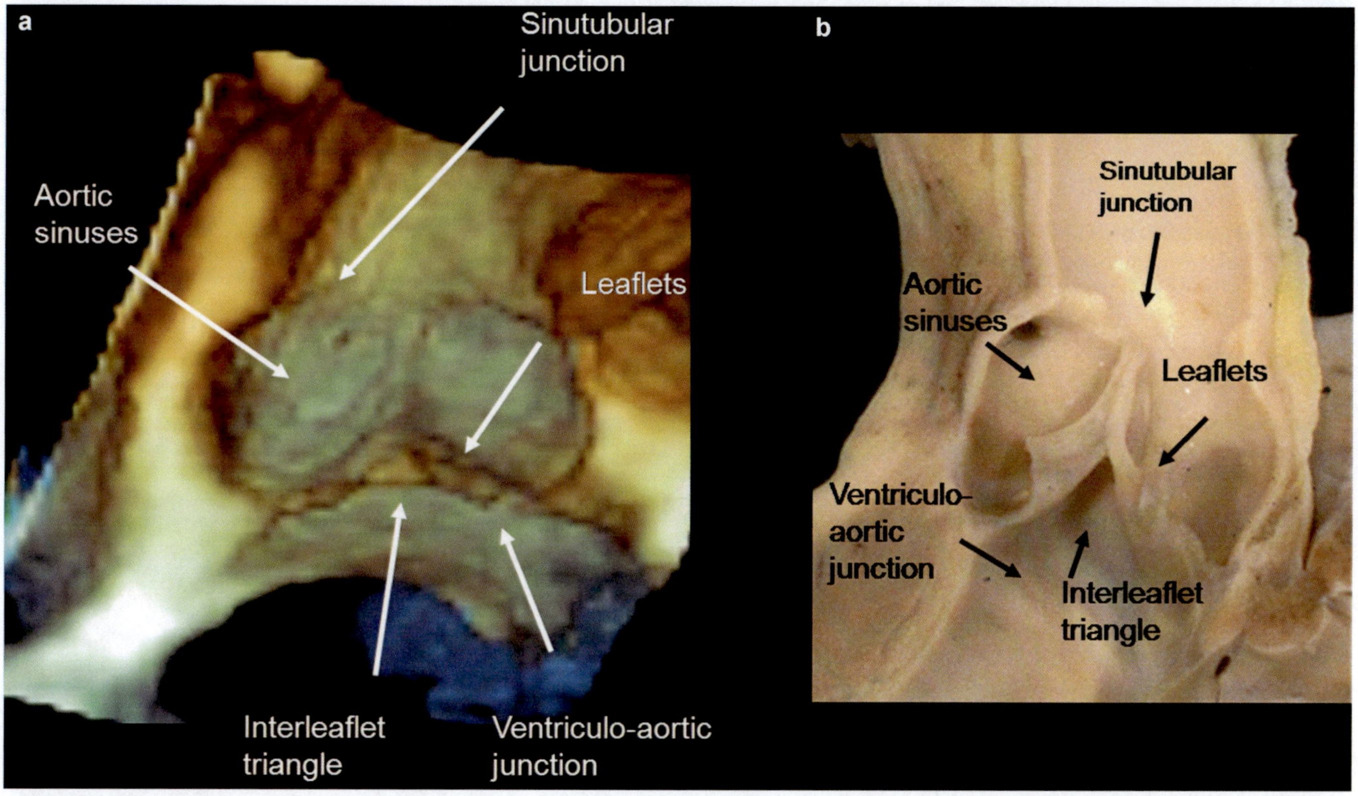

FIGURE 4.3 Real-time 3D TEE image of the aortic root in zoom modality. By cropping the aortic root longitudinally (a), the ventriculo-aortic junction, interleaflet triangles, leaflets, sinuses and sinutubular junction can be visualized in a single image. This is due to the perception of space in the *z*-axis direction given by different color variations. (b) The corresponding anatomical specimen.

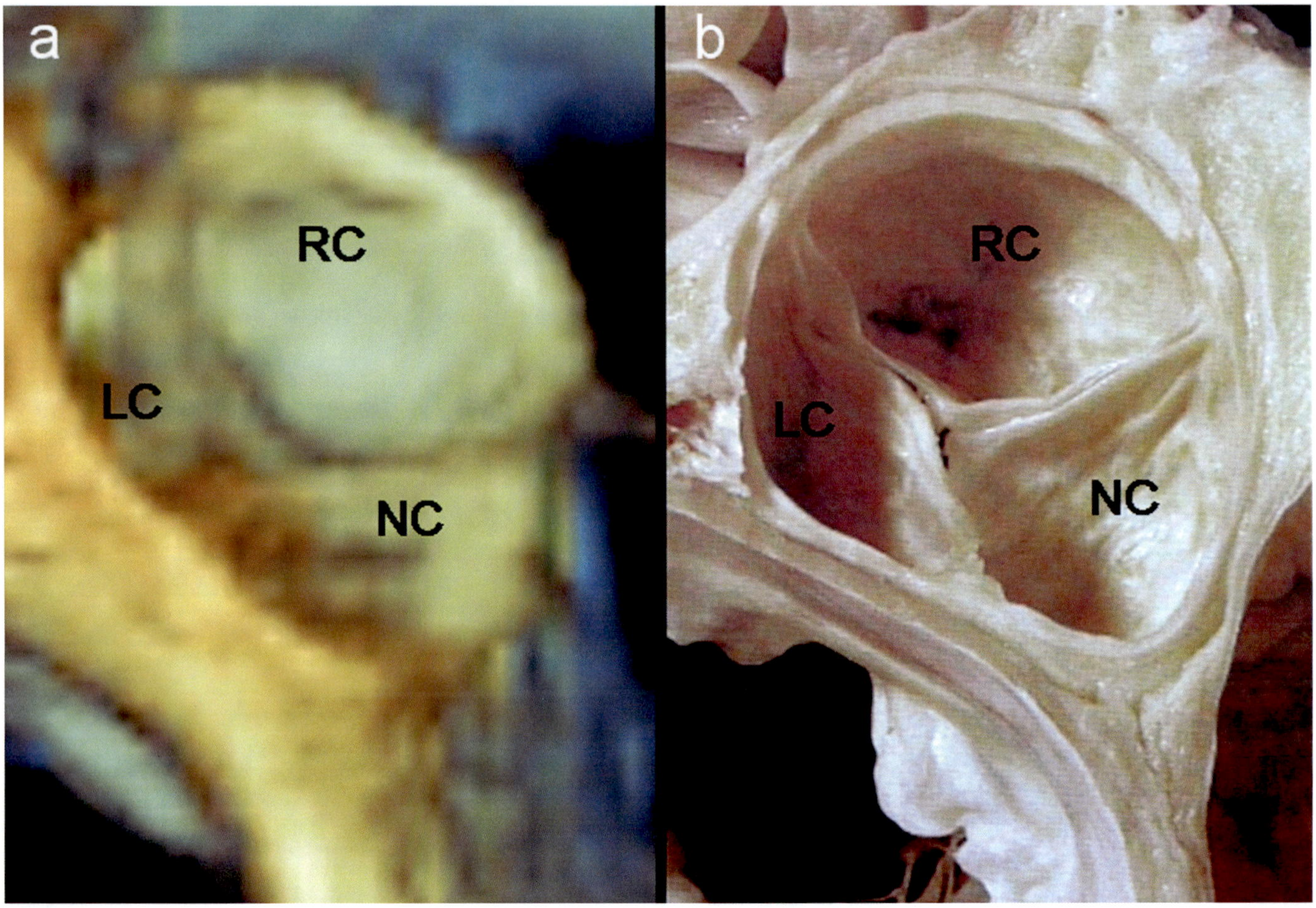

FIGURE 4.4 (a) Details of a real-time 3D TEE image and (b) the corresponding anatomic specimen showing the three leaflets in closed position. The three leaflets meet centrally. *LC* left coronary sinus; *RC* right coronary sinus; *NC* noncoronary sinus.

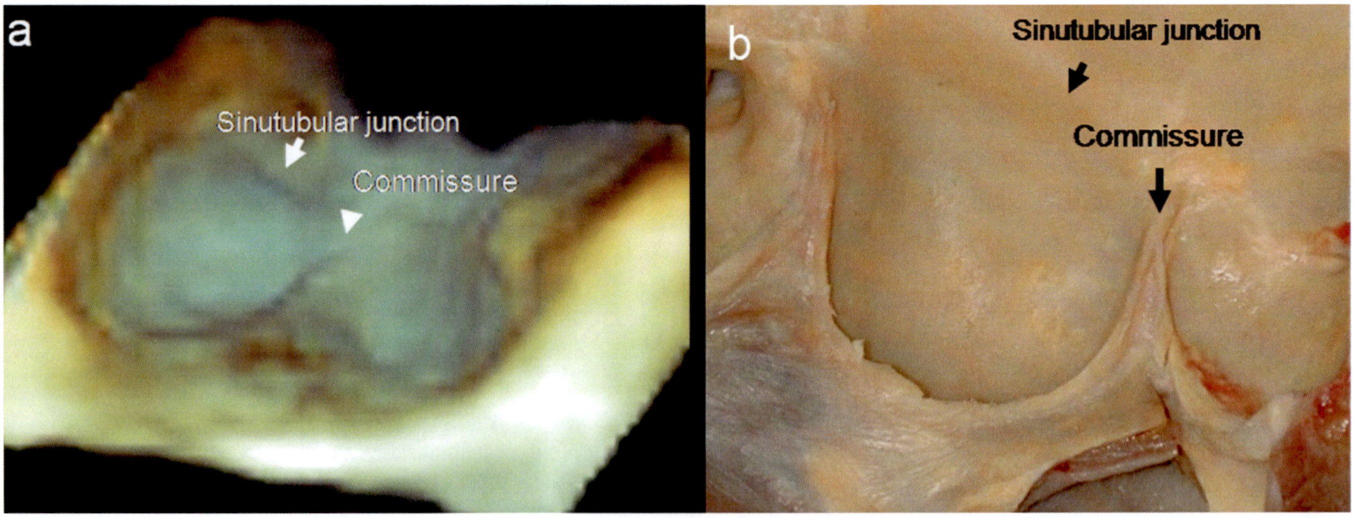

FIGURE 4.5 (a) Details of a real-time 3D TEE image and (b) the corresponding anatomical specimen. By cropping the aortic root longitudinally, commissures can be visualized. The hingeline of collagenous tissue where leaflets are anchored has a crown-shaped configuration.

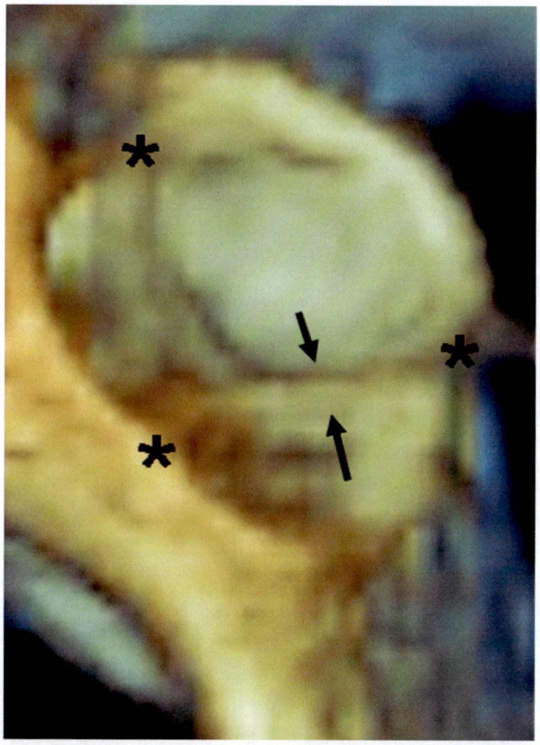

FIGURE 4.6 The same real-time 3D TEE image as in Fig. 4.4. The angulation highlights the coaptation zone between the right coronary and noncoronary leaflets (*arrow*). The *asterisks* indicate the positiono ft het hreec ommissures.

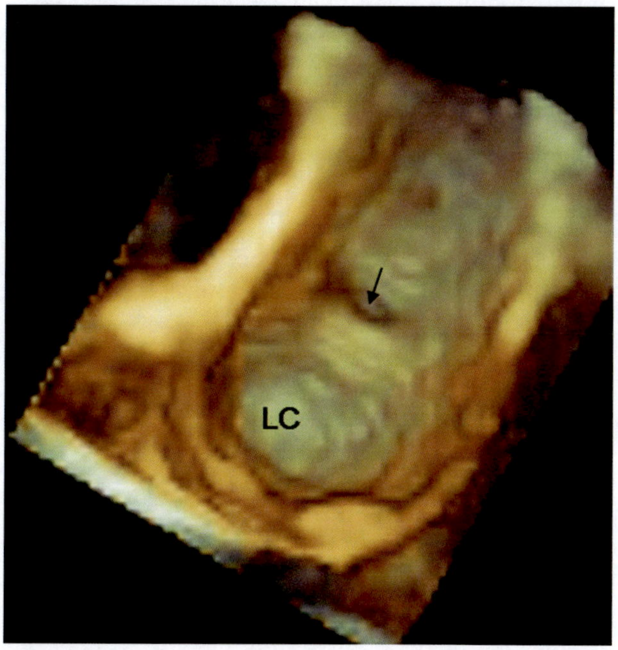

FIGURE 4.7 Details of a real-time 3D TEE image showing the left coronary sinus (LC) and the ostium of the left main coronary artery (*arrow*). This electronic "piece" of heart can be obtained by cropping the surrounding structures. The shape of the sinus and the leaflett ogetherr esemblea swa llow'sn est.

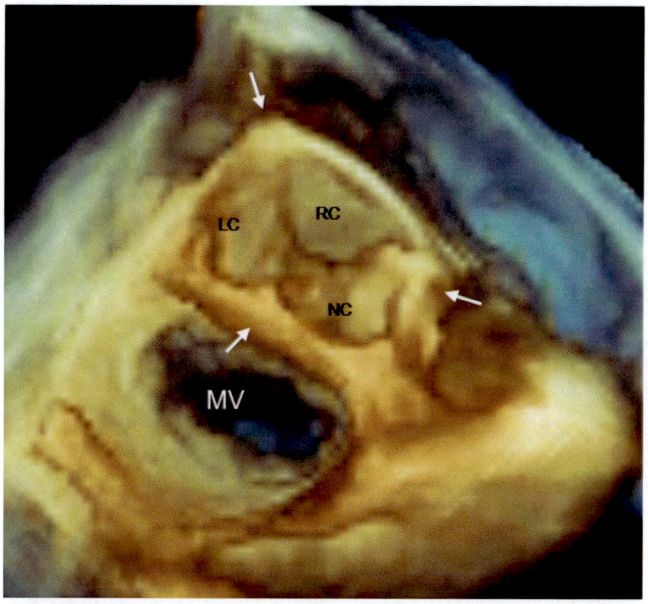

FIGURE 4.8 3D TEE image in full volume modality showing the position of the interleaflet triangles (*arrows*). *LC* left coronary leaflet; *RC* right coronary sinus; *NC* noncoronary sinus; *MV* mitral valve.

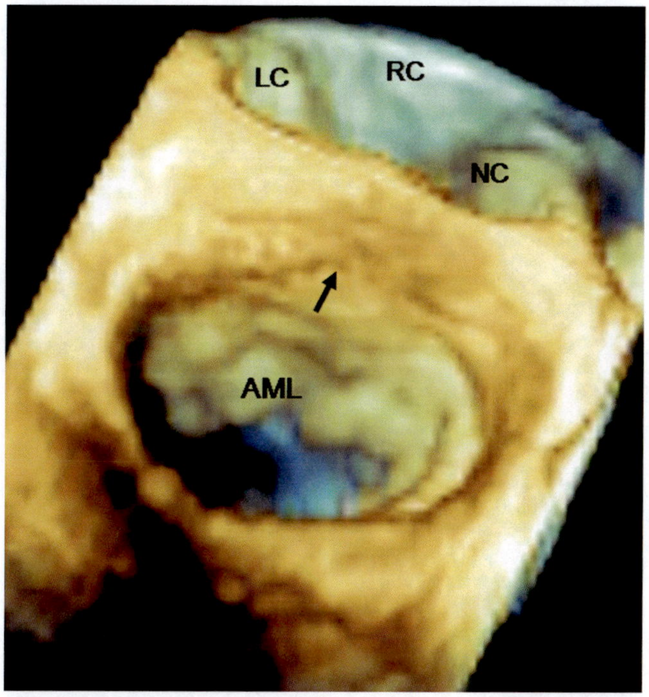

FIGURE 4.9 Real-time 3D TEE image in zoom modality showing the position of the interleaflet triangle (*arrow*) between the left (LC) and noncoronary sinus (NC). This triangle forms part of the mitral-aortic curtain. This triangle can be more easily recognized than others because it is an extension of the anterior mitral leaflets (AML). In this case, the resolution power in the *z*-axis of the system is able to depict the triangle by registering a slight difference in color. *RC* right coronary sinus.

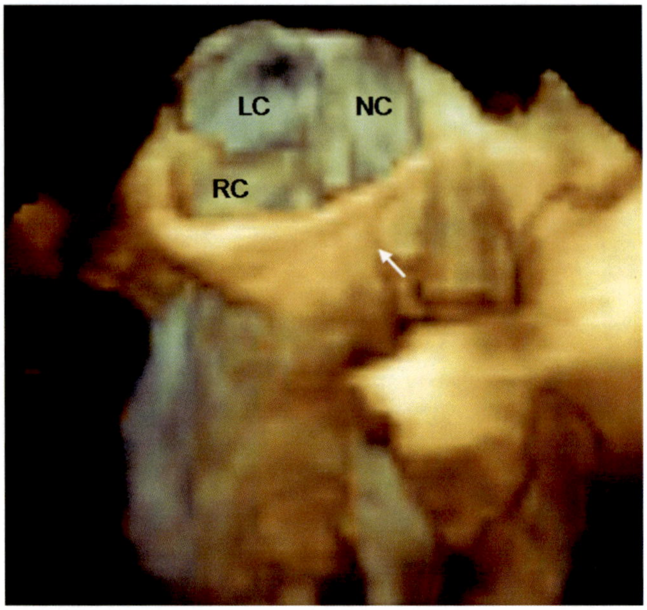

FIGURE 4.10 Real-time 3D TEE image in zoom modality showing the position of the interleaflet triangle (*arrow*) between the right (RC) and noncoronary sinuses (NC). This figure has been obtained by cropping the lateral wall of the right ventricle. This triangle adjoins the membranous part of the ventricular septum. The *z*-axis resolution of the system is not sufficient to image the slight external bulge of the sinuses and the triangle in between them. *LC* left coronary sinus.

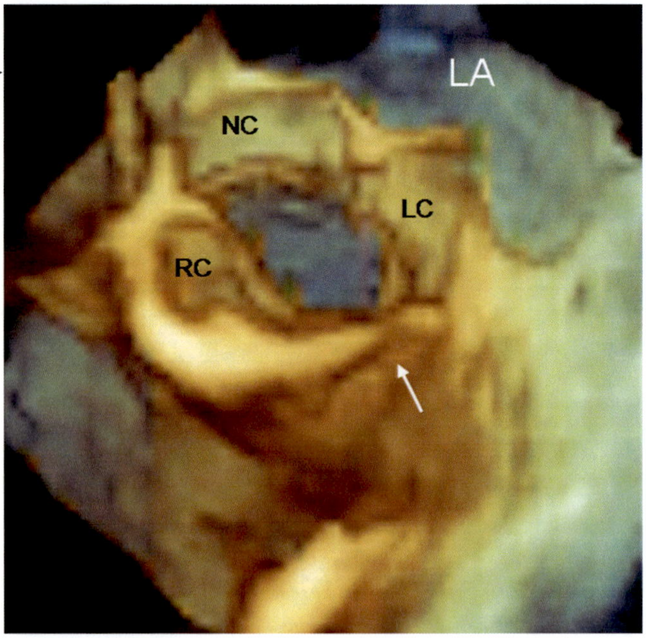

FIGURE 4.11 Real-time 3D TEE image in zoom modality showing the position of the interleaflet triangle (*arrow*) between the right (RC) and left coronary sinuses (LC). The figure has been obtained by cropping the anterior wall of the right ventricle. This triangle is the only one adjoining purely muscular tissue at its base. As in the previous image, the resolution power in the *z*-axis is not sufficient to image the slight depression in between the two coronary aortic sinuses. *NC* noncoronary sinus; *LA*l efta trium.

4.1 3D TEE EXAMPLES OF AORTIC VALVE DISEASE

4.1.1 Aortic Stenosis

The suboptimal visualizations of the aortic valve structures raise the question of whether real-time 3D TEE offers any additional information when compared to 2D TEE in the assessment of aortic valve disease. Some additional data in individual patients can sometimes be obtained with real-time 3D TEE, when live modality is used. Aortic valve stenosis is one of the aortic diseases best studied with live 3D modality. One of the reasons is that stenotic aortic leaflets are thicker than normal leaflets. Figure 4.12 shows a patient with severe aortic stenosis. It is likely that the aortic valve area planimetry will be more accurate with real-time 3D TEE than with 2D TEE (Movie 4.3).

4.1.2 Aortic Regurgitation

Aortic regurgitation results from malcoaptation of the aortic leaflets due to abnormalities in the aortic leaflets, their supporting structures (the aortic root and annulus), or both. Diseases that primarily affect the leaflets include bicuspid aortic valve and other congenital abnormalities, atherosclerotic degeneration, infective endocarditis, rheumatic heart disease, connective tissue or inflammatory diseases, antiphospholipid syndrome, and the use of anorectic drugs. Diseases that primarily affect the annulus or aortic root include idiopathic aortic root dilation, aortic anuloectasia, Marfan syndrome, Ehlers–Danlos syndrome, osteogenesis imperfecta, aortic dissection, syphilitic aortitis, or various connective tissue diseases. Figure 4.13 shows a regurgitant orifice resulting from dilation of the aortic root (Movie 4.4).

4.1.3 Bicuspid Valve

One of the most useful applications of real-time 3D TEE is in the assessment of the bicuspid valve. Images derived with this technique are probably the most accurate ever for determining the size of the leaflets and the presence of a raphe. Figure 4.14 shows a bicuspid valve and a corresponding anatomical specimen (Movie 4.5).

4.1.4 Supravalvular Aortic Stenosis

Supravalvular aortic stenosis is a fixed form of congenital obstruction of the left ventricular outflow tract that occurs as a localized or diffuse narrowing of the ascending aorta beyond the superior margin of the sinuses of Valsalva. This congenital anomaly has three commonly recognized morphological forms. An external hourglass deformity, with a corresponding luminal narrowing of the aorta immediately distal to the coronary artery ostia, is present in 50–75% of patients. In approximately 25% of patients, a fibrous diaphragm is immediately distal to the coronary artery ostia. In

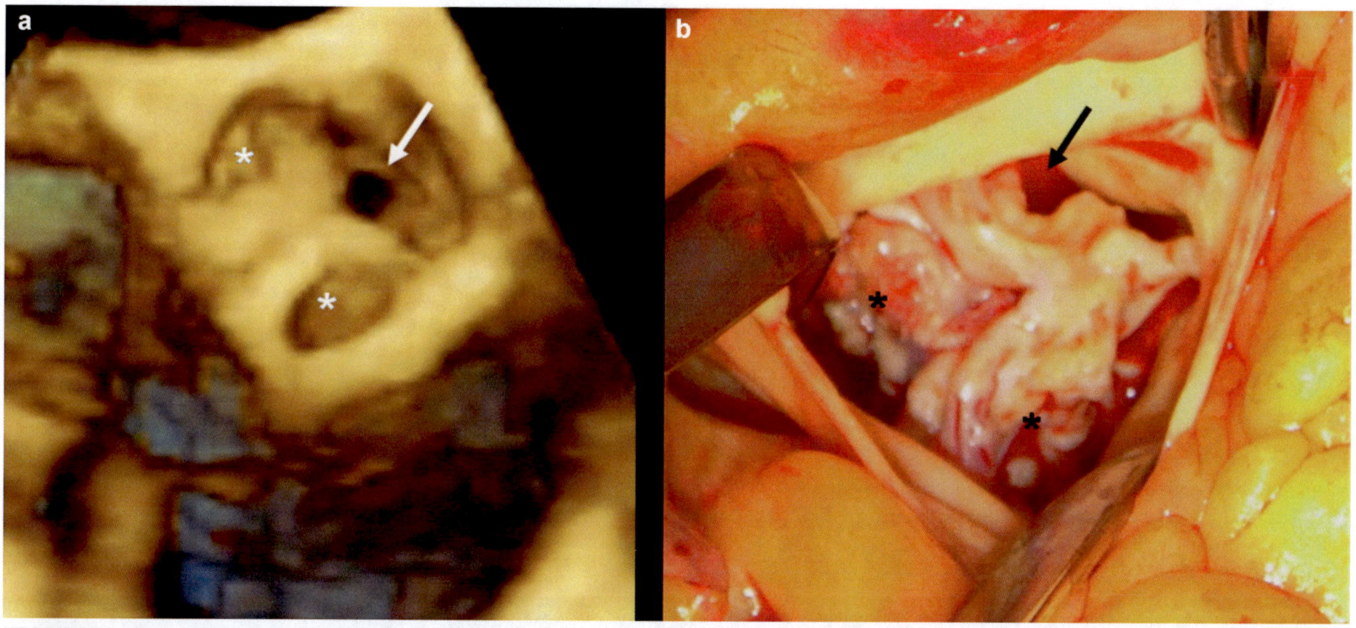

FIGURE 4.12 (a) Real-time 3D TEE image in live modality showing severe aortic stenosis. The noncoronary leaflet and the right coronary cusp (*asterisks*) are fused and immobile. The *arrow* points to the small aortic orifice caused by a limited excursion of the left coronary leaflet. (b)T hec orresponding surgical anatomy.

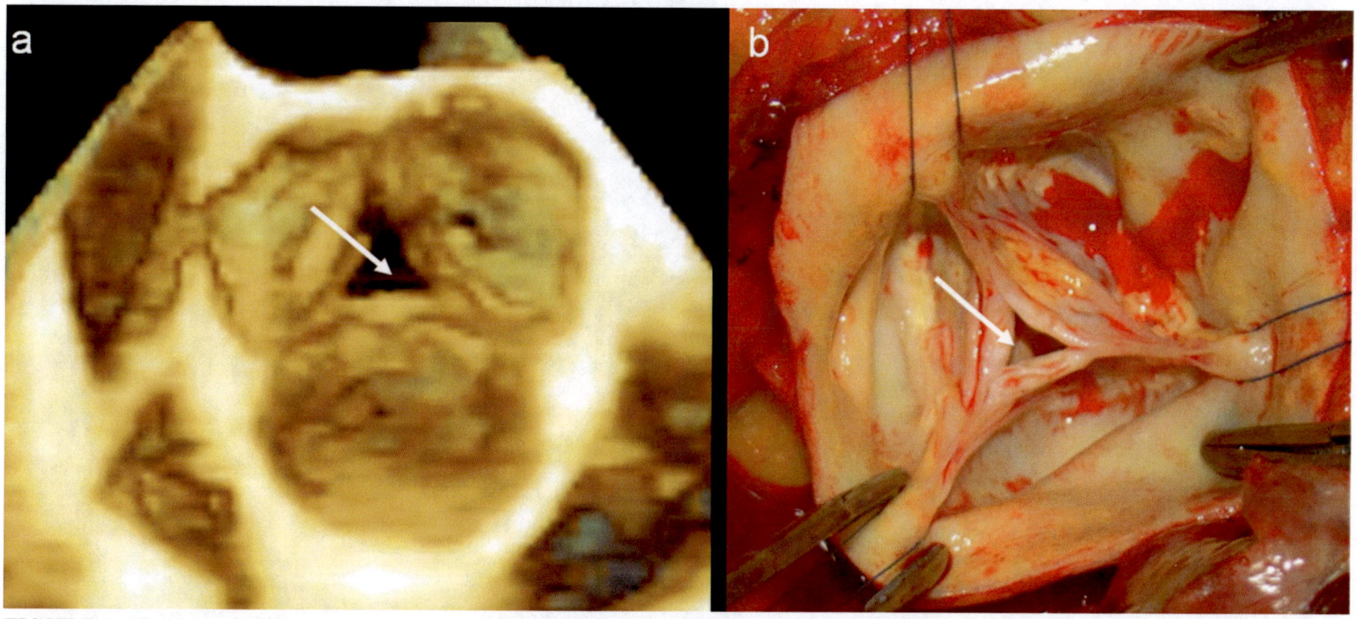

FIGURE 4.13 (a) Real-time 3D TEE image in zoom modality showing annuloectasia resulting in inadequate aortic valve coaptation and severe aortic regurgitation. The *arrow* indicates the regurgitant orifice. (b) The corresponding surgical anatomy.

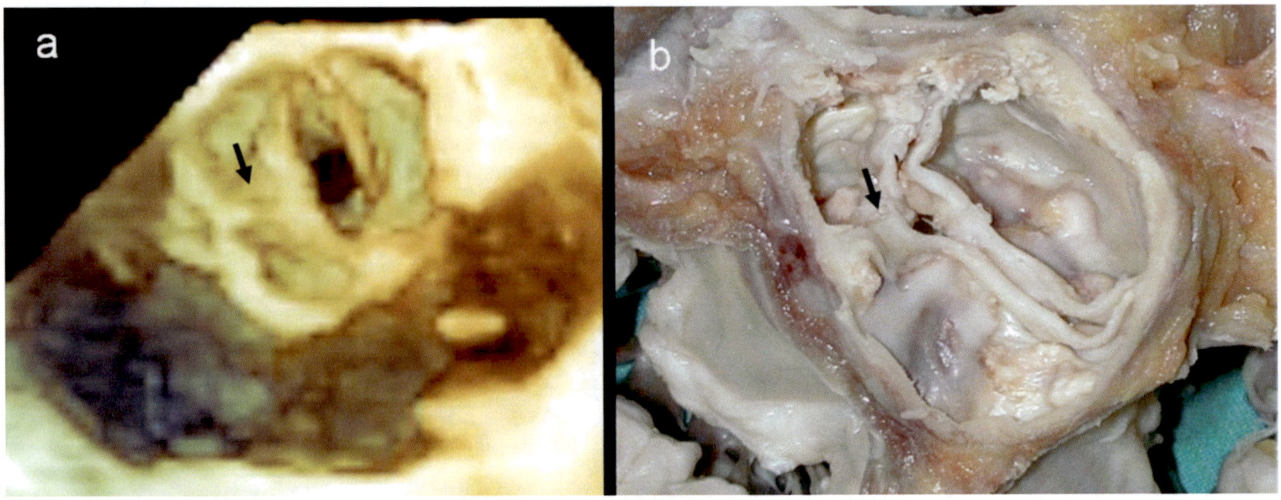

FIGURE 4.14 (a) Real-time 3D TEE image showing a bicuspid aorta and (b) a corresponding anatomic specimen. The *arrow* indicates the raphe.

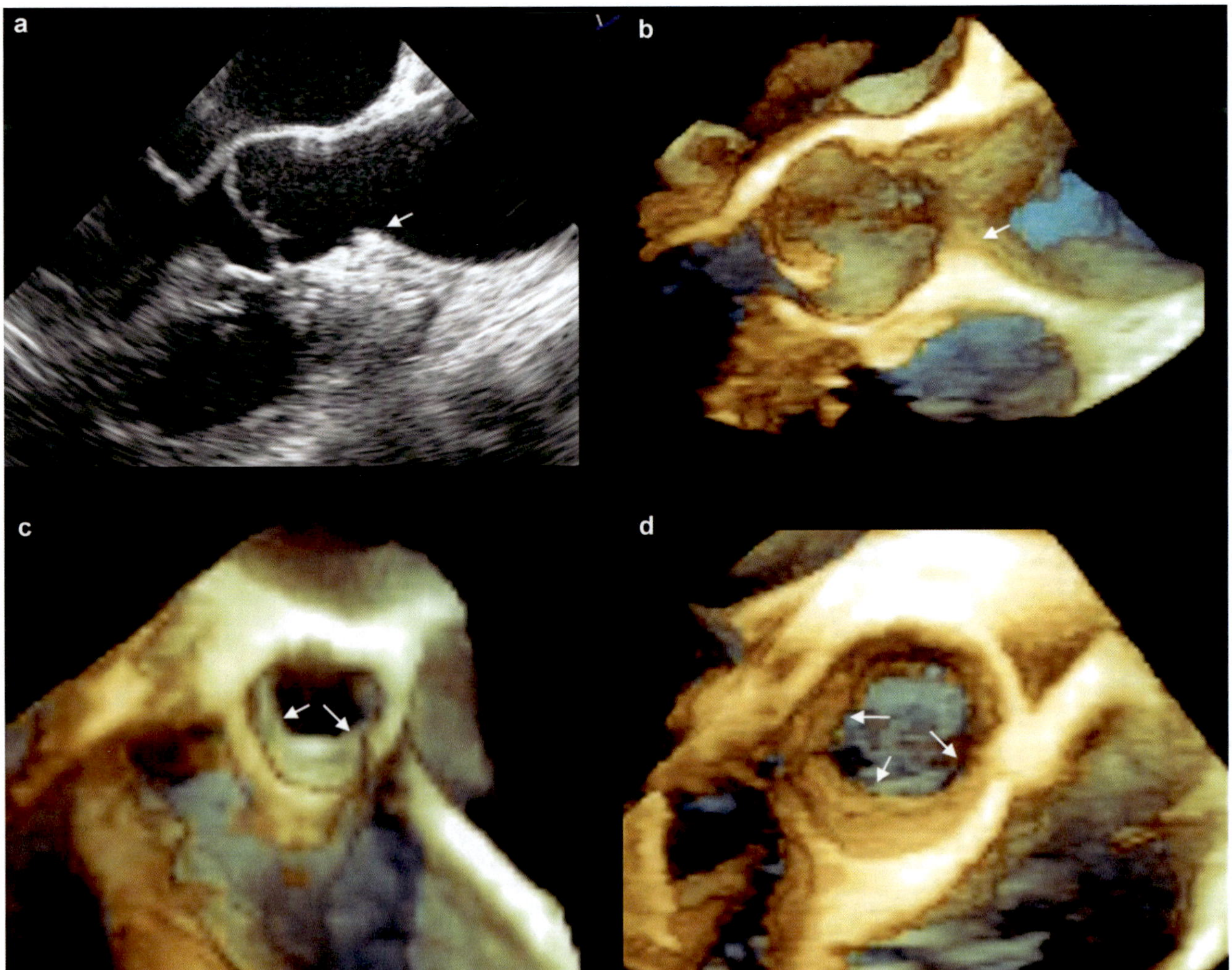

FIGURE 4.15 A composite image of a supravalvular aortic stenosis. (a) 2D TEE shows a supravalvular ridge (*arrow*). (b) Real-time 3D TEE shows the same long axis view. However, the variations in color reveal the *z*-axis showing the semicircle shape of the ridge. (c, d) Images of the ridge from the ventricular and aortic perspectives (*arrows*). From the latter viewpoints, the ridge has a semilunar configuration.

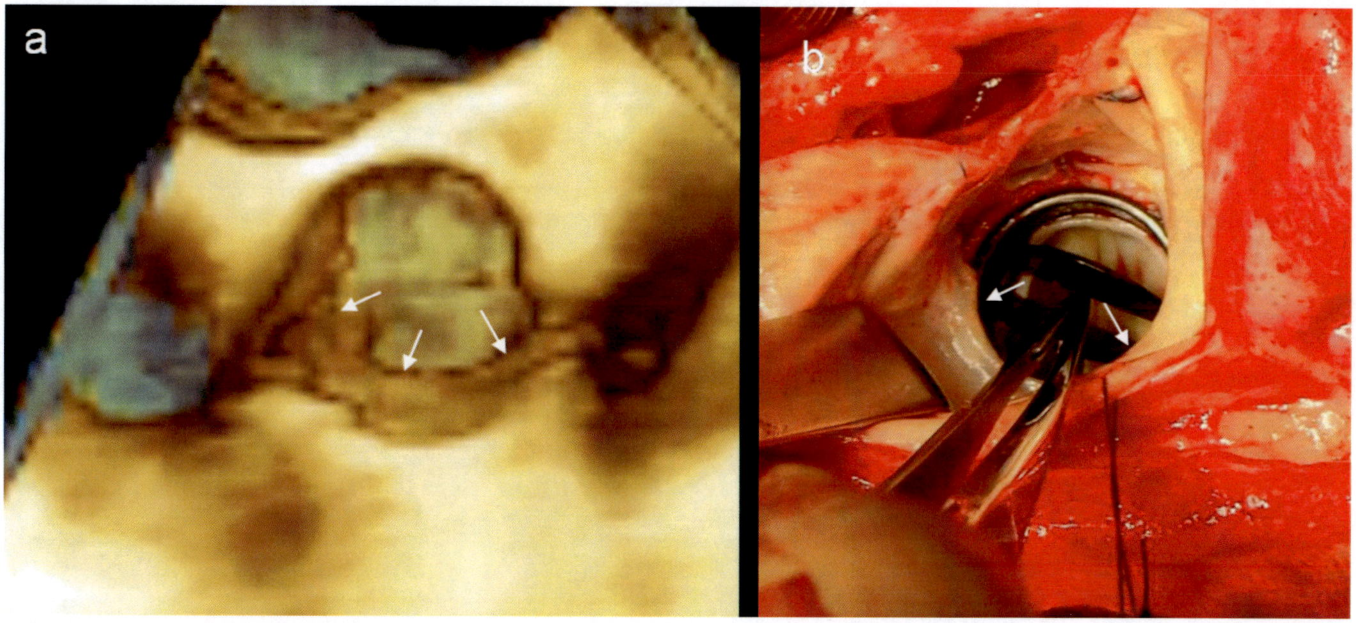

FIGURE 4.16 (a) Real-time 3D TEE image in zoom modality from the aortic perspective showing a semilunar-shaped fibrotic pannus (*arrows*). (b) The corresponding surgical image showing the pannus partially covering the mechanical prosthesis (*arrow*).

fewer than 25% of patients, a diffuse narrowing along a variable length of the ascending aorta is present. Real-time 3D TEE may enhance the diagnostic accuracy of 2D TEE showing the obstruction not only in long axis view but also from the ventricular and aortic perspective (Fig. 4.15).

A fibrotic tissue growing around an aortic prosthetic valve is a rare complication that may cause prosthetic obstruction. Figure 4.16 refers to a patient with a high transprosthetic gradient where real-time 3D TEE enabled an accurate diagnosis of supraprosthetic fibrotic pannus.

4.1.5 Atherosclerotic Plaques

The ascending aorta and aortic arch are visualized in detail with 2D TEE. Large, protrusive atherosclerotic plaques in the ascending aorta, aortic arch, and descending aorta, moving freely with the blood flow, could cause embolic syndromes, especially after catheter manipulation in the aorta. Real-time 3D TEE offers new perspectives, providing a "geographic distribution" of the protruding plaques (Figs.4. 17a nd 4.18).

4.1.6 AorticDi ssection

The classic aortic dissection is a longitudinal split of the aorta wall when a small tear occurs in the intima layer allowing the blood to reach the medial layer and form a false lumen. The original lumen (true lumen) continues to be lined by intima, while the false lumen is lined by media. Typically, the false lumen often becomes aneurysmal when subjected to systemic pressure. Aortic dissection is the most common catastrophe of the aorta. When left untreated, about 33% of patients die within the first 24 h and 50% die within 48 h. The 2-week mortality rate approaches 75% in patients with undiagnosed ascending aortic dissection. The Stanford classification divides dissections into two types: type A and type B. Type A includes the ascending aorta (DeBakey types I and II); type B does not involve this portion (DeBakey type III). This system also helps delineate treatment. Usually, type A dissections require surgery, while type B dissections may be managed medically under most conditions.

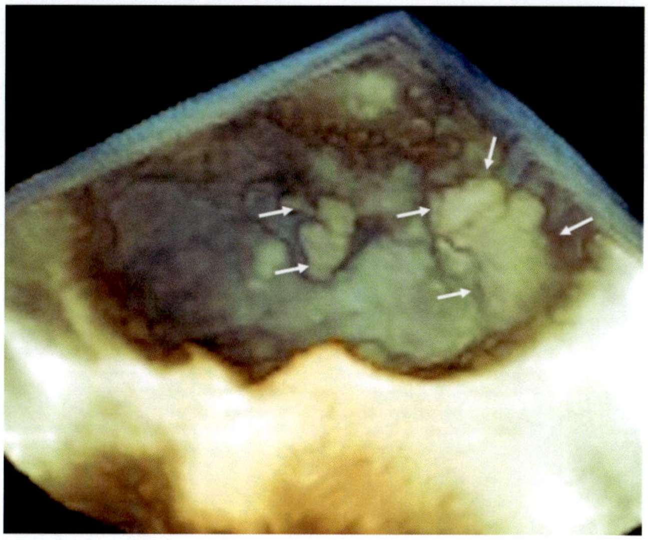

FIGURE 4.17 Real-time 3D TEE image in zoom modality showing two large protruding plaques (*arrows*) in the aortic arch.

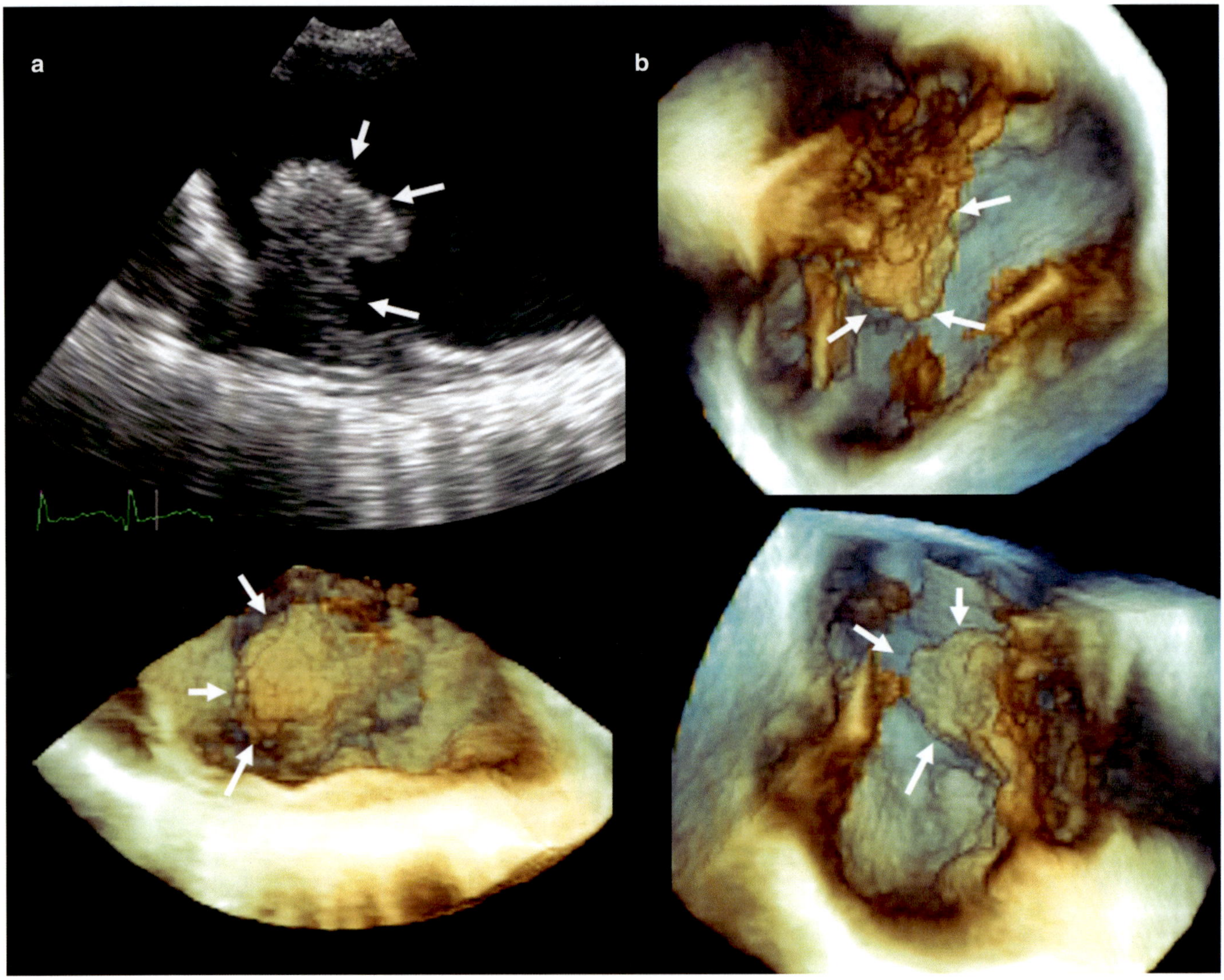

FIGURE 4.18 (a) 2D TEE and (b–d) real-time 3D TEE image in zoom modality showing different perspectives of a large protruding irregular plaque in the descending aorta (*arrows*).

MOVIE 4.3 An example of severe aortic stenosis from aortic perspective.

MOVIE 4.4 An example of severe dilatation of the aortic root with the central regurgitant orifice.

MOVIE 4.5 An example of a bicuspid aortic valve.

MOVIE 4.6 An example of a stenosis of a bicuspid aortic valve with central raphe on the anterior leaflet.

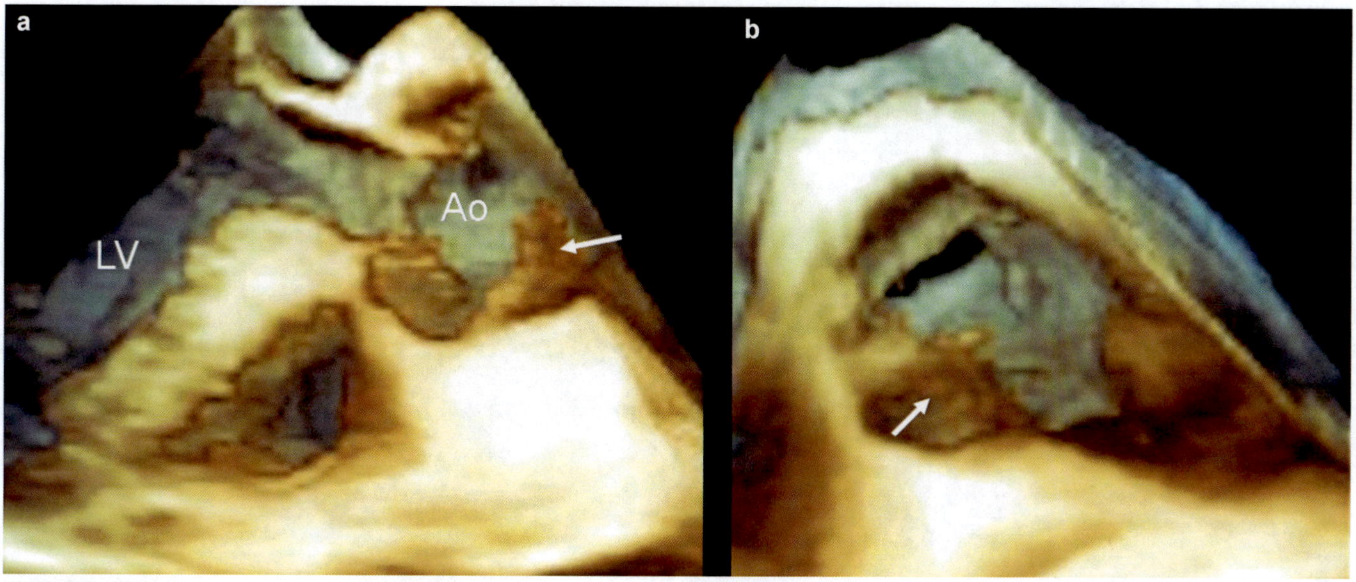

FIGURE 4.19 (a) RT 3D TEE image showing the dissection of the aortic wall (*arrow*) in longitudinal view and (b) from the aortic perspective. *Ao* aorta; *LVl* eftv entricle.

Patients with suspected thoracic aortic dissection require early and accurate diagnosis. Conventional aortography has been completely replaced in the last decade by less invasive imaging techniques including TEE, computed tomography, and magnetic resonance imaging. All three diagnostic approaches yield comparable, clinically reliable diagnostic value for confirming or excluding thoracic aortic dissection. Again, real-time 3D TEE has the advantage of imaging the dissection from different perspectives(Fig.4 .19).

Because of the ability of 3D to explore the *z*-dimension, this technique provides a more comprehensive view of the pathology and a simpler method of detection of intimal tears (Fig. 4.20) (see also Movie 4.7).

MOVIE 4.7 An example of aortic dissection clearly showing the tear on the intimal layer dividing the true lumen from the false lumen.

4.1.7 Percutaneous, Catheter-Based Aortic Valve Implantation

This is a promising technique that can be performed either by the transfemoral or transapical approach and may offer an alternative to conventional surgery for high-risk patients with aortic stenosis. It is still in its early days and there are many unanswered questions regarding safety and long-term durability. Currently, a retrograde approach via the femoral artery is preferred. Recently, an alternative, transapical approach has been proposed in patients with extensive ilio femoral artery disease: after an intercostal incision, direct puncture of the apical portion of the left ventricular free wall is performed to gain catheter access to the left ventricle and aortic valve.

Two types of implantable prosthesis have been used: a balloon-expandable aortic valve prosthesis and a self-expanding valve prosthesis. The balloon-expandable aortic valve implantation is performed under general anesthesia, with fluoroscopic and TEE guidance. After retrograde crossing and predilation of the native valve, the prosthesis is pushed by a flexible catheter, positioned within the aortic valve, and then delivered by balloon-inflation under rapid ventricular pacing. The self-expanding valve prosthesis consists of a trileaflet bioprosthetic porcine pericardial tissue valve, which is mounted and sutured in a self-expanding nitinol stent. The procedure of implantation is similar to that used for balloon-expandable device: the prosthesis is deployed retrogradely under fluoroscopic and TEE guidance. Further technical details are beyond the scope of this chapter.

Two-dimensional TEE allows accurate assessment of the aortic annulus size, continuous visualization of intracardiac catheters and devices, immediate evaluation of the result of the procedure, as well as assessment of the patency of the left main coronary artery at the completion of the procedure. Equally reliable data can be obtained with real-time 3D TEE. However, the ability to switch from biplane to 3D imaging instantaneously might increase confidence and safety during the procedure (Figs. 4.21–4.25).

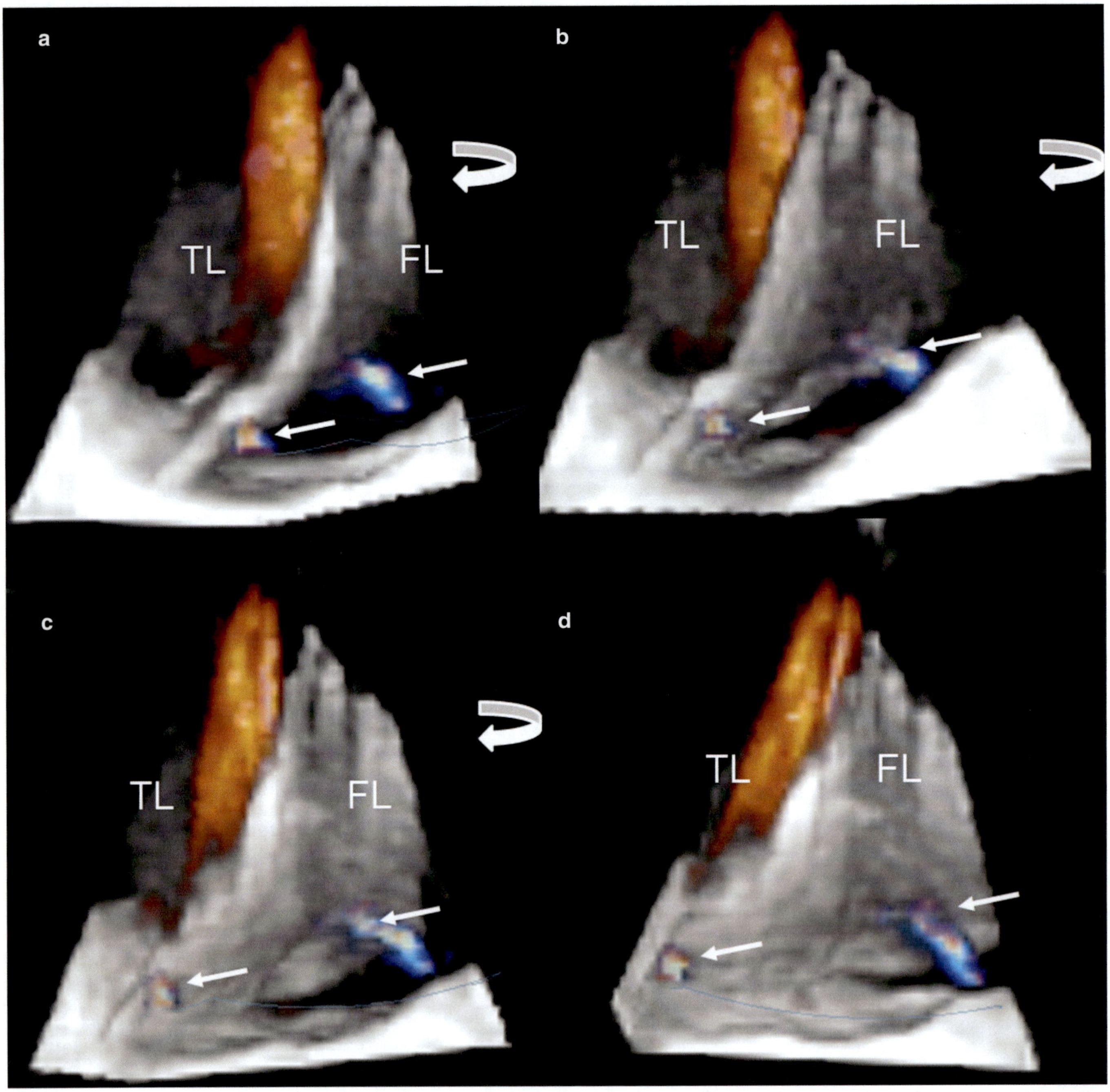

FIGURE 4.20 (a–d) 3D TEE images showing two intimal tears (*arrows*). A progressive right-to-left rotation (*curved arrows*) provides an "en face" image of the aortic wall dividing the true lumen (TL) from the false lumen (FL).

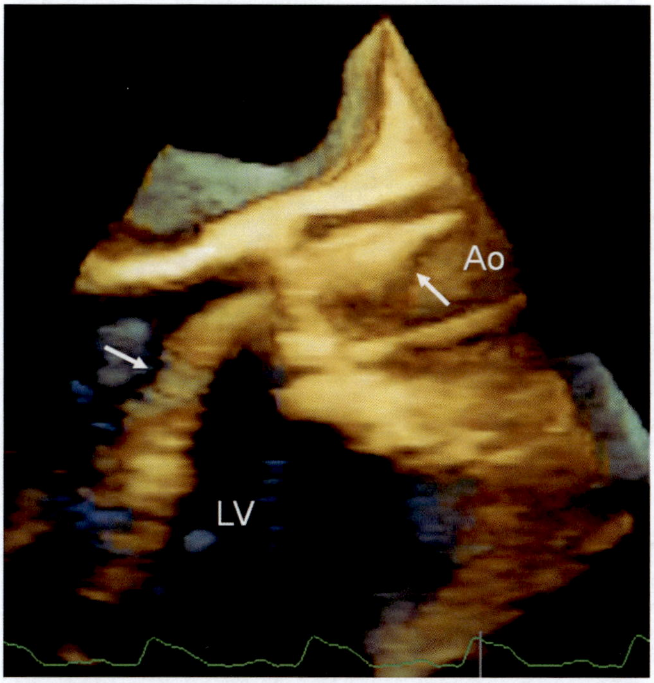

FIGURE 4.21 Real-time live 3D TEE showing guiding catheter passing through the aortic valve (*arrows*). *Ao* aorta; *LV* left ventricle.

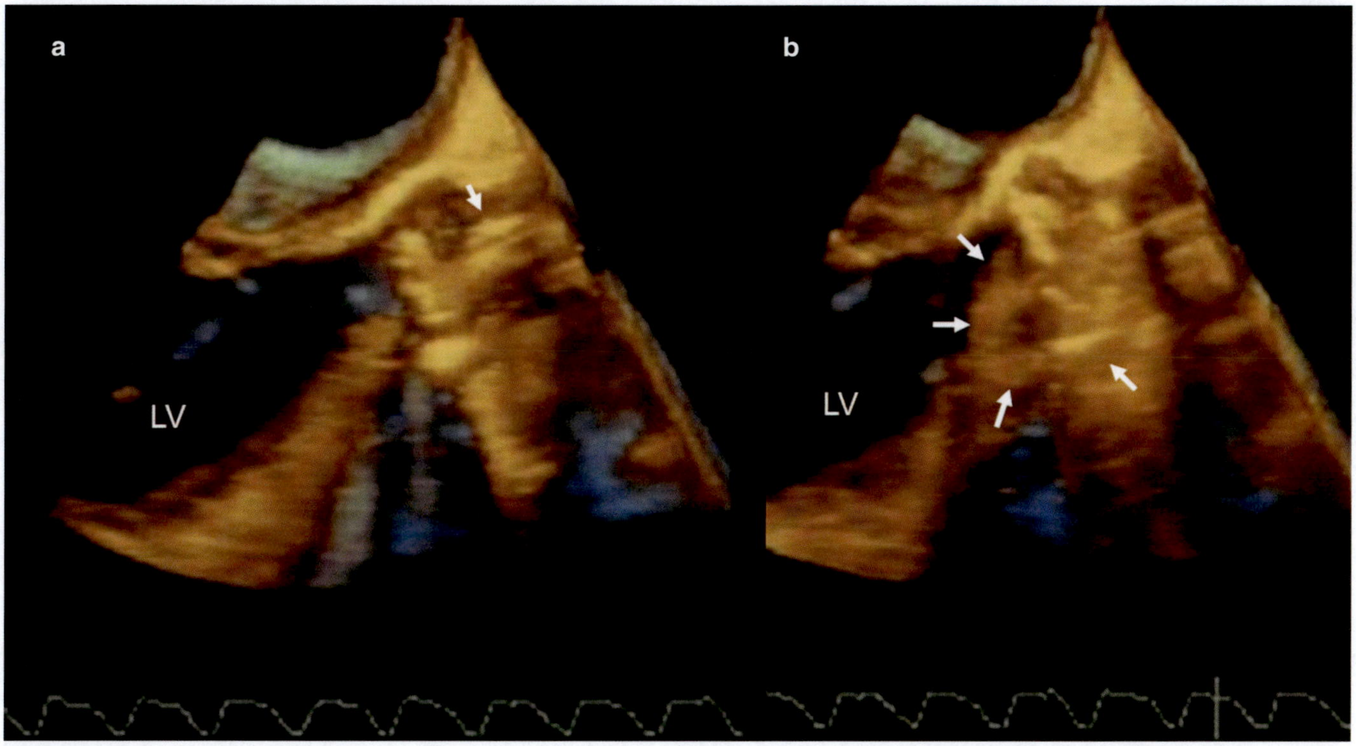

FIGURE 4.22 (a) Real-time live 3D TEE showing a guiding catheter passing through the aortic valve (*arrows*) and (b) during balloon-inflation. *LV*,l eftv entricle.

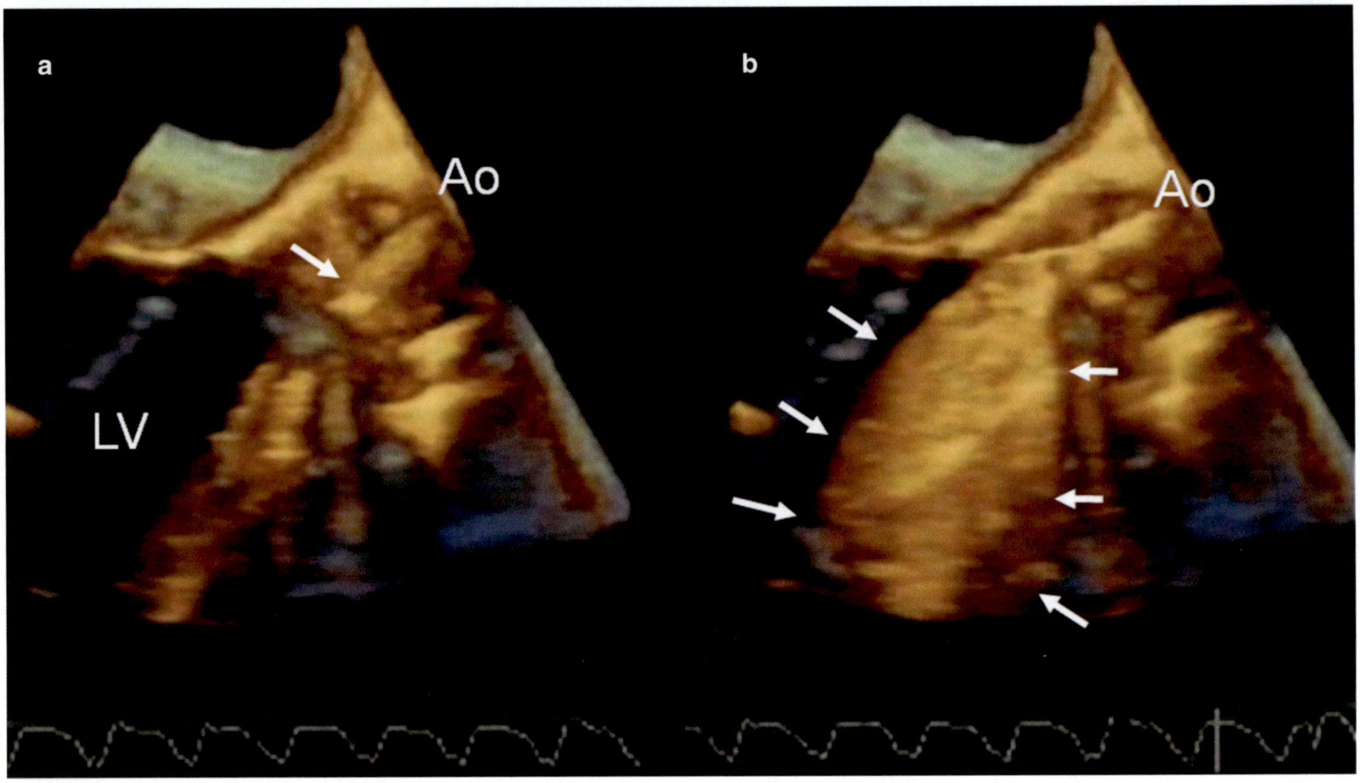

FIGURE 4.23 (a) Real-time live 3D TEE showing a guiding catheter passing through the aortic valve (*arrow*) and (b) the "wrong" position of the delivery system in the left ventricular outflow tract. *Arrows* mark the inflated balloon. *Ao* aorta; *LV* left ventricle.

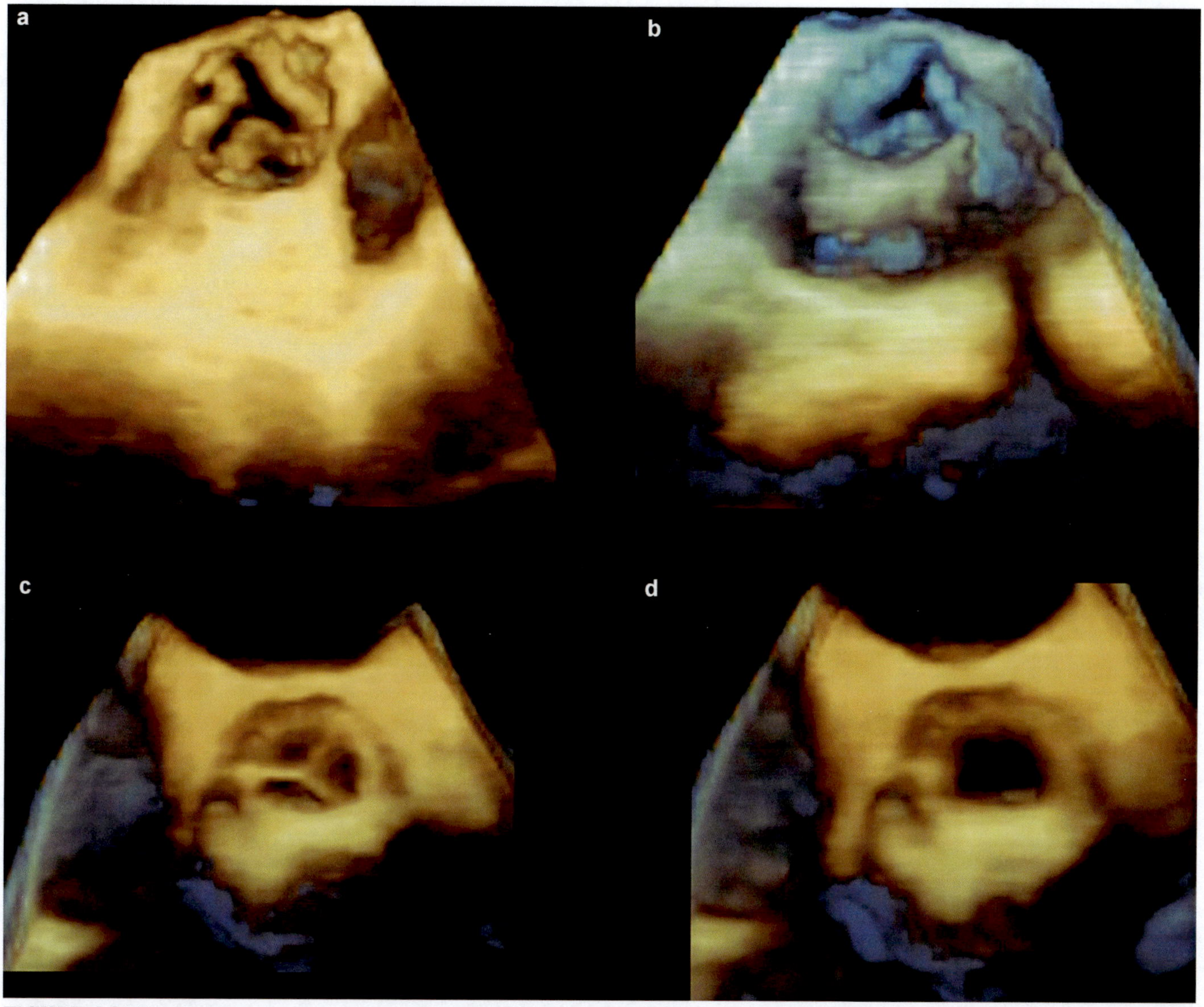

FIGURE 4.24 (a) Real-time live 3D TEE showing a systolic frame from the aortic and (b) the left ventricular perspective of a patient with severe aortic stenosis; (c) diastolic and (d) systolic frames as seen from aortic perspective in the same patient after percutaneous valve implantation.

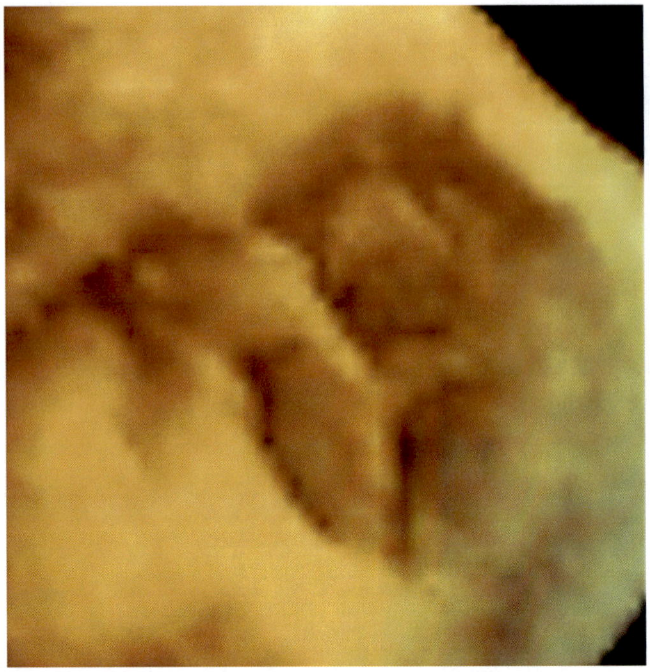

FIGURE 4.25 Magnified image of the leaflets of a percutaneously implanted aortic valve in real-time live 3D TEE from the aortic perspective. A slight angulation helps to minimize drop-out artifacts.

CHAPTER5

Tricuspida nd Pulmonic Valves

5.1 THE TRICUSPID VALVE

Imaging of the tricuspid valve in real-time 3D TEE produces consistently suboptimal results. The reasons for this substantial failure are (a) the oblique plane of the valve in relation to the ultrasound pyramidal beams and (b) the thinness of the leaflets that makes it difficult to find the appropriate gain setting to remove noises but not structures. In Fig. 5.1a, a near perfect image of the base of the heart, seen from the atrial perspective, is obtained. But the image of the tricuspid valve is poor, and unlike the nearby mitral valve, part of the tissue at the base of the leaflets and along their free margins is missing because of the inadequate gain level. However, even a small increase in gain [in Figure 5.1b] causes noise that obscures both the mitral and tricuspid leaflets.

In some patients, because of its favorable orientation in relation to ultrasound pyramidal beams, the tricuspid valve is well imaged. We have used images derived from these patients to describe the normal appearance of the tricuspid valve.

The tricuspid valve comprises of an annulus, leaflets, tendinous chords, and papillary muscle The annulus has an elliptical shape that nearly mirrors the mitral annulus

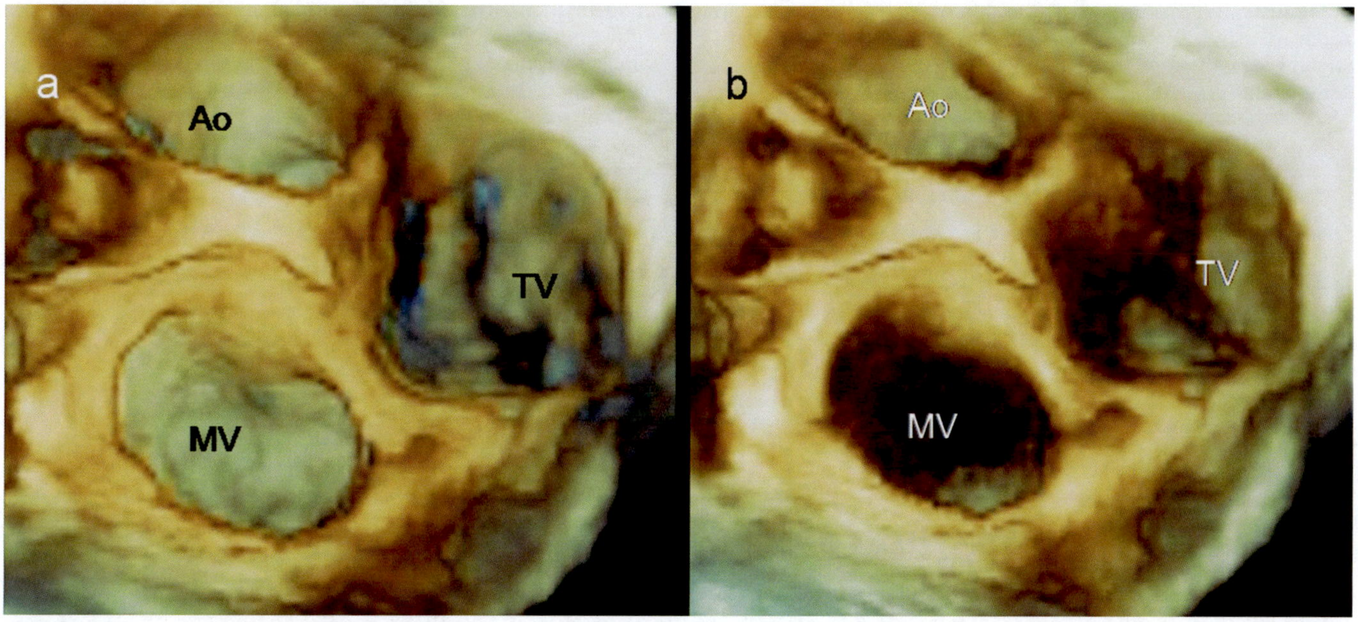

FIGURE 5.1 (a) 3D TEE of the base of the heart in full volume modality. The gain setting is at the right level for the mitral valve (MV), but it is not adequate for the tricuspid valve (TV), resulting in parts of the tissue of the tricuspid leaflets being lost. (b) The same image with only a slight increase of the gain resulting in the leaflets of both valves being obscured by noise. *Ao* aorta.

with a straight septal component and a curved mural component (Figs. 5.2 and 5.3). Usually, the valve has three leaflets: the septal, the antero-superior, and the posterior (inferior) (Figs.5. 4a nd 5.5).

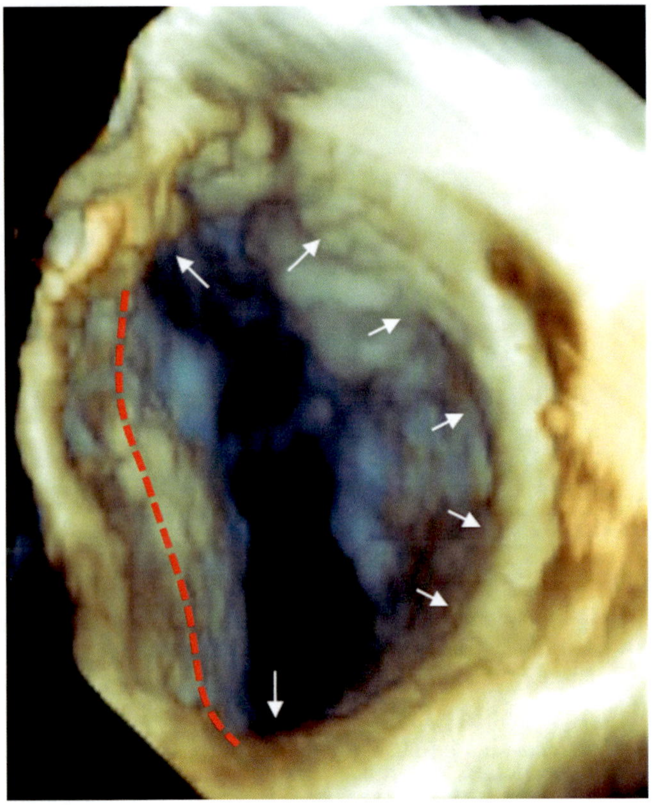

FIGURE 5.2 Real-time 3D TEE image of the tricuspid valve in zoom modality. The annulus has a roughly elliptical shape with a straight septal component (*red dotted line*) and a curved mural component (*arrows*).

Different perspectives can optimize the visualization of the leaflets (Fig. 5.6). As with the mitral valve, tricuspid leaflets may have further subdivisions consisting of scallops (Fig. 5.7).

Sometimes, the division between the antero-superior and posterior leaflets is not so clear, and surgeons consider the two leaflets to be a single unique structure, the so-called "mural" leaflet (Fig. 5.8).

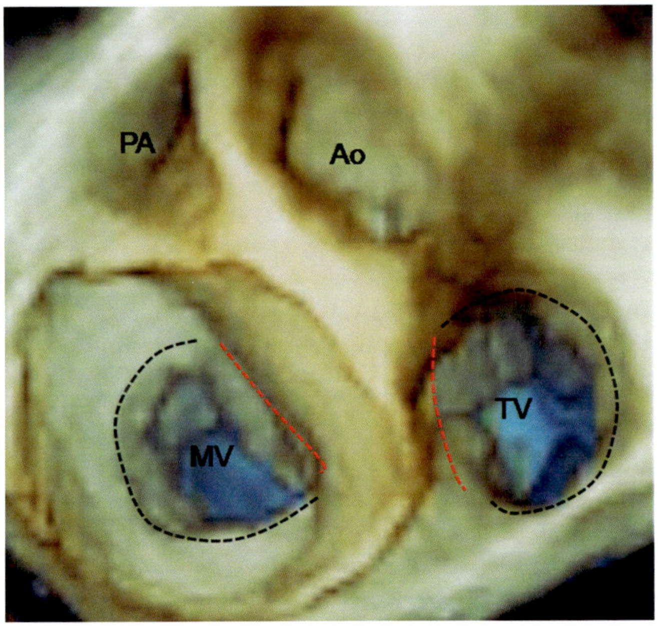

FIGURE 5.3 3D TEE image of the base of the heart in full volume modality. The shape of the tricuspid annulus roughly mirrors that of the mitral annulus with a straight septal component (*red dotted line*) and a curved mural component (*black dotted line*). *PA* pulmonary artery; *Ao* aorta; *MV* mitral valve; *TV* tricuspid valve.

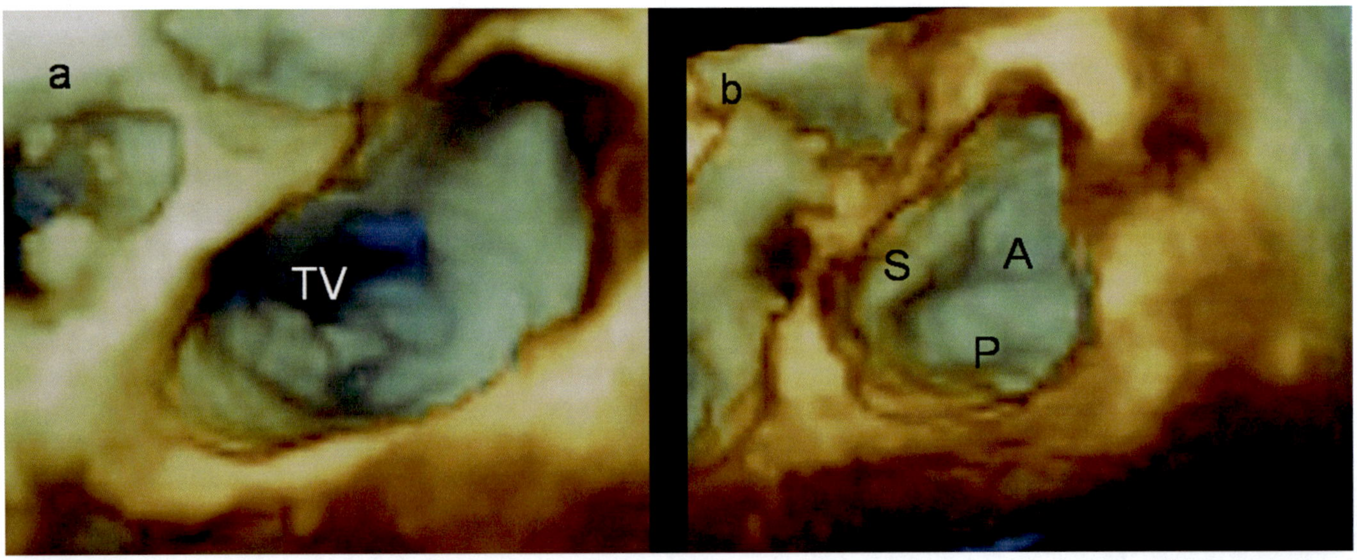

FIGURE 5.4 Real-time 3D TEE images of the tricuspid valve in zoom modality. (a) The tricuspid valve (TV) in diastole and (b) in systole viewed from the atrial perspective. The septal (S), posterior (P), and antero-superior (A) leaflets can be recognized in systole, but not in diastole.

Functional tricuspid regurgitation owing to annular dilatation, without organic leaflet disease, is a commonly encountered tricuspid disease. Very often, functional tricuspid regurgitation is caused by left-side heart disease such as mitral stenosis, mitral regurgitation, or severe left ventricular dysfunction associated with elevated pulmonic pressure. More rarely, tricuspid annular dilatation is caused by long-standing atrial fibrillation with normal left-sided structures. Figures 5.9 and 5.10 show the case of a 65-year-old patient with long-standing atrial fibrillation who developed severe tricuspid regurgitation as a result of annular dilatation. Notably, in daily clinical practice, the tricuspid valve is more visible when the right-sided chambers are enlarged. There are two possible reasons: (a) the valve becomes more perpendicular to the ultrasound pyramidal beams and (b) the enlarged right atrium leaves more space for complete visualization of the valve.

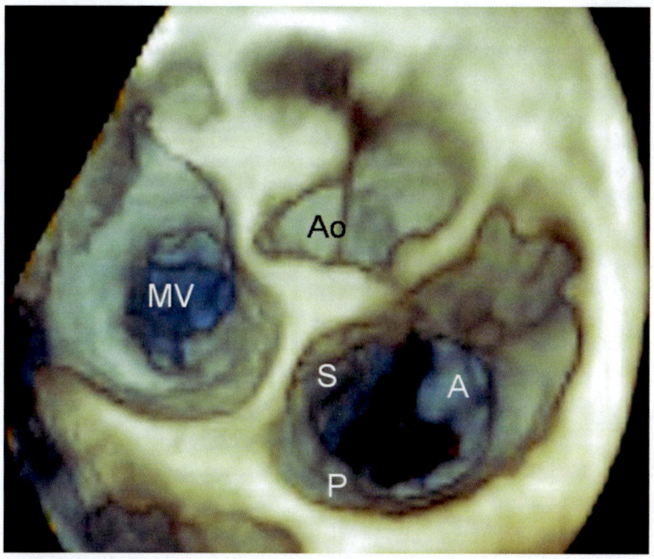

FIGURE 5.5 3D TEE image of the tricuspid valve in full volume modality. The tricuspid valve in diastole is seen from the atrial perspective. The septal (S), posterior (P), and antero-superior (A) leaflets can be recognized. *MV* mitral valve; *Ao*a orta.

5.2 THE PULMONIC VALVE

The pulmonic valve is identical in design to the aortic valve. However, pulmonic leaflets are slightly thinner than the aortic ones. This thinness makes it more difficult to set the gain correctly and distinguish from other noise. Moreover, the long distance between the transducer and the pulmonic leaflets causes a deterioration in image quality. As the ultrasound beams diverge, the resolution power decreases resulting in the pulmonic leaflets appearing thick and hard to discern (Fig. 5.11). Occasionally, by rotating the image, the interaction between shadow and colors makes the leaflets more visible (Fig. 5.11b).

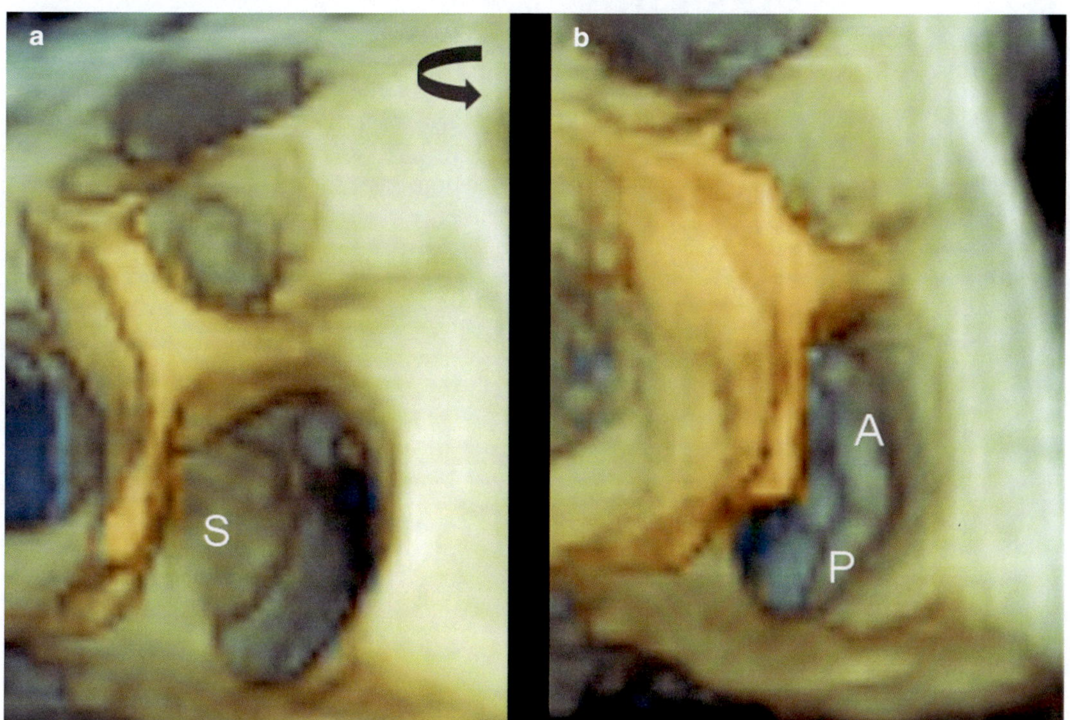

FIGURE 5.6 3D TEE image of the tricuspid leaflets in full volume modality. (a) the septal (S) leaflet. (b) A slight rotation of the image (*black curved arrow*) reveals the antero-superior (A) and posterior (P) leaflets.

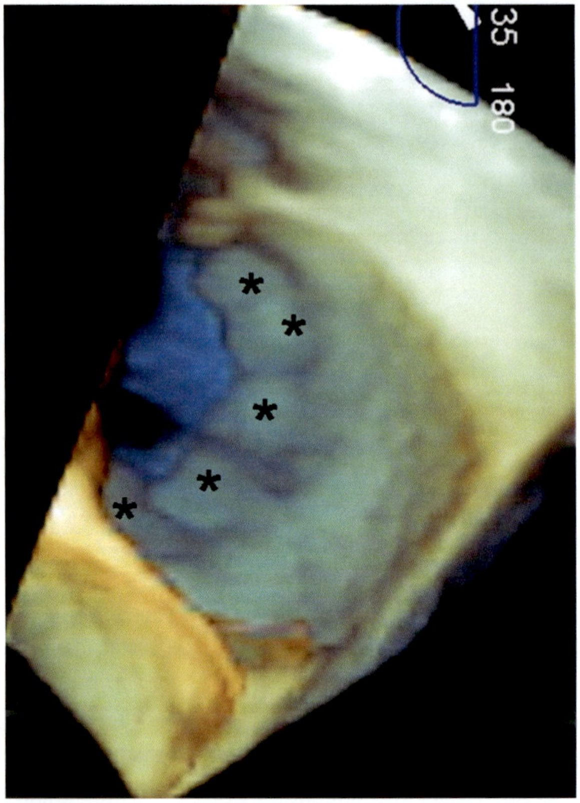

FIGURE 5.7 Real-time 3D TEE image of antero-superior and posterior leaflets in zoom modality. The two leaflets have several scallops (*asterisks*).

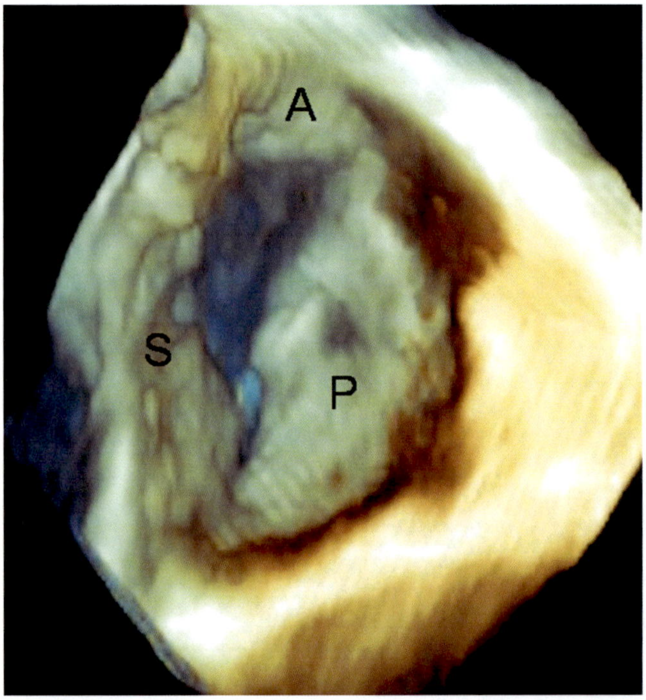

FIGURE 5.8 Real-time 3D TEE image of the tricuspid valve in zoom modality. A large posterior leaflet (P) hinging on almost all of the mural annulus can be observed. *S* septal; *A*a ntero-superior.

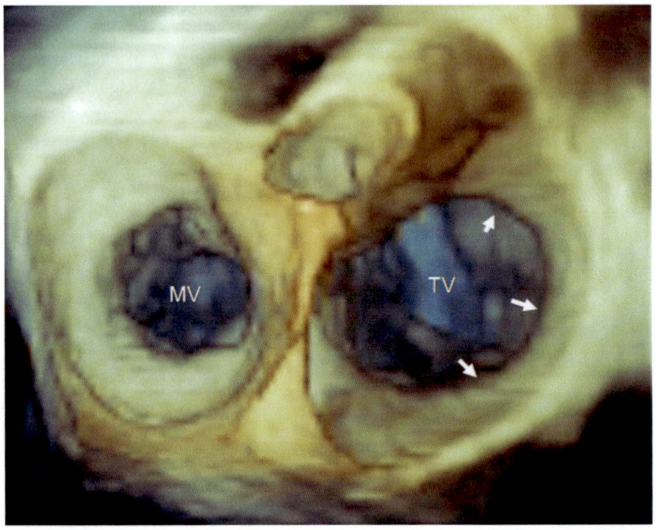

FIGURE 5.9 3D TEE in full volume modality showing an enlarge tricuspid annulus. The shape of the annulus is circular instead of ellipsoidal. Dilatation is caused mainly by an increase in the medio-lateral diameter owing to the remodeling of the "mural" component of the annulus (*arrows*). *MV* mitral valve; *TV* tricuspid valve.

Like the aortic valve, pulmonic valve leaflets are better imaged in systole than in diastole since the leaflets are perpendicular to the ultrasound pyramidal beams. In diastole, most of the leaflets disappear, leaving only some parts of the coapting surface (which remains perpendicular to the ultrasound beams) (Fig. 5.12). On the other hand, when the gain is slightly increased, the noise appears and the leaflets are no longer discernible (Fig. 5.13).

The same difficulties are encountered when the leaflets are imaged "en face" (Fig. 5.14).

In rare cases, under the circumstances of a favorable orientation of the ultrasound pyramidal beams, pulmonic leaflets can also be imaged in diastole (Fig. 5.15).

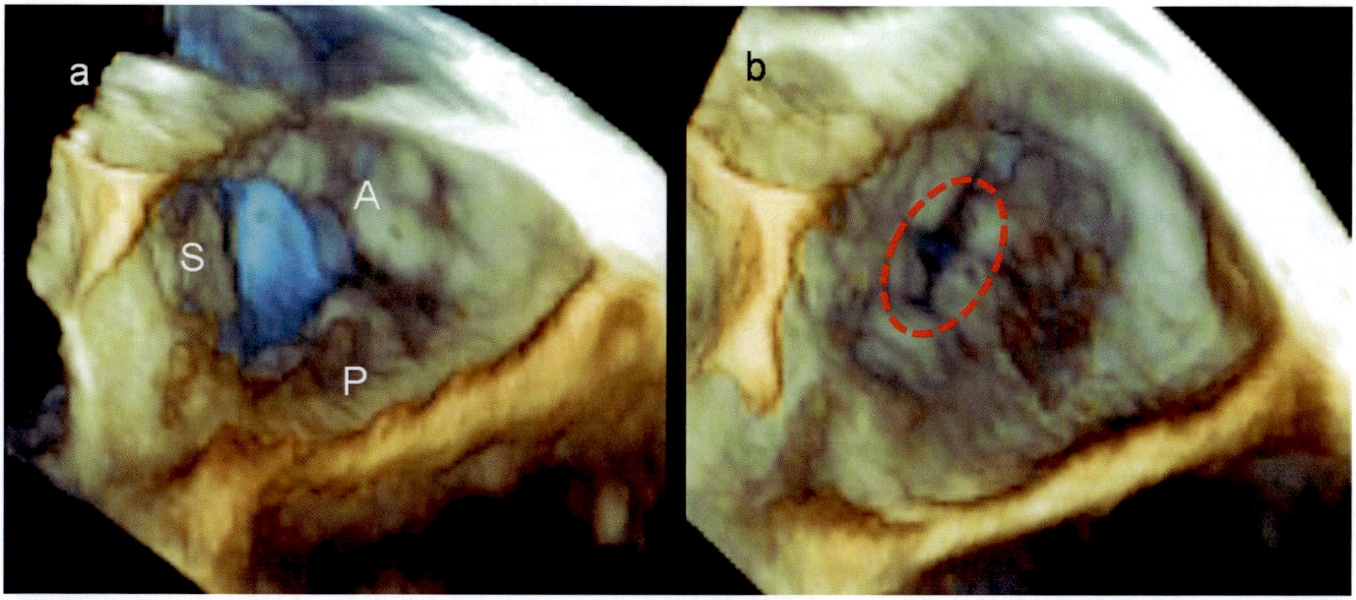

FIGURE 5.10 (a) RT 3D TEE in zoom modality showing the tricuspid leaflets in diastole and (b) in systole. A large regurgitant orifice (indicated by the *red dotted ellipse*) due to annular dilatation causes severe tricuspid regurgitation. To avoid drop-out artifacts on the tricuspid leaflets, the gain was slightly increased and small areas of noise can be observed. *A* antero-superior leaflet; *P* posterior leaflet; *S* septal leaflet.

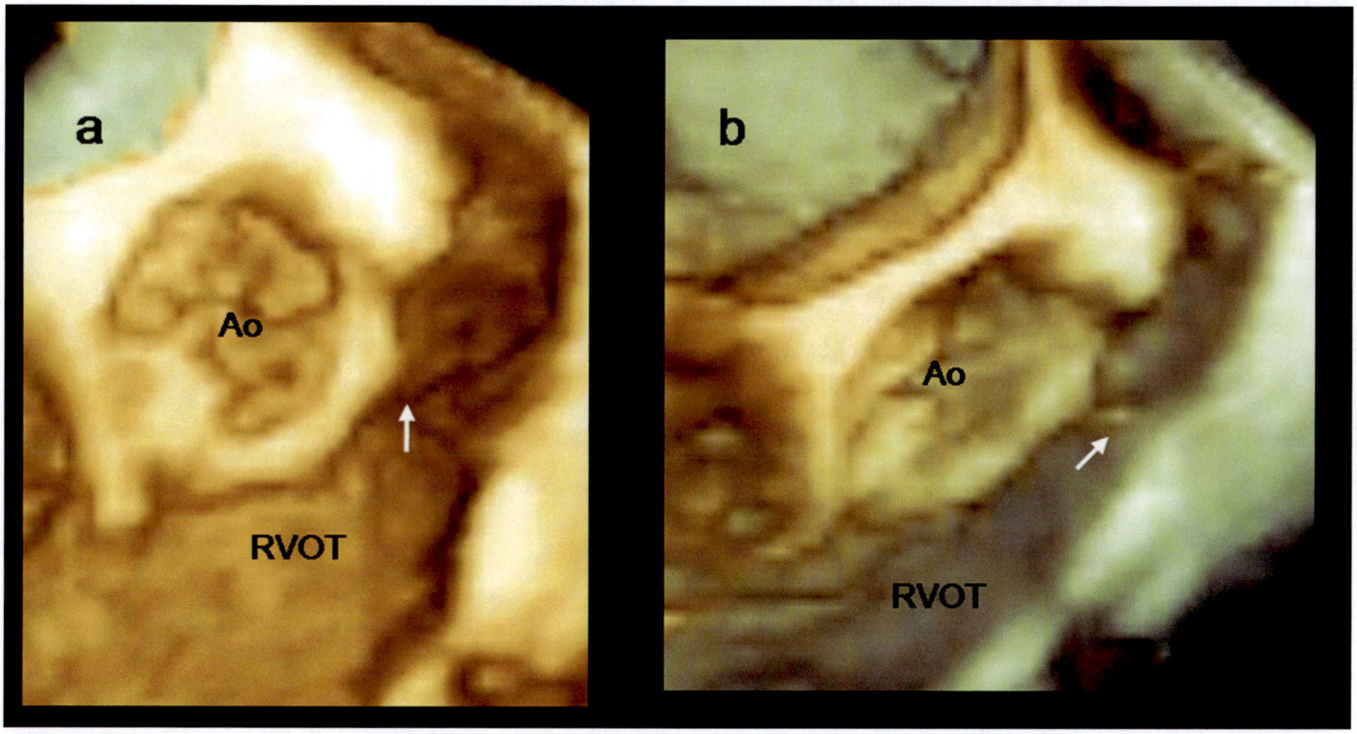

FIGURE 5.11 3D TEE image of right ventricular outflow tract (RVOT) and pulmonary artery after cropping a full volume data set. The pulmonic valve leaflets are seldom visible. In (a) leaflets are shown, as is more commonly the case, as thick protuberances (see *arrow*). (b) With a slight rotation of the 3D image, the interaction between shadow and colors occasionally makes the leaflets more visible (see *arrow*). *Ao* aorta.

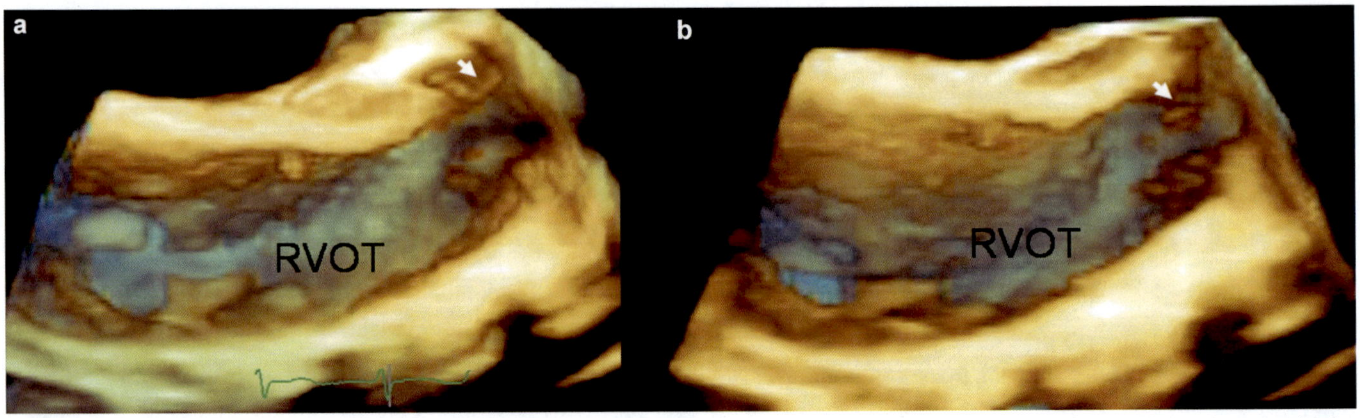

FIGURE 5.12 Real-time 3D TEE image of right ventricular outflow tract (RVOT) and pulmonic valve in zoom modality. (a) In systole, the posterior leaflets are acceptably defined (*arrow*). (b) In the closed position, most of the leaflets are parallel to the ultrasound beams; thus echoes returning from these parts are weak. When the gain is lowered to separate noise from structures, they tend to disappear leaving only small spots corresponding to the coapting surface (*arrow*).

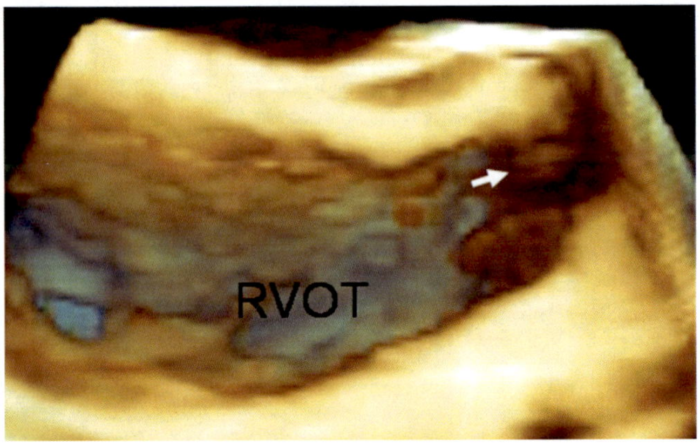

FIGURE 5.13 Same image as in Fig. 5.10. A sligh increase in the gain produces noise that blocks out the image of the leaflets. *RVOT* right ventricle outflowt ract.

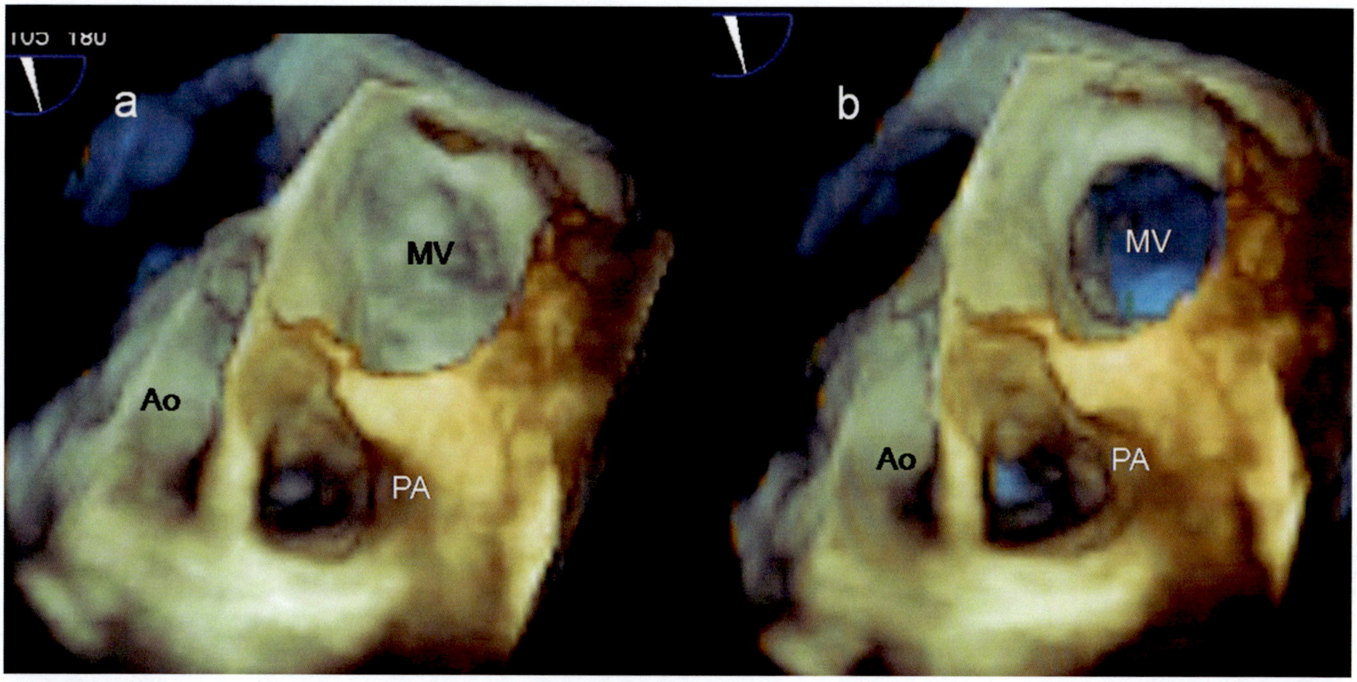

FIGURE 5.14 Real-time 3D TEE of the pulmonic valve seen "en face" (a) in systole and (b) in diastole. In systole (note the mitral valve is closed), the image of the pulmonic leaflets is coherent (the leaflets in open position adhere to the wall). In diastole (note the mitral valve opened), the central hole seen in the middle of the pulmonic valve (the leaflets are supposed to be in a closed position) is clearly a drop-out artifact. *Ao* aorta; *PA* pulmonary artery; *MV*m itralv alve.

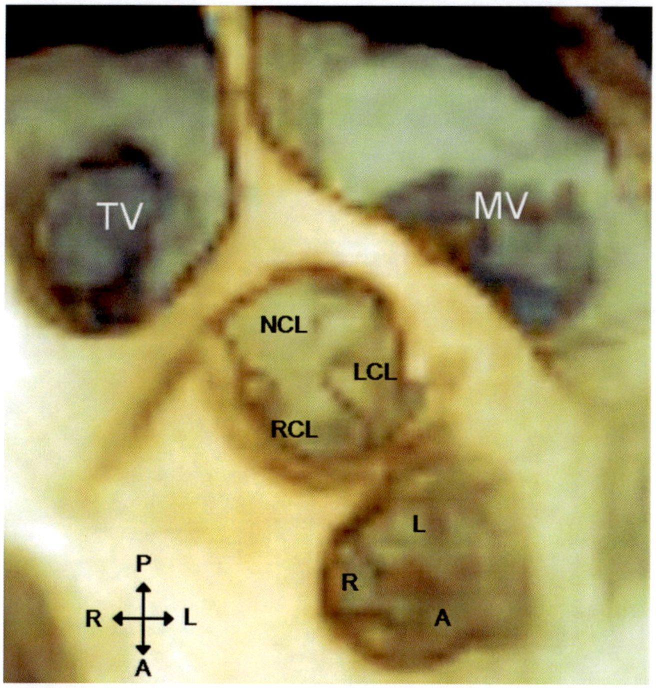

FIGURE 5.15 3D TEE of the base of the heart showing the four valves: the right (R) and left pulmonic leaflet (L) "face" the right coronary (RCL) and left coronary (LCL) aortic leaflets. *NCL* non-coronary leaflet; *A* anterior pulmonic leaflet; *TV* tricuspid valve; *MV*m itralv alve.

CHAPTER6

Atriala nd Ventricular Septa

6.1 THE ATRIAL SEPTUM

The atrial septum is the wall between the left atrium and the right atrium. Real-time 3D TEE has the potential to visualize the atrial septum "en face" both from the right andt hel efts ides(Figs. 6.1–6.3).

Figure 6.4 shows the antero-medial wall of the left atrium. From this unique perspective, the atrial septum appears as an extensive area of potential communication between the atria. However, from a strictly anatomical point of view, only the region within the dotted line is the true atrial septum. The supero-anterior region communicates with the aortic sinus through the atrial wall and transverse pericardial sinus, while the supero-medial region communicates with the superior vena cava.

Figure 6.5 shows the atrial septum from a slightly different perspective. The wall of the vena cava entering the right atrium joins with the enfolded wall of the right atrium on the septal side. A perspective from above (Fig. 6.6) shows further details of the anatomy of the atrial septum. Quite often, it is possible to distinguish the septum secundum from the septum primum. While the right side of the septum is often characterized by the crater-like structure of the fossa ovalis (Fig. 6.7), when viewed from

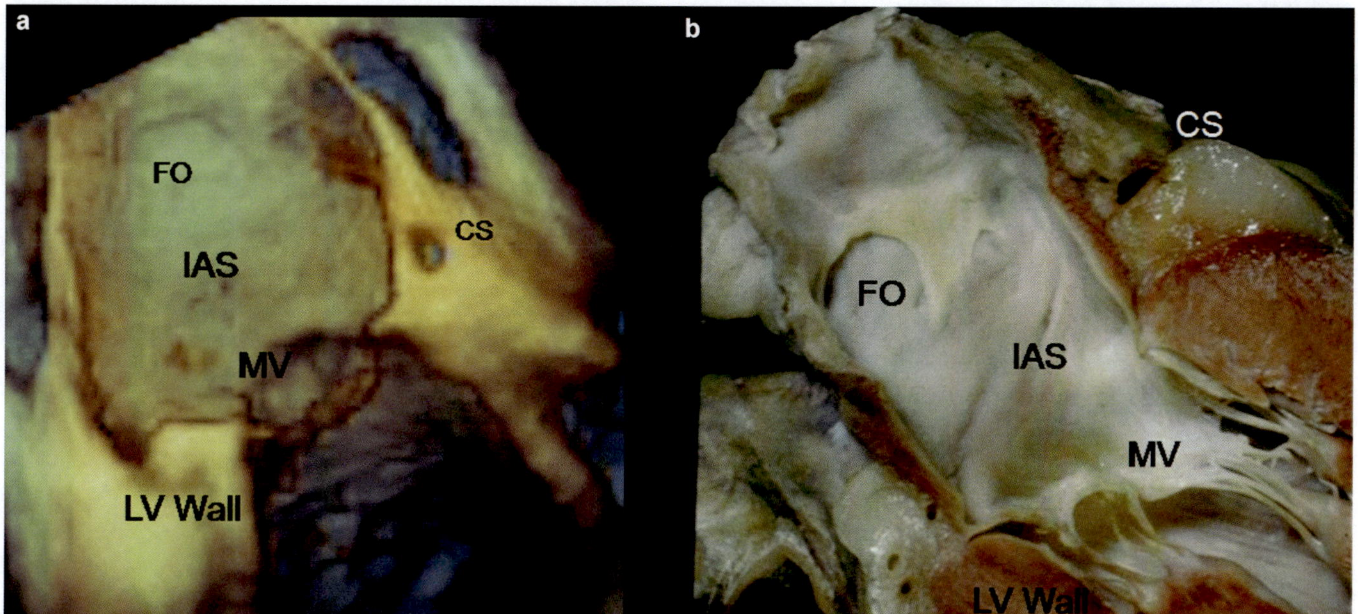

FIGURE 6.1 (a) 3D TEE of the septal surface from the left-sided perspective after cropping the full volume data set and (b) the corresponding anatomical specimen. The slight depression in the center of the septum is most likely due to the fossa ovalis (FO). *IAS* interatrial septum; *LV* left ventricle; *MV* mitral valve; *CS*c oronary sinus.

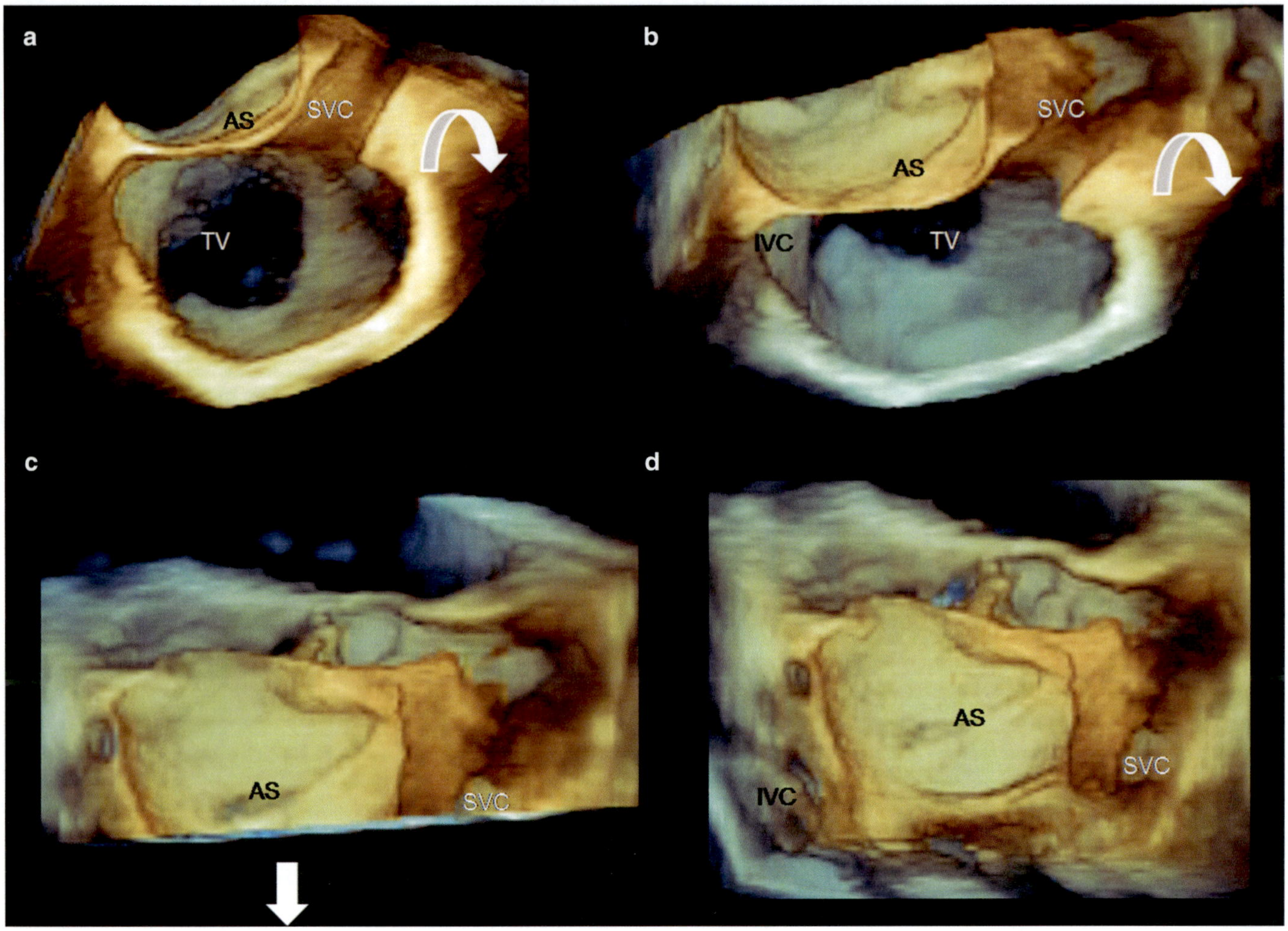

FIGURE 6.2 3D TEE in full volume modality shows (a) an image similar to a bicaval view in 2D TEE; (b, c) "up–down" rotations in the direction of *curved arrows* in (a, b); (d) expanded image in the direction of the *arrow* in (c) showing the entire left-sided surface of the atrial septum (AS). *SVC* superior vena cava; *IVC* inferior vena cava; *TV* tricuspid valve.

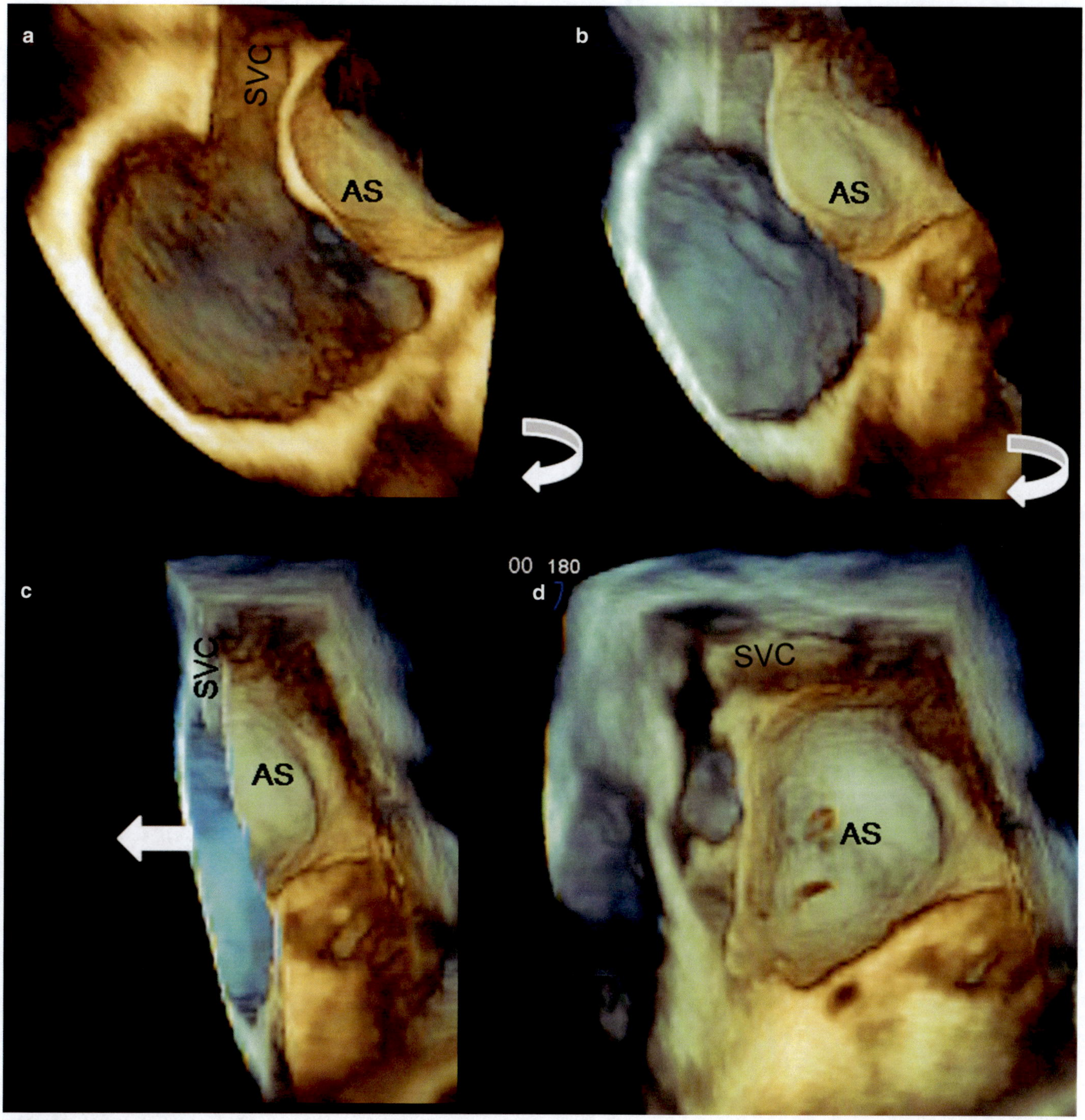

FIGURE 6.3 3D TEE in full volume modality. (a) The superior vena cava (SVC) is seen in its long axis view from the right-sided perspective; the atrial septum (AS) is cut perpendicularly to its surface. With a right-to-left rotation (a, b) (*curved arrows*) and expanded image in the direction of the arrow in (c), the entire atrial septum is imaged (d).

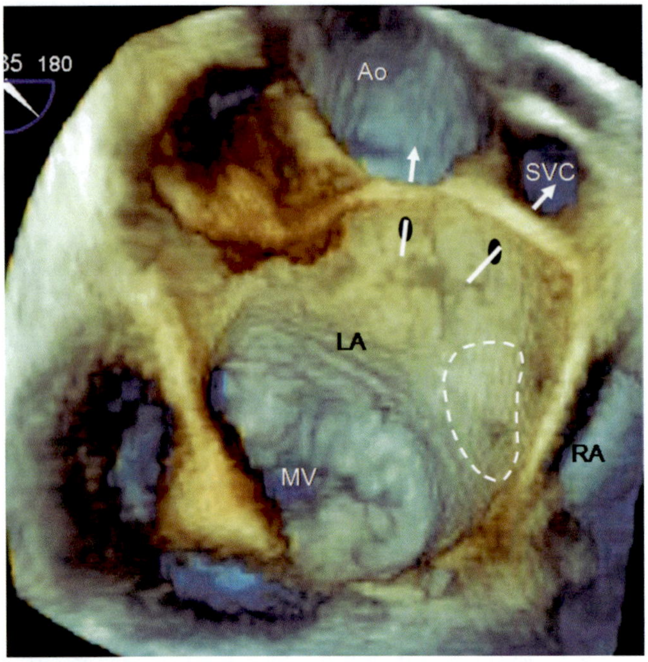

FIGURE 6.4 3D TEE of the septal surface from a slightly modified atrial perspective obtained with 3D zoom: only the region within the *dotted line* is the true atrial septum. In the antero-superior region, the "electronic probes" (*arrows*) demonstrate the close anatomic relations between the left atrium and the aorta (Ao) and the superior vena (SVC) cava, respectively. *MV* mitral valve; *LA* left atrium; *RA*r ighta trium.

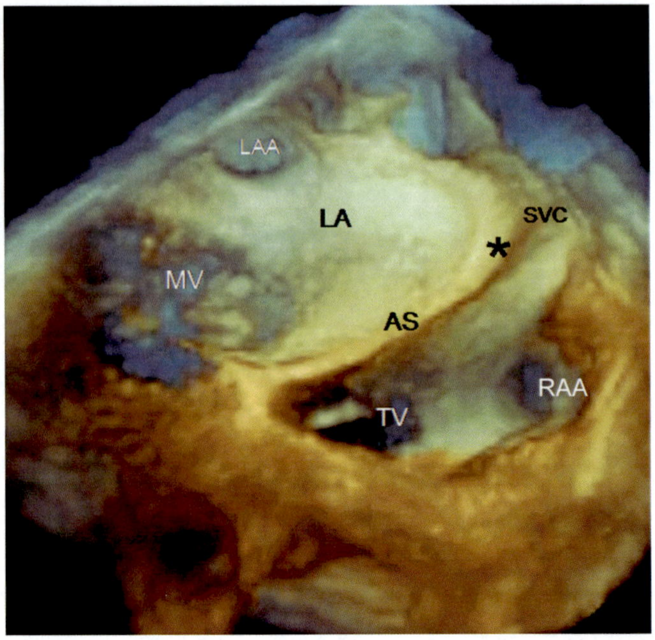

FIGURE 6.5 Real-time 3D TEE in zoom modality of the atrial septum (AS) from a slightly modified atrial perspective after having properly cropped the data set. The *asterisk* marks the enfolded atrial wall (septum secundum) in between the left atrium (LA) and the superior vena cava (SVC). From an anatomical point of view, this region is not a true atrial septum. Mal-development of this region leads to a sinus venous defect. *LAA* left atrial appendage; *MV* mitral valve; *TV* tricuspid valve; *IVC* inferior vena cava.

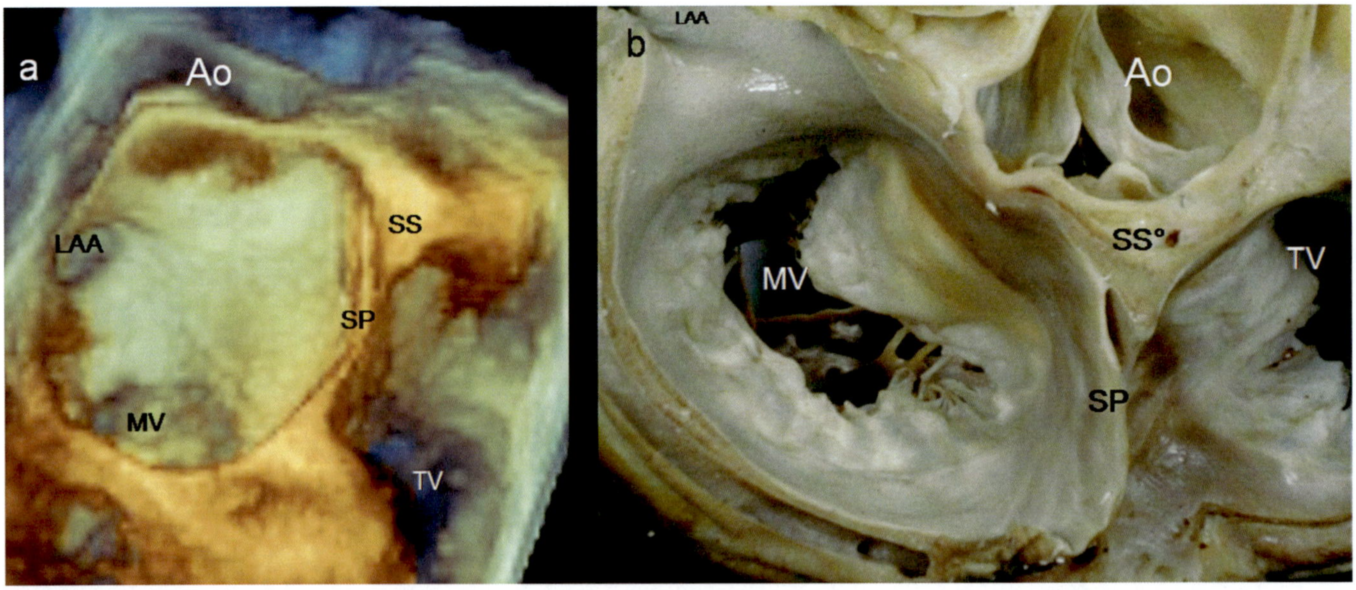

FIGURE 6.6 (a) Real-time 3D TEE of the septum viewed from a slightly modified atrial perspective and (b) the corresponding anatomical specimen. The septum primum (SP) and septum secundum (SS) are easily distinguished. The SP overlaps the SS and in about two third of adults anatomic fusion of these structures occurs, firmly closing the foramen ovale. This enfolded atrial wall is filled with extracardiac adipose tissue. *Ao* aorta; *LAA* left atrial appendage; *MV* mitral valve; *TV* tricuspid valve.

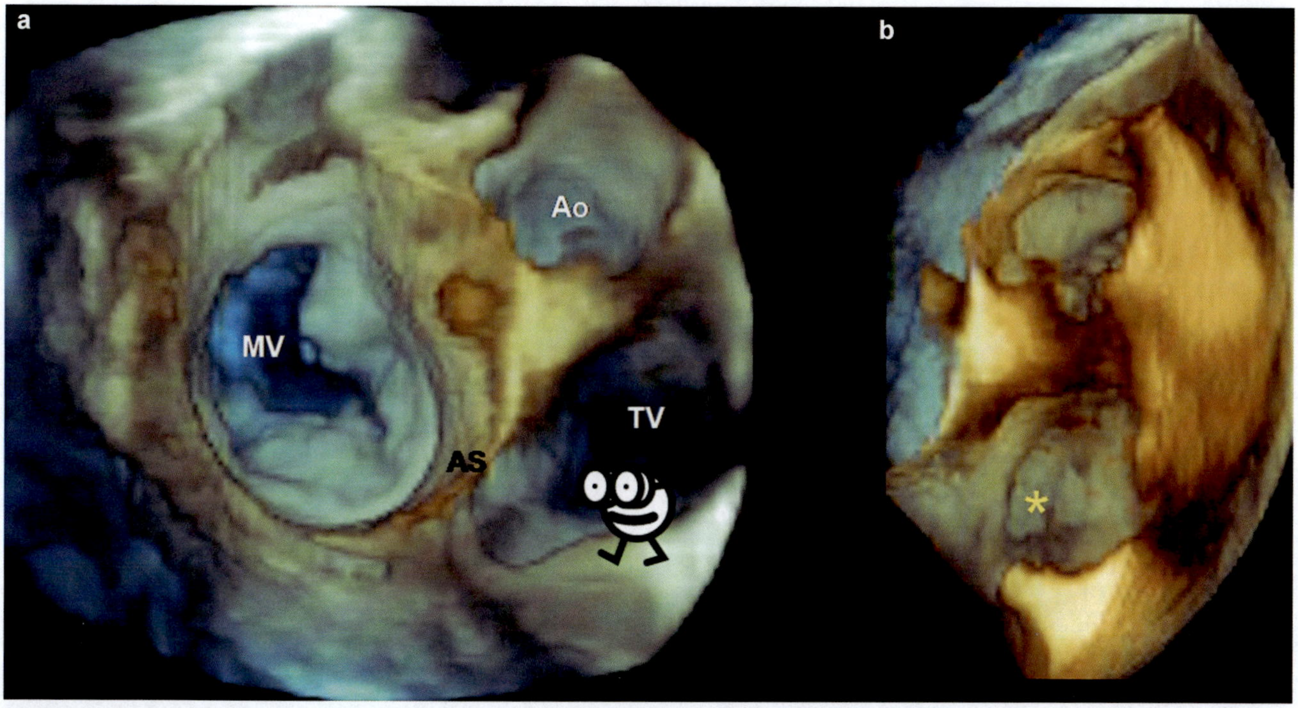

FIGURE 6.7 3D TEE in full volume modality from (a) above and (b) from right-sided perspective. This perspective is obtained by cropping the lateral wall of the right ventricle. The image obtained is that seen by the "homunculus" in (a). In some cases, when viewed from the right-sided perspective, changes in color define the position of the crater-like structure of the fossa ovalis (*asterisk*). *MV* mitral valve; *TV* tricuspid valve; *AS* atrial septum; *Ao*a orta.

the left-sided perspective, the septum is rather featureless (Fig. 6.8).

6.2 3D TEE EXAMPLES OF ATRIAL SEPTAL ANOMALIES

6.2.1 Patent Foramen Ovale

A patent foramen ovale (PFO) is a flap-like opening between the atrial septa primum and secundum in the area of the fossa ovalis. In utero, the foramen ovale serves as a physiological conduit for right-to-left shunting. Once the pulmonic circulation is established after birth, left atrial pressure increases, allowing the functional closure of the foramen ovale. Anatomical closure usually occurs within 12 months after birth but may persist permanently. The prevalence of PFO as detected by pathological studies is in the range of 30–35%. With increasing evidence that PFO is the etiopathogenetic lesion in paradoxical embolic events, the relative importance of this anomaly has being reevaluated. Any condition that pathologically increases right atrial pressure more than the left atrial pressure can induce right-to-left shunting and may result in a paradoxical embolic event. 2D TEE with saline contrast injection is an established modality of diagnosing PFO, while real-time 3D TEE may allow a detailed anatomical imaging of PFO, comparable to pathological specimens (Fig. 6.9).

6.2.2 Atrial Septal Defects

There are four major types of atrial septal defects (ASD): ostium secundum, ostium primum, sinus venous, and coronary sinus septal defects. Echocardiography is a well-established technique to provide diagnosis of all types of ASD as well as their hemodynamic consequences. While the lesions are identified as interruptions in the linear image of the atrial septum in 2D echocardiography, the additional value of 3D techniques is to display the hole in the septum "en face" and from both the right and left-sides. Real-time 3D TEE, because of its superior image quality, can better visualize the "dynamic" geometry (systole and diastole) of the defect and its surrounding rims (Figs. 6.10–6.13). Moreover, the "en face" defect area can be measured (Fig. 6.14) permitting a better informed choice regarding therapeutic strategy: percutaneous or surgical closure (see Movies 6.1 and 6.2).

MOVIE 6.1 An example of an ostium secundum atrial septal defect imaged from the left atrial perspective.

MOVIE 6.2 An example of an ostium secundum atrial septal defect imaged from right atrial perspective.

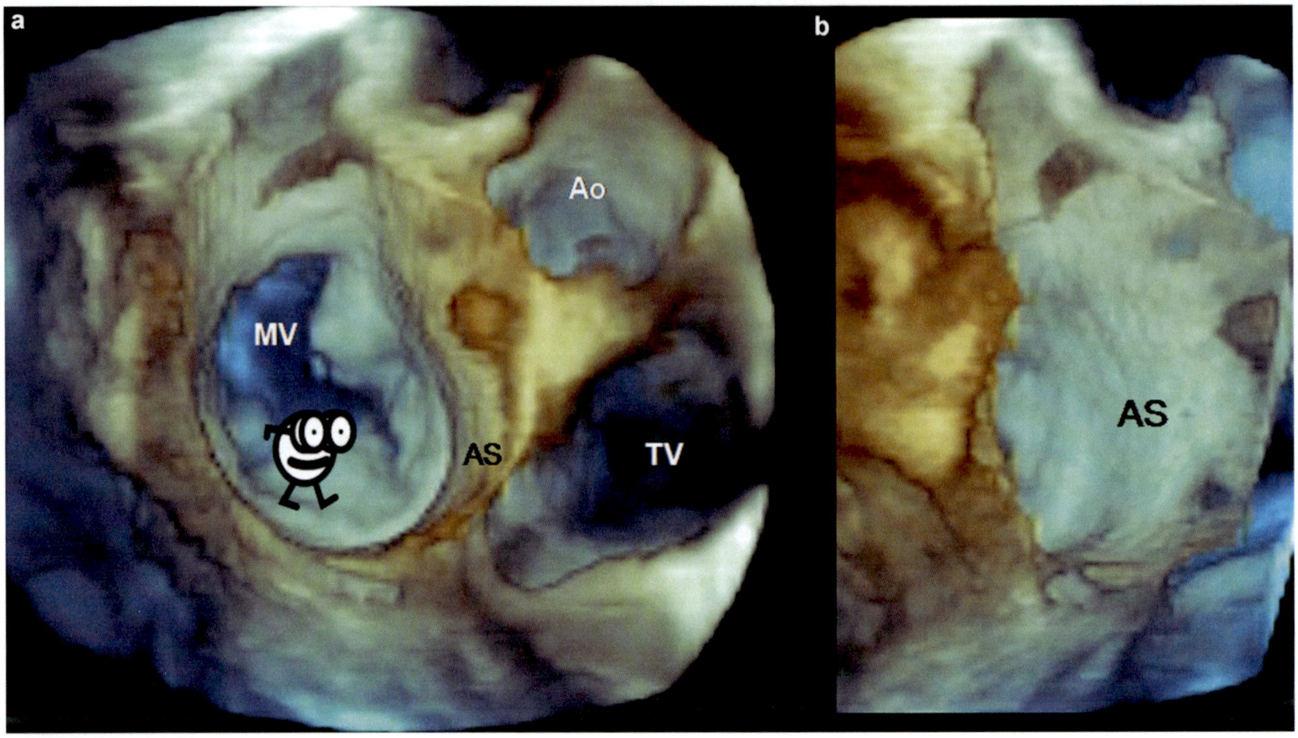

FIGURE 6.8 Real-time 3D TEE from (a) above and (b) from left-sided perspective. Viewed from the left perspective, the atrial septum (AS) is rather featureless. *MV* mitral valve; *TV* tricuspid valve; *Ao* aorta.

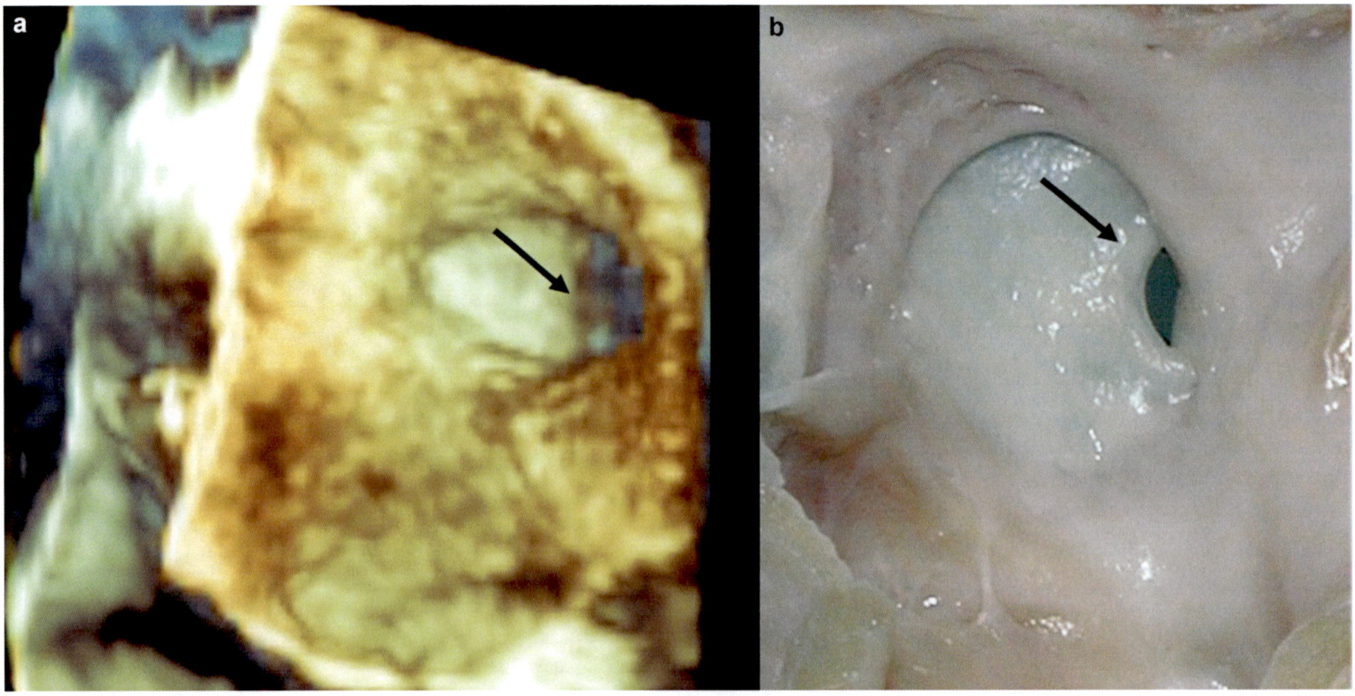

FIGURE 6.9 (a) Real-time 3D TEE image of a PFO and (b) the corresponding anatomical specimen. The *arrow* points to the PFO opening froma l eft-sidedp erspective.

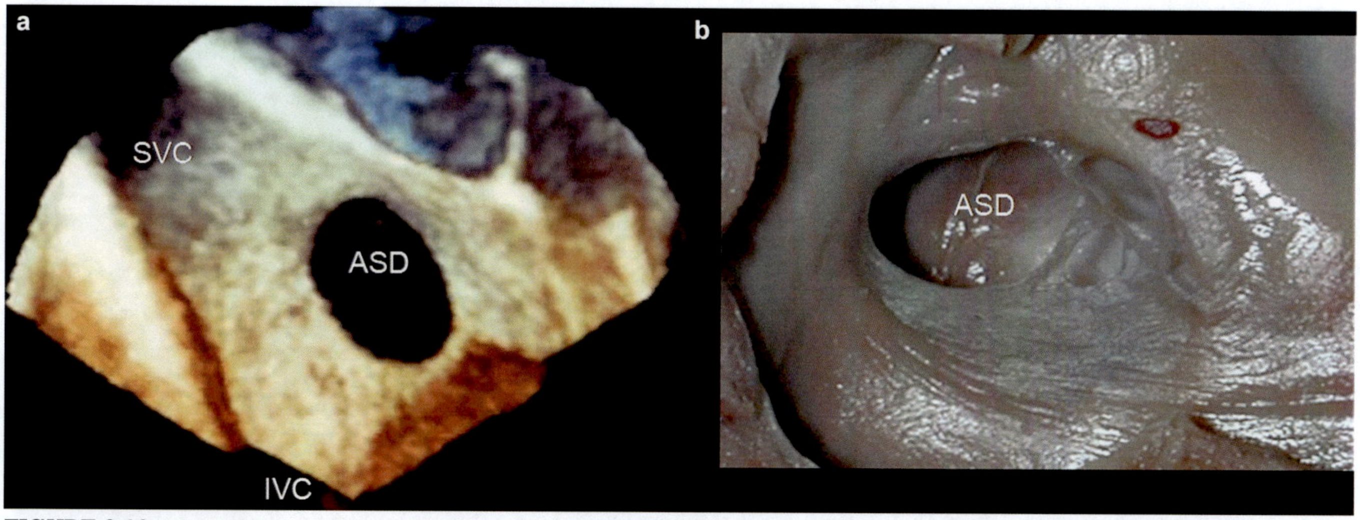

FIGURE 6.10 (a) Real-time 3D TEE image of an *ostium secundum* defect in zoom modality and (b) the corresponding anatomical specimen from the right-sided perspective. *ASD* atrial septal defect; *SCV* superior vena cava; *IVC* inferior vena cava.

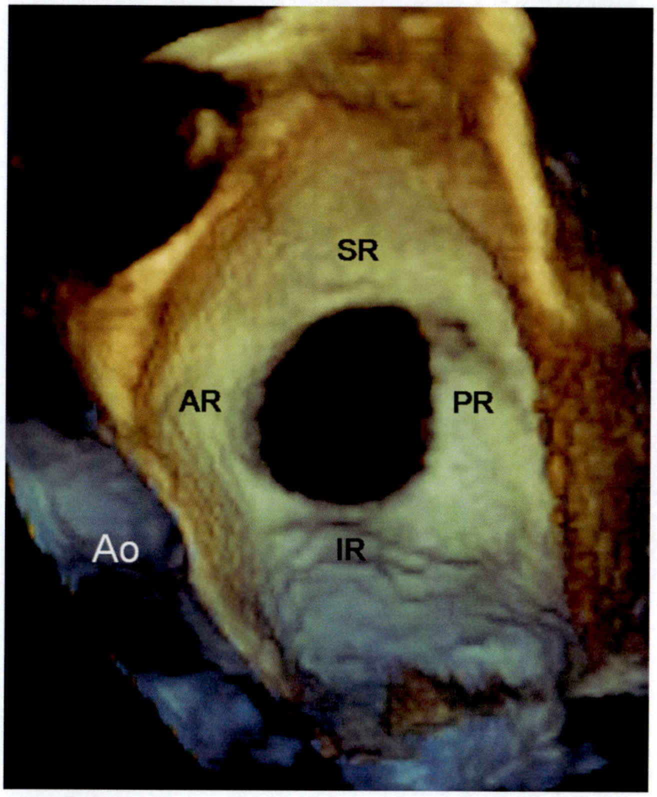

FIGURE 6.11 3D TEE images of an *ostium secundum* defect from a left-sided perspective in zoom modality. Inferior (IR), posterior (PR), anterior (AR) and superior (SR) rims can be imaged. A comprehensive evaluation of the site, size, and shape of the ASD and its rims can be obtained in one shot. *Ao*a orta.

6.2.3 Percutaneous Closure of PFO and ASD

Because of its ability to display the long segments of the catheter and its relationship to adjacent and surrounding anatomical structures, real-time 3D TEE is increasingly used as a "guide" for monitoring percutaneous closure of *ostium secundum* ASDs and PFOs. The procedure is performed via central venous access using a guiding catheter that is passed though the ASD (or the PFO). Real-time 3D TEE allows continuous visualization of the tip of catheter, (Figs. 6.15 and 6.16) postprocedural results, and potential complications (Fig. 6.17). See also Movies 6.3–6.6.

MOVIE 6.3 The clip shows the catheter passing through atrial septal defect seen from the left atrial perspective during a percutaneous closure of an ASD.

MOVIE 6.4 The clip shows the catheter passing through atrial septal defect seen from the right atrial perspective.

MOVIE 6.5 The clip shows the expansion and deployment of the left disc of the occluder.

MOVIE 6.6 The clip shows successful positioning of the occluder device from left atrial perspective.

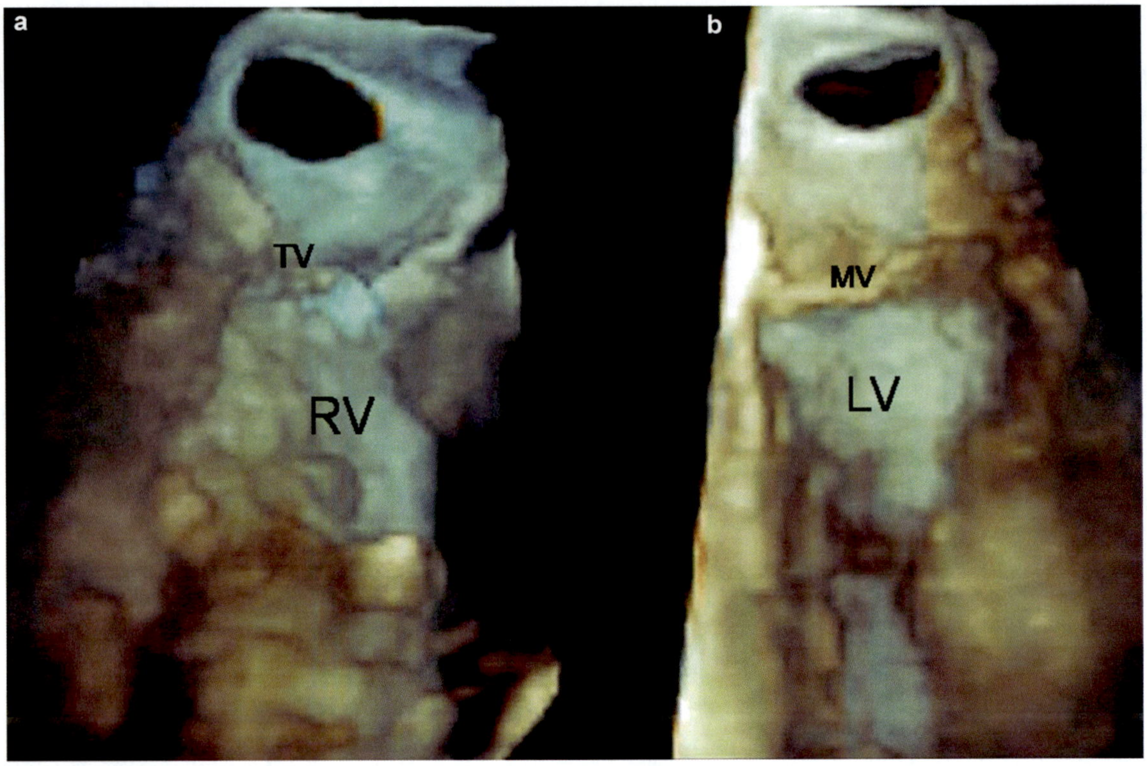

FIGURE 6.12 3D TEE images of a large *ostium secundum* defect seen from (a) the right-sided and (b) the left-sided perspective. *RV* right ventricle; *LV* left ventricle; *TV* tricuspid valve; *MV* mitral valve.

6.3 THE VENTRICULAR SEPTUM

The ventricular septum is a complex nonplanar structure (Fig. 6.18). It has inlet, outlet, and apical trabecular portions with the membranous septum at the pivot. Owing to the acute angulation between the inflow and outflow tracts of the left ventricle, the inlet portion of the septum in the right ventricle does not correspond to the inlet portion of the septum in the left ventricle. It is for this reason that naming of the septal portions (and therefore the locations of ventricular septal defects) should be done only from the right ventricular aspect. The hingeline (annulus) of the septal leaflet of the tricuspid valve bisects the membranous septum into atrioventricular and interventricular components. The membranous septum, a part of the central fibrous body, is an anatomical landmark for the atrioventricular conduction bundle. Hence, the categorization of ventricular septal defects into muscular and perimembranous types highlights the proximity of the conduction tissues in the latter type. Another common misinterpretation is the assignment of an outlet septum in the normally structured heart. Owing to the difference in levels between the aortic root and the pulmonic valve, the muscular flange of the sub-pulmonic infundibulum interposes between the aortic valve and the right ventricular outflow tract. *This is not a septal structure.* In congenitally malformed hearts (i.e., Tetralogy of Fallot or complete transposition) however, defects involving the outflow tracts can produce an outlet ventricular septal defect. In these instances, the outlet septum can also be the substrate of the right ventricular outflow tract obstruction because it is misaligned from the rest of the ventricular septum.

When viewed from the right ventricular aspect, the inlet portion of the septum is taken to be that containing the tricuspid valve and its apparatus from the hingeline to the insertions of the papillary muscles. The outlet portion is proximate to the pulmonic valve while the trabecular portion is also the apical portion. These designations are arbitrary since there are no clear anatomic demarcations. Normally, the ventricular septum is curved (Fig. 6.18). Consequently, the inlet portion and the outlet portion are on completely different planes to one another.

The inlet portion is infero-posterior to the membranous septum. It must be emphasized that the inlet portion in the right ventricle relates to the tricuspid valve, but on the left side, the same portion relates to the overlapping left ventricular inlet and outlet (Fig. 6.19).

The outlet (or infundibular) portion separates the right and left ventricular outflow tracts. On the right side, it extends from the membranous septum to the medial

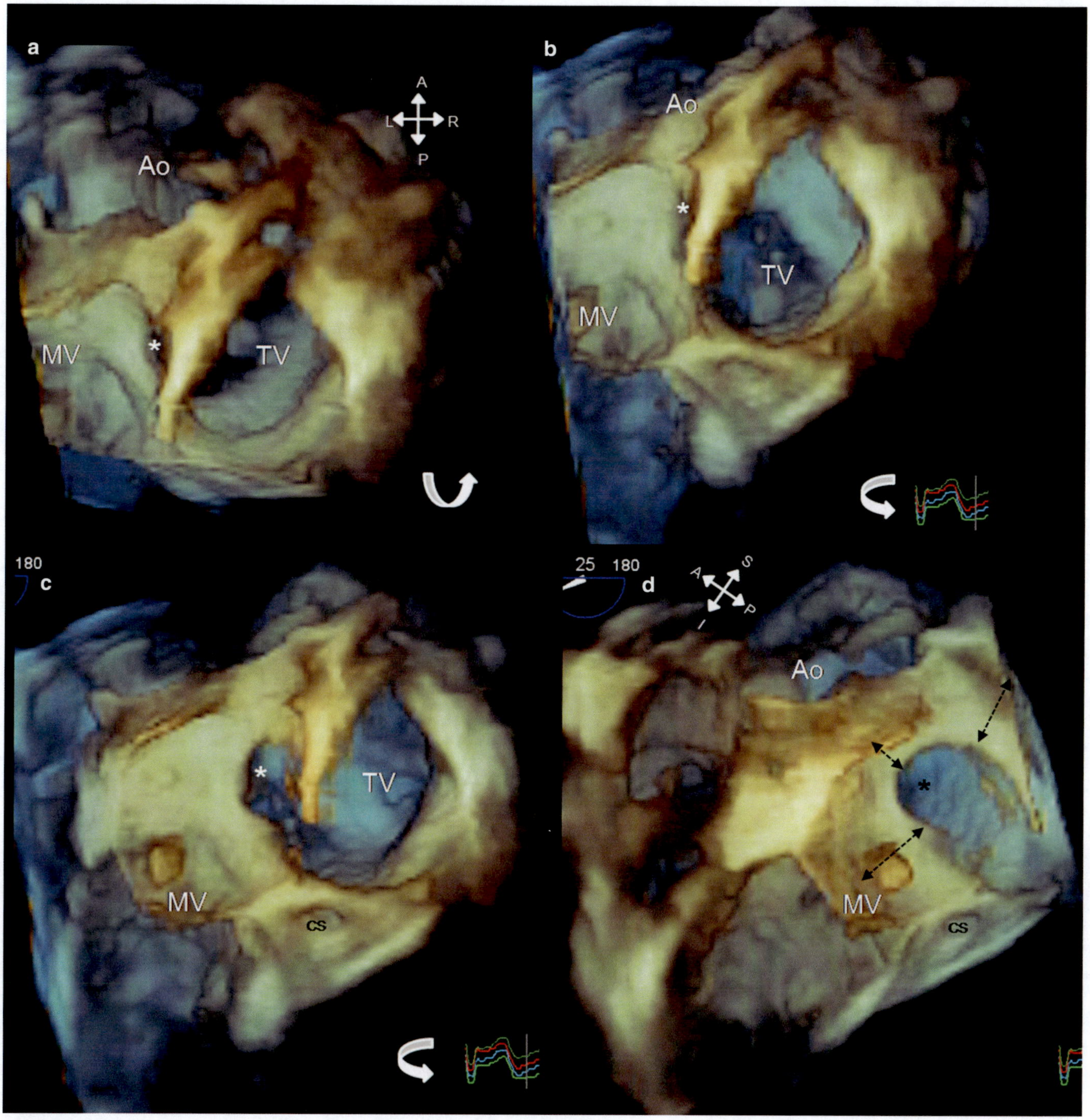

FIGURE 6.13 3D TEE images of an *ostium secundum atrial septal defect.* The entire contour of the defect cannot always be visualized in one image. (a) The base of the heart as seen from the atrial perspective. The ASD is partially hidden (*asterisk*); (b–d) down–up and left-to-right rotations (*curved arrows*) progressively disclose the defect. However, while the anterior, superior, and inferior rims are easily imaged (*arrows*), the posterior rim is not visualized. *MV* mitral valve; *TV* tricuspid valve; *Ao* Aorta; *CS* coronary sinus.

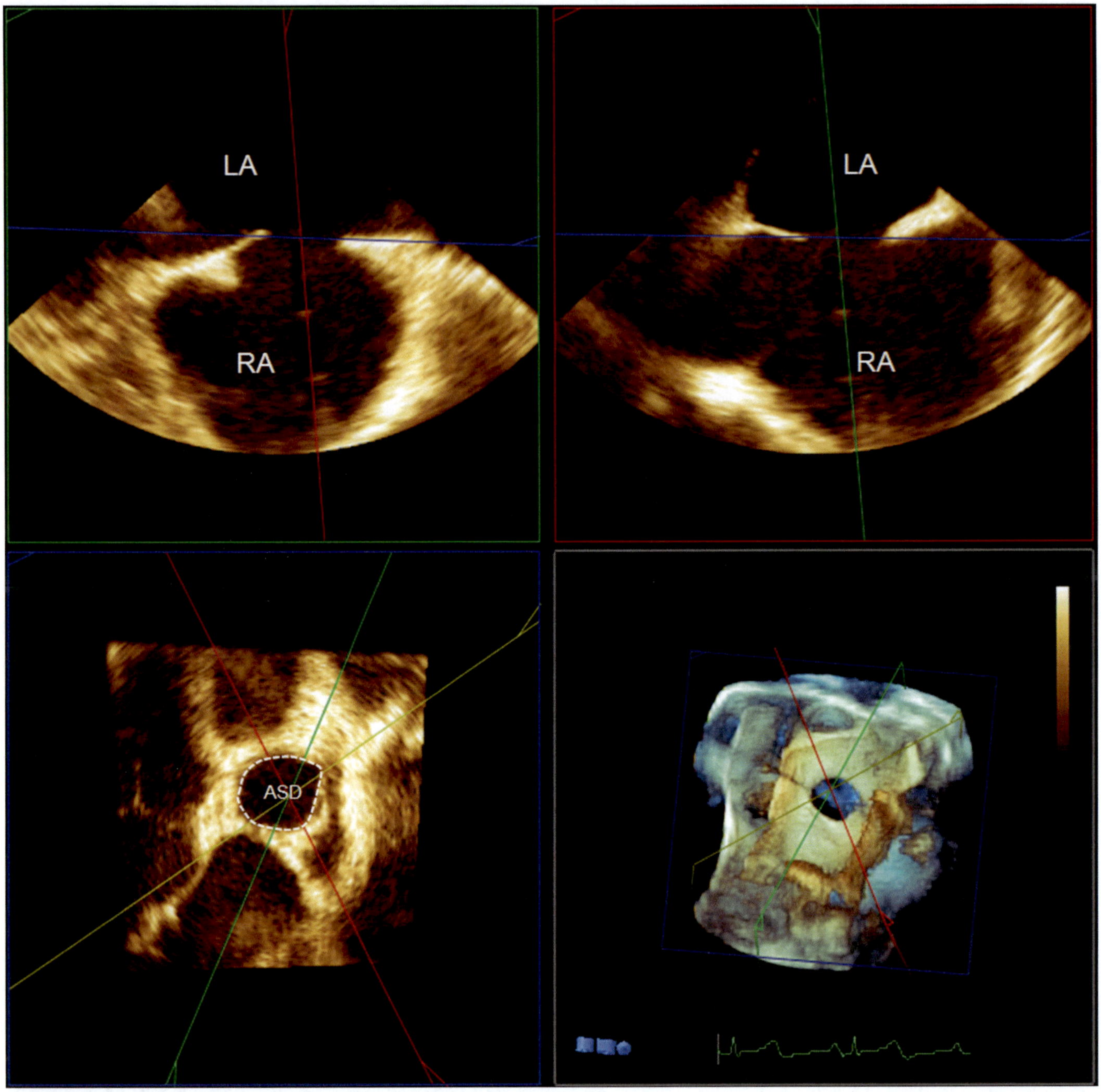

FIGURE 6.14 3D TEE demonstrates an *ostium secundum* atrial septal defect (ASD) en face. The size of the ASD can be easily measured. *LA* left atrium; *RA*r ighta trium.

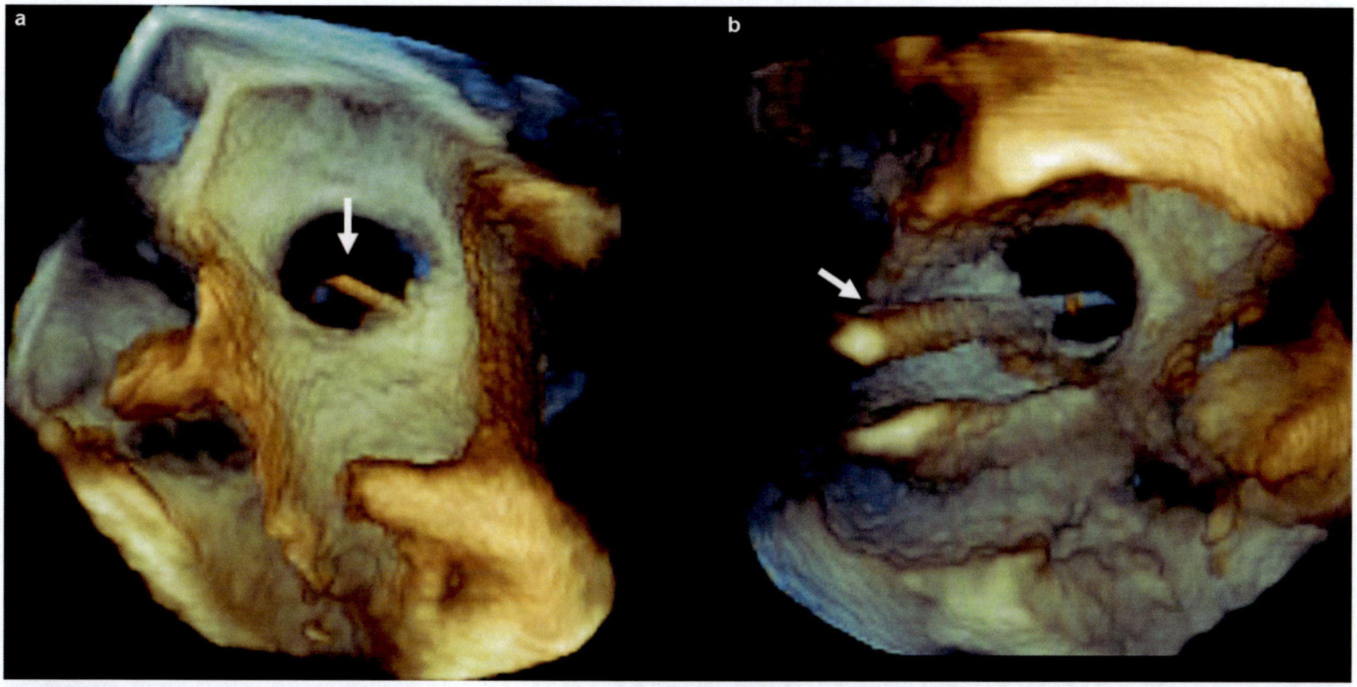

FIGURE 6.15 (a) Real-time 3D TEE in zoom modality from a left-sided perspective and (b) a right-sided perspective showing the catheter (*arrow*)pa ssingt hrough thea trial septal defect.

papillary muscle (muscle of the conus) below and to the semilunar valves above. The upper part of the right aspect of the outlet portion is actually the subpulmonic muscular infundibulum and not a septal structure (Fig. 6.20).

The trabecular portion is the largest part of the ventricular septum. It extends from the membranous septum to the apex and above to the outlet portion. It is characterized by irregularly arranged trabeculations compared to other portions of the septum (Fig. 6.21).

The membranous septum is a small component of the ventricular septum, but is important on account of its central location in the heart. It is a part of the central fibrous body; the other part is the right fibrous trigone. Since the atrioventricular bundle of the conduction system usually passes between the membranous septum and the crest of the muscular septum, the membranous septum is a useful landmark for its location. The membranous septum is located immediately below the right and noncoronary aortic sinuses (Figs. 6.22 and 6.23).

The annular attachment of the septal leaflet of the tricuspid valve is anchored more caudally than that of the anterior mitral leaflet. As a consequence, a portion of the septum lies between the right atrium and the left ventricle. This segment is the so-called muscular *atrioventricular septum*. Above, the "atrioventricular septum" adjoins the atrioventricular part of the membranous septum that lies above the hinge line of the tricuspid leaflet (Fig. 6.24). Although the muscular component of the so-called atrioventricular septum separates the left ventricle from the right atrium on account of the "offset" between the septal insertions in the tricuspid and mitral leaflets, it is not a true septum. Detailed anatomy reveals it to be composed in the form of a sandwich with the atrial septum on one side, the crest of the ventricular septum on the other, and the fibro-fatty tissue plane of the inferior atrioventricular groove in between making up the filling.

6.4 3D TEE EXAMPLES OF VENTRICULAR SEPTUM ANOMALIES

6.4.1 Ventricular Septal Defect

The ventricular septal defect (VSD) is one of the most common of all congenital cardiac malformations. VSDs are the result of failure of growth and alignment or fusion of one or more septal components. According to the relationship between its borders and surrounding structures, VSDs may be classified as *muscular* when the defect is completely surrounded by a muscular rim,

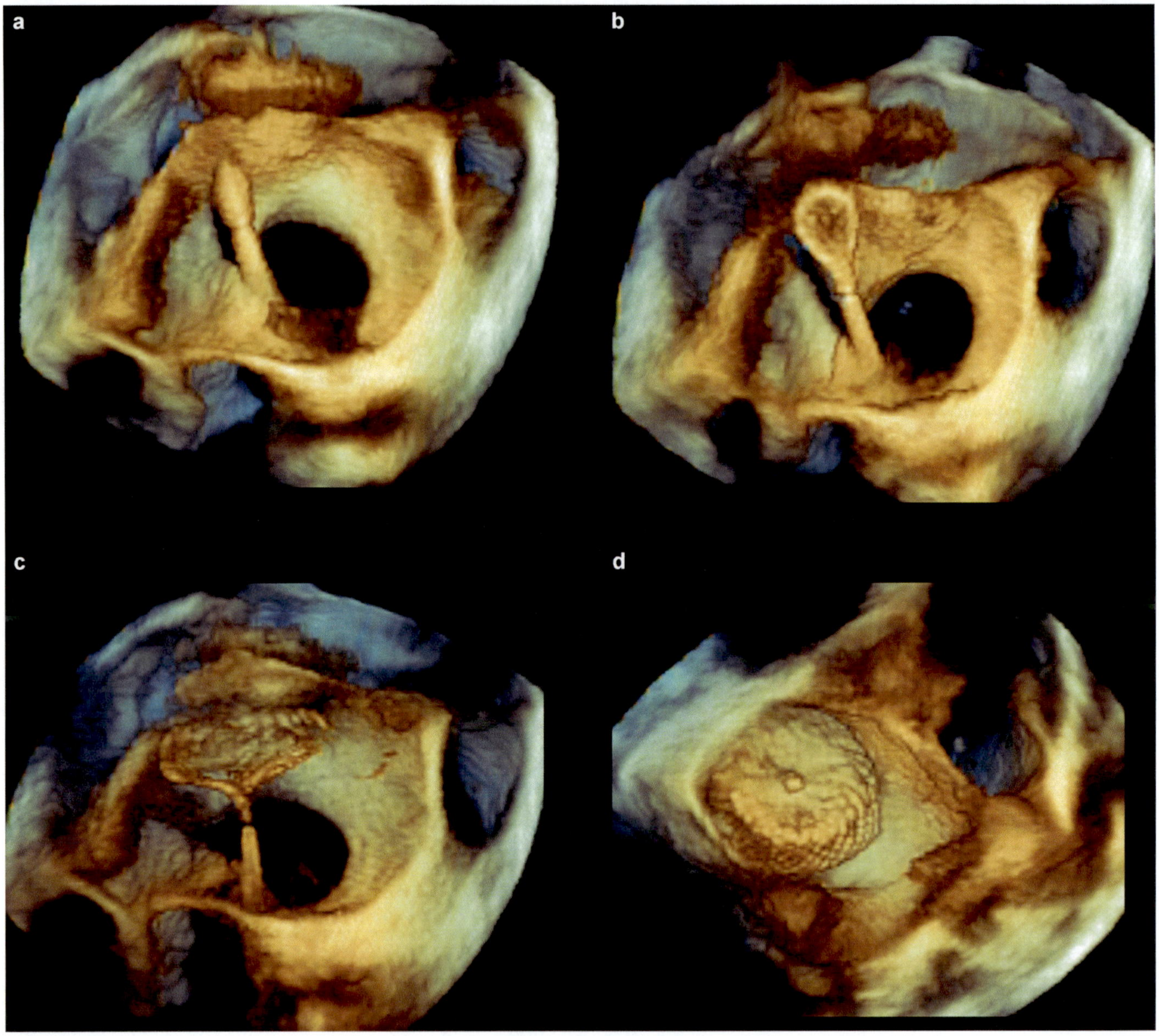

FIGURE 6.16 Real-time 3D TEE in zoom modality showing different steps in the ASD closure. (a) A preexpanded device is visualized; (b, c) two moments in the expansion of device; (d) the device is deployed in a correct position.

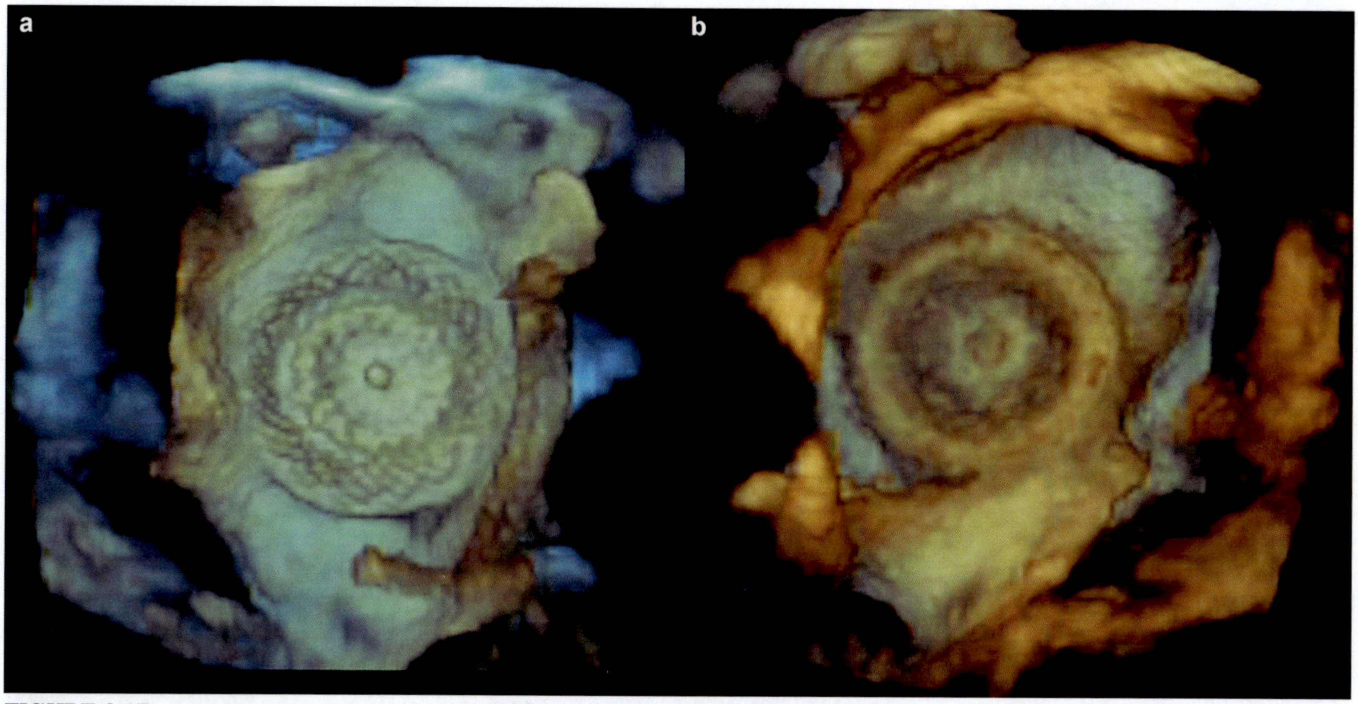

FIGURE 6.17 Real-time 3D TEE in zoom modality showing (a) the left side and (b) the right side of the device.

perimembranous when part of its border is in fibrous continuity with the membranous septum, or *double committed subarterial* when the border of the defect is formed by a fibrous continuity between the aortic and pulmonic valves. The last category can be further described as either muscular or perimembranous depending on the morphology of its posterior inferior rim. Like ASD, real-time 3D TEE can image VSD "en face" both from a right and left-sided perspective (Fig. 6.25).

6.4.2 The Atrioventricular Septal Defect

The hallmark of the atrioventricular septal defect (AVSD) is the absence of atrioventricular septation resulting in a common atrioventricular junction. It is associated with a common atrioventricular valve. It is the morphology of the common valve that allows this malformation to be further described as having a common valvular orifice (so-called *complete AVSD*) or separate right and left valvular orifices (so-called *partial AVSD*, often referred to as the "primum defect" when the communication is at the atrial level only). Typically, the atrioventricular valve consists of five leaflets: the superior and the inferior bridging (both cross the ventricular septum and are anchored to the right and left ventricles), the left mural, the right antero-superior, and the right inferior leaflets. Therefore in AVSD, the right-sided component of the common valve has four leaflets, whereas the left-sided component has three leaflets. Thus, the atrioventricular valve cannot be described as a tricuspid or a mitral valve since it resembles neither. An important distinguishing feature from the normal heart is the lack of septal "offset" between the hingelines of the left and right components of the valve. Furthermore, because of the common atrioventricular junction, the aortic valve is not lodged in its usual position between the mitral and tricuspid valves but is displaced anteriorly (Fig. 6.26). There is also a disproportion between inlet and outlet lengths of the left ventricle, the outlet being elongated relative to the inlet in hearts with AVSD.

In a partial AVSD the crest of the ventricular septum is covered by both the superior and inferior bridging leaflets which are joined by a tongue of leaflet tissue. This arrangement results in the following anatomical features:

(a) two separate atrioventricular valvular orifices (Fig. 6.26); (b) a characteristic tri-leaflet appearance of the left atrioventricular valve (which is formed by the left part of the superior bridging leaflet, the left mural leaflet, and the left part of the inferior bridging leaflet) (Fig. 6.27). The closure line between the two bridging leaflets (erroneously known as a mitral cleft) may be imperfect leaving a regurgitant orifice; (c) an interatrial communication called "ostium primum" ASD (Fig. 6.28). See also Movies 6.7 and 6.8.

A Complete AVSD usually consists of a) a large ventricular communication between the crest of ventricular septum

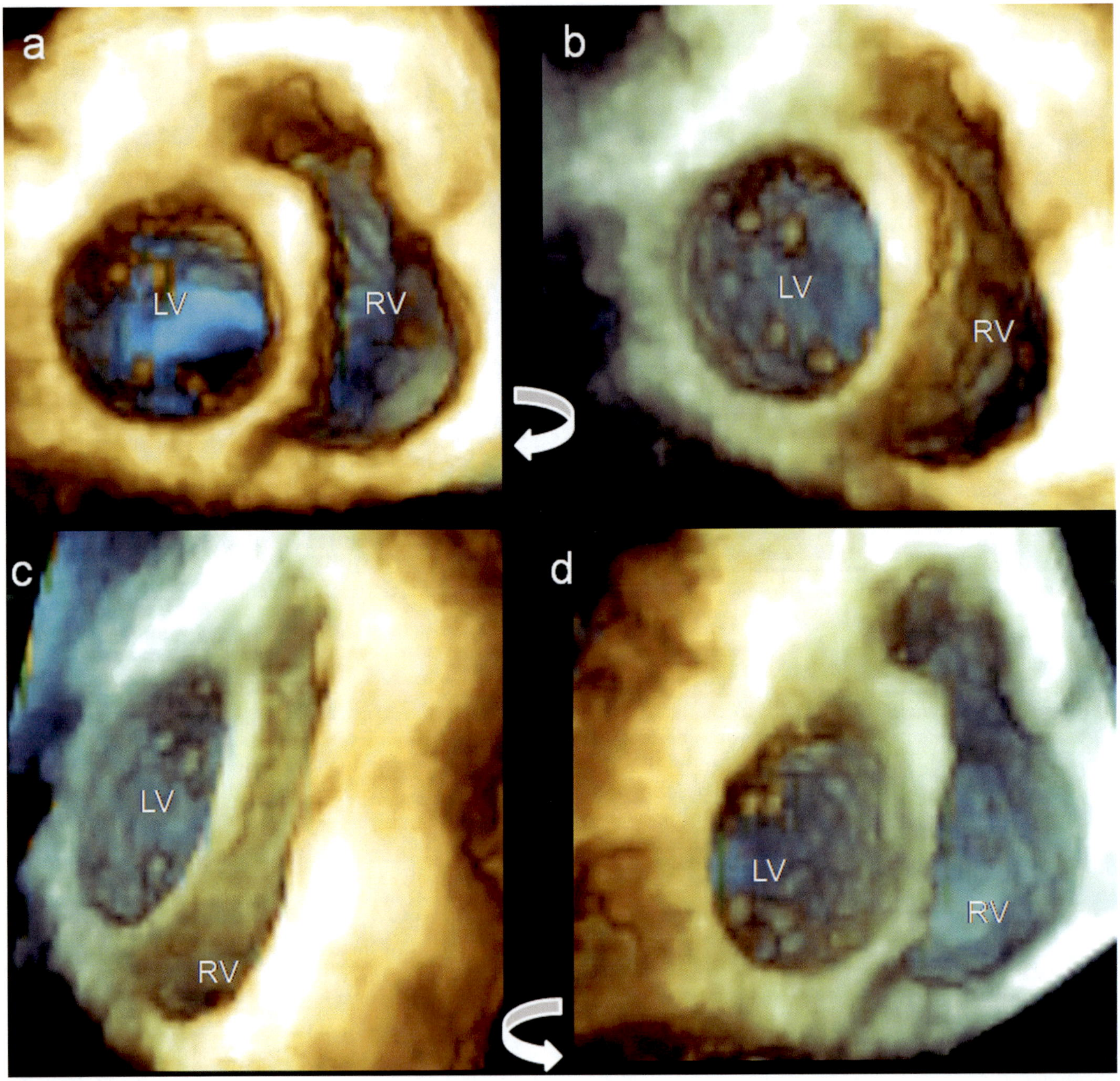

FIGURE 6.18 3D TEE in full volume modality. Overhead perspective following a transverse cut perpendicular to the long axis of the left ventricle. *Curved arrows* indicate leftward rotations (a, b) and rightward rotations (c, d). The images clearly show the nonplanarity of the septum. *LV* left ventricle; *RV* rightv entricle.

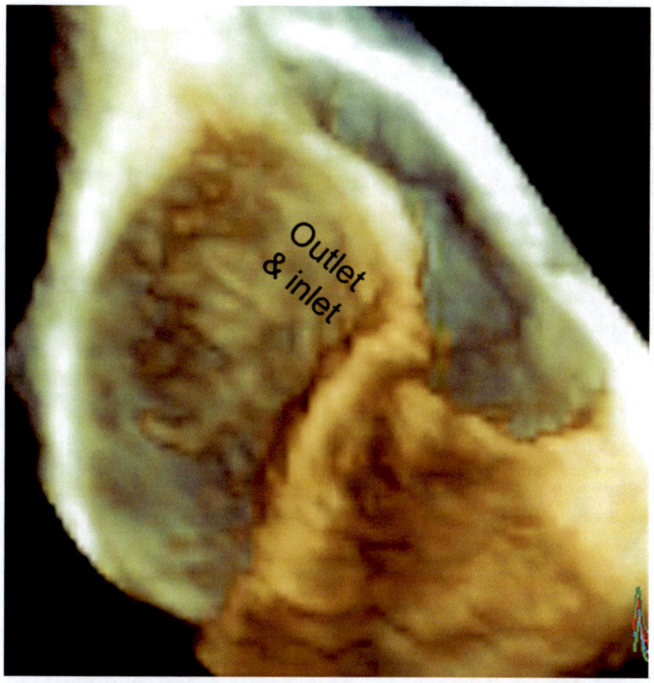

FIGURE 6.19 3D TEE in full volume modality. The image shows the adjoining outlet and inlet portions of the septum viewed through a cut in the left ventricle. These left ventricular portions correspond to the inlet portion on the right ventricular side. The image is obtained after having removed the antero-lateral wall of the left ventricle. The concavity of the septum is evident when imagedf roma l eft-sidedper spective.

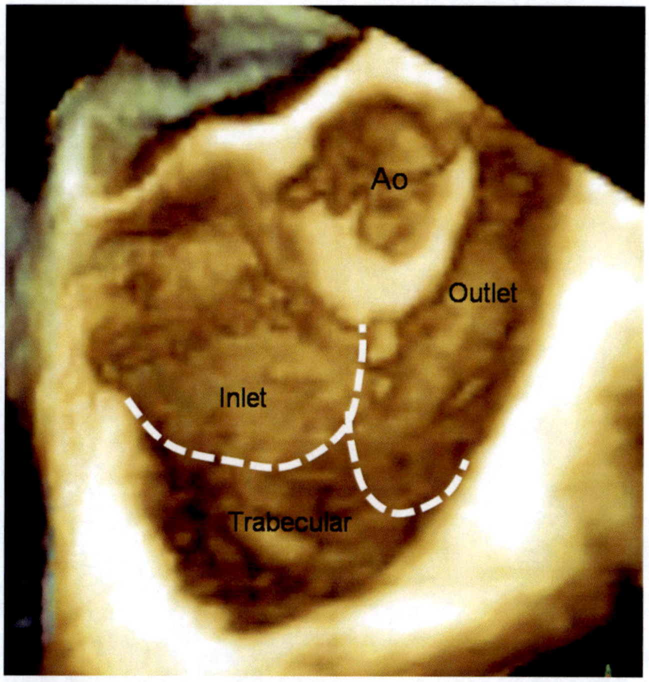

FIGURE 6.20 Real-time 3D TEE in full volume modality. Right ventricular perspective of the septum, after removing right ventricular antero-lateral wall. The *curved dotted lines* arbitrarily mark the boundaries of the three parts of the muscular septum on the right side. From this perspective, the upper portion of the outlet is not a septal structure. Note the aorta (Ao) interposing between the inlet and outlet portions.

MOVIE 6.7 A large atrioventricular septum defect from left Perspective.

MOVIE 6.8 A large atrioventricular septum defect from right perspective.

and the ventricular surface (underside) of the bridging leaflets, and with b) an interatrial component (or ostium primum ASD) between the atrial surface of the bridging leaflets and the free edge of the atrial septum.

In between these forms, there are variants ranging from the small ventricular defect partially or completely closed by chordal of tissue of the right atrioventricular valve (Fig. 6.29), to the absence of interatrial communication. In the latter case, the atrial septum is partly fused with the atrial surface of the bridging leaflets such that the leaflets are lifted up to the level of the atrial septum when the valve closes, obliterating any potential for interatrial communication. Very rarely, both atrial and ventricular components of the defect are obliterated, leaving an AVSD with an intact septum but still having all the anatomical features such as common atrioventricular junction, tri-leaflet left atrioventricular valve and inlet-outlet disproportion. Such rare entities may be mistaken for isolated "mitral cleft". With both common and divided orifices the right and left components of the atrioventricular valve are always at the same level (Fig. 6.30), i.e. loss of "offset".

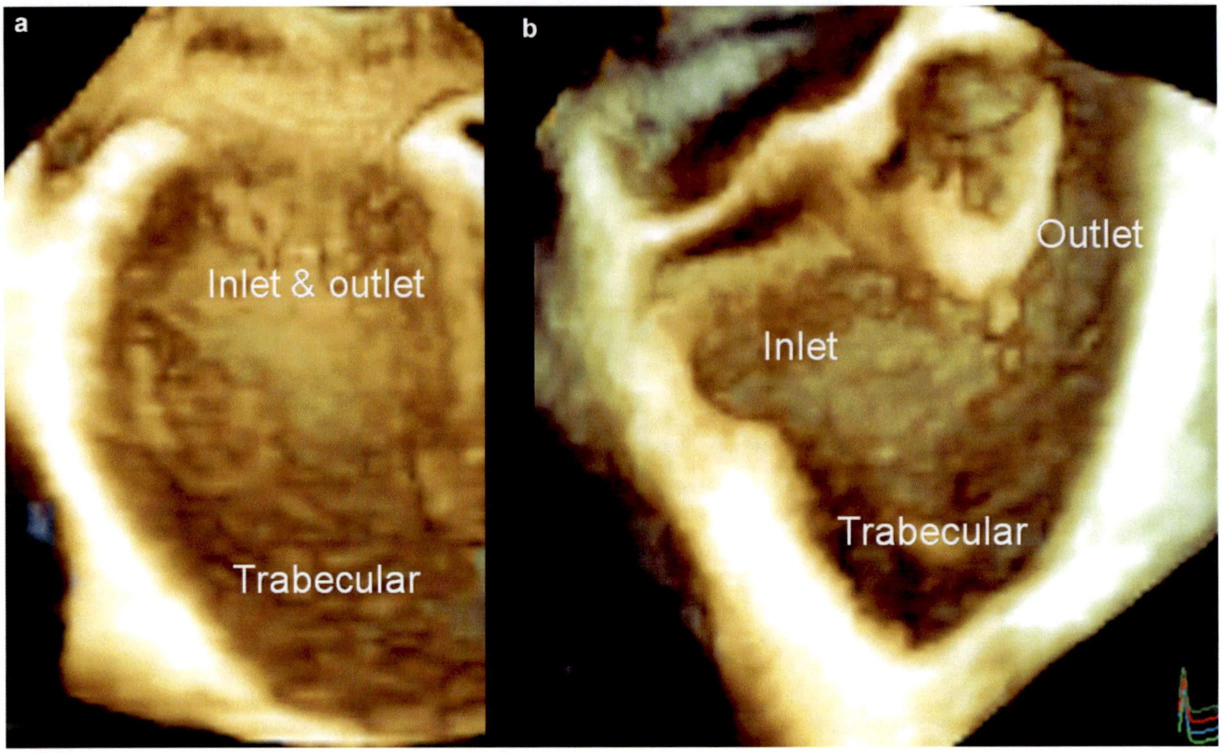

FIGURE 6.21 3D TEE in full volume modality. The septum is viewed from (a) the left ventricular perspective and (b) the right ventricular perspective after removing the parietal walls from each chamber. The trabecular apical septum can be recognized.

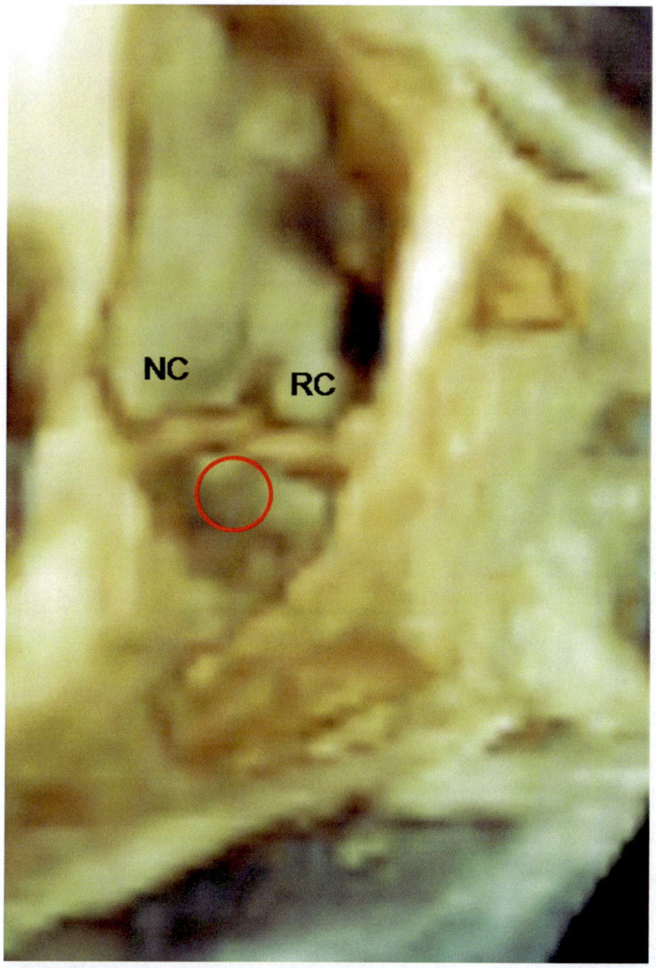

FIGURE 6.22 3D TEE in full volume modality after cropping the aorta to expose the right (RC) and noncoronary (NC) sinuses. The *red circle* marks the position of the membranous septum from the left-sided perspective.

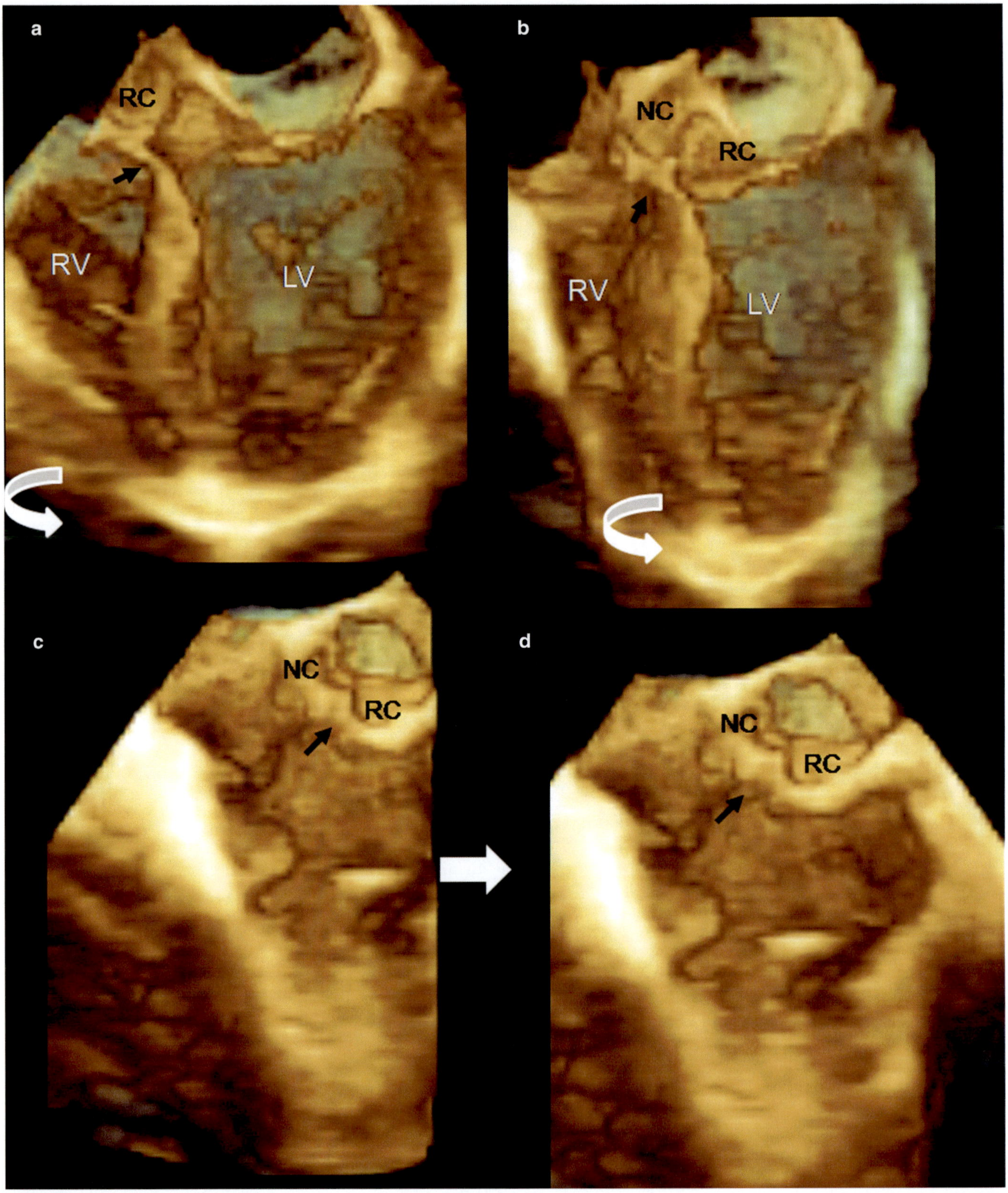

FIGURE 6.23 3D TEE in full volume modality. (a) The membranous septum can be recognized as the thinnest part of the septum (*arrow*). The cut plane of the image is equivalent to the long axis in 2D TEE. (a, b) A leftward rotation (*curved arrows*) progressively reveals the position of membranous septum on the right side of the septum. (d) An expansion of the image in the direction of the straight arrow shown in (c). *LV* left ventricle; *RV* right ventricle; *RC* right coronary sinus; *NC* noncoronary sinus.

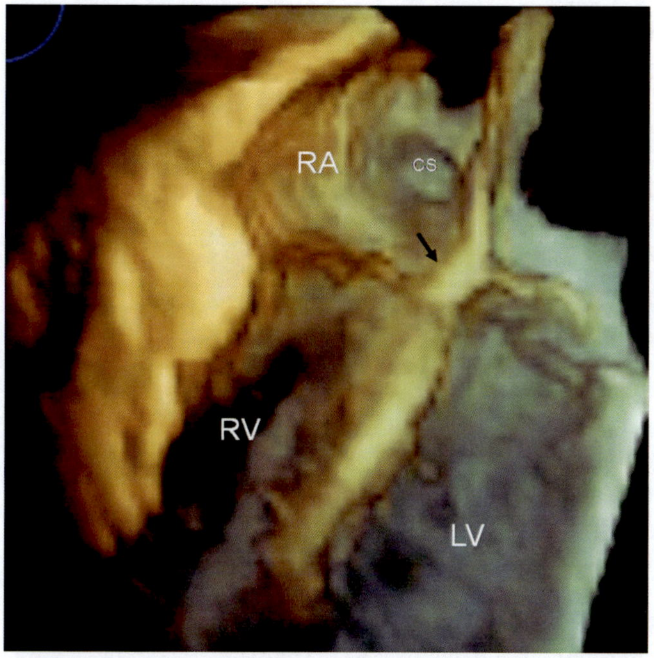

FIGURE 6.24 3D TEE in full volume modality. The *arrow* points to the atrioventricular septum. *RV* right ventricle; *LV* left ventricle; *RA* right atrium; *CS*c oronarysi nus.

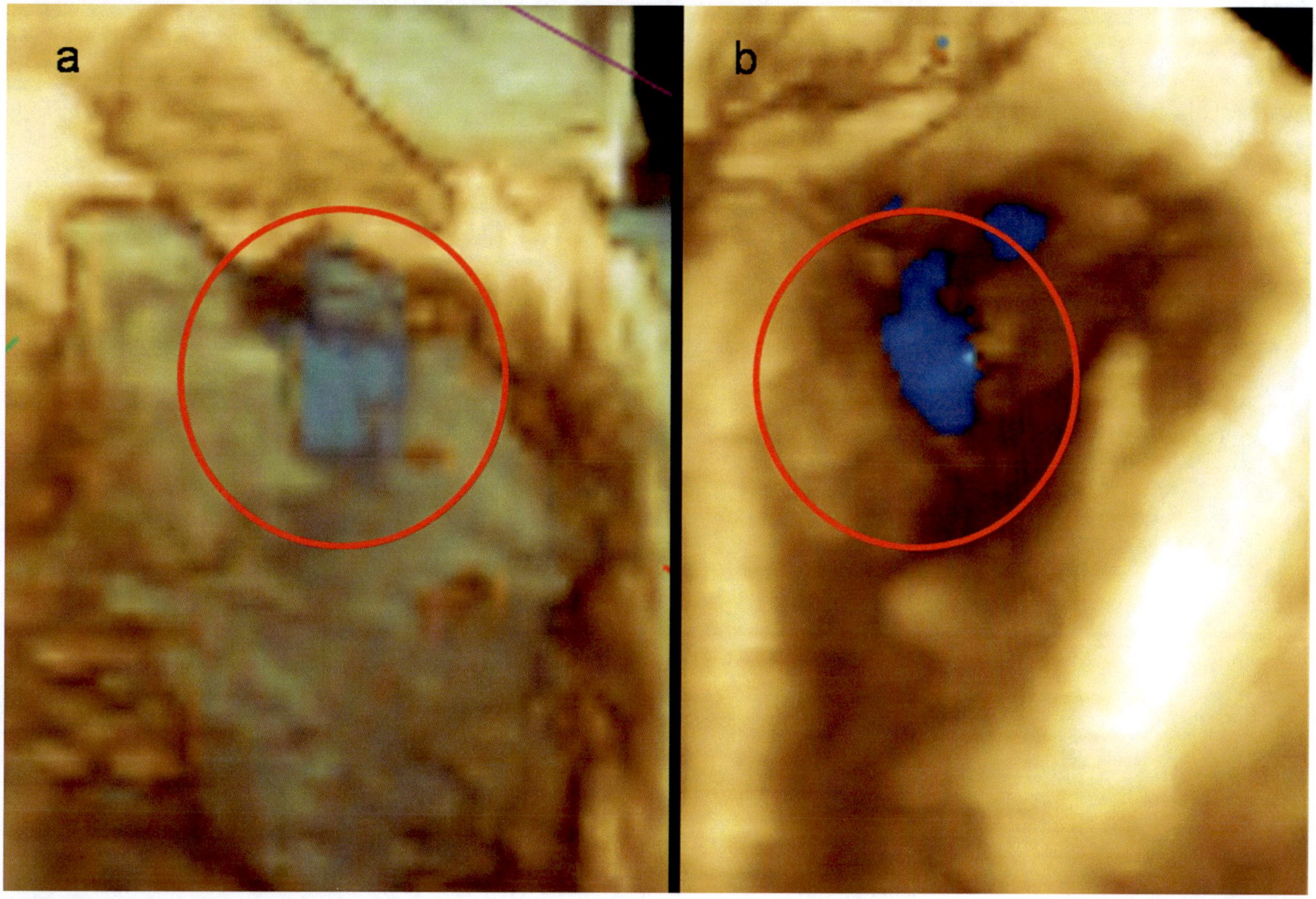

FIGURE 6.25 (a) Muscular VSD (*red circle*) imaged from a left-sided perspective and (b) in 3D TEE color modality from a right-sided perspective.

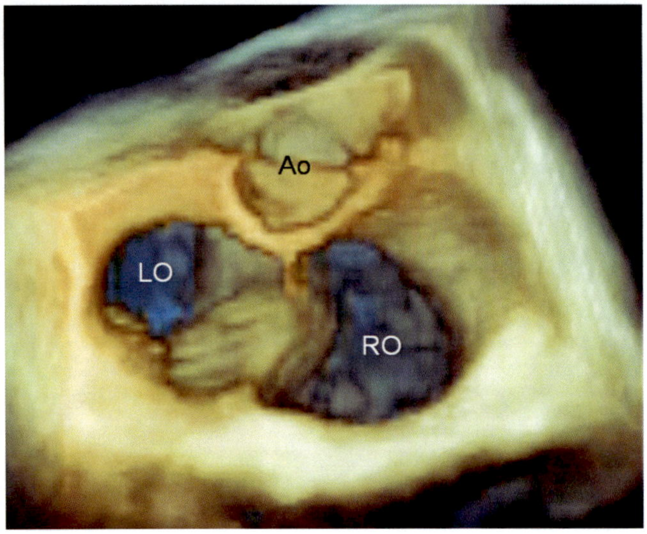

FIGURE 6.26 3D TEE in full volume modality showing an AVSD with two divided valvular orifices. Note the un-wedged position of the aorta (Ao). *LO* left orifice; *RO* right orifice.

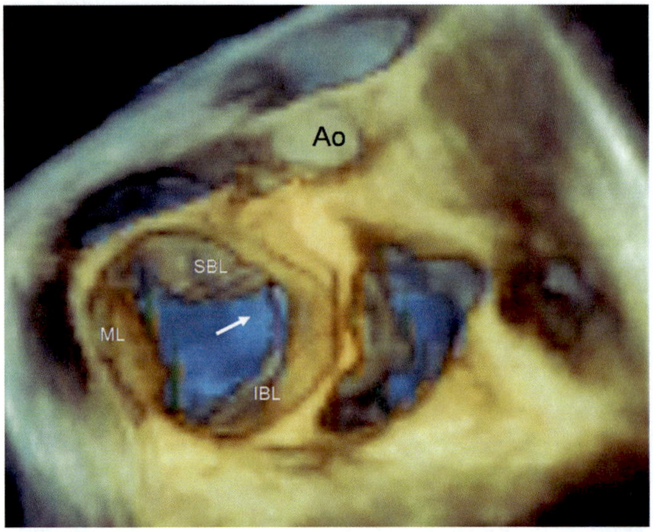

FIGURE 6.27 3D TEE in full volume modality showing a three-leaflet configuration of the left atrioventricular valve. The *arrow* points to the so-called "mitral cleft." Note: the valve does not resemble a mitral valve at all. *SBL* superior bridging leaflet; *IBL* inferior bridging leaflet; *ML* mural leaflet; *Ao* aorta.

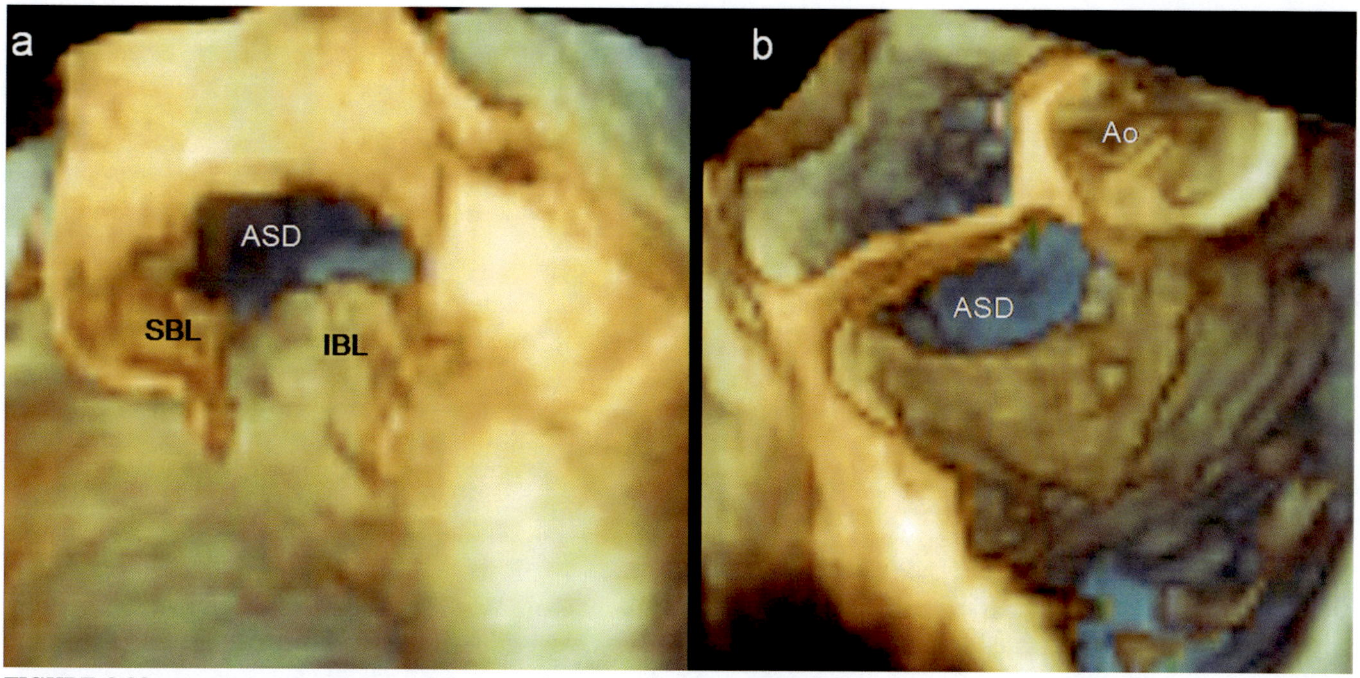

FIGURE 6.28 3D TEE in full volume modality showing "en face" a large *ostium primum* atrial septum defect (ASD) from (a) a left-sided perspective and (b) a right-hand perspective. The bridging leaflets have joined together to obliterate any potential for interventricular shunting, leaving the communication at interatrial level only. *SBL* superior bridging leaflet; *IBL* inferior bridging leaflet.

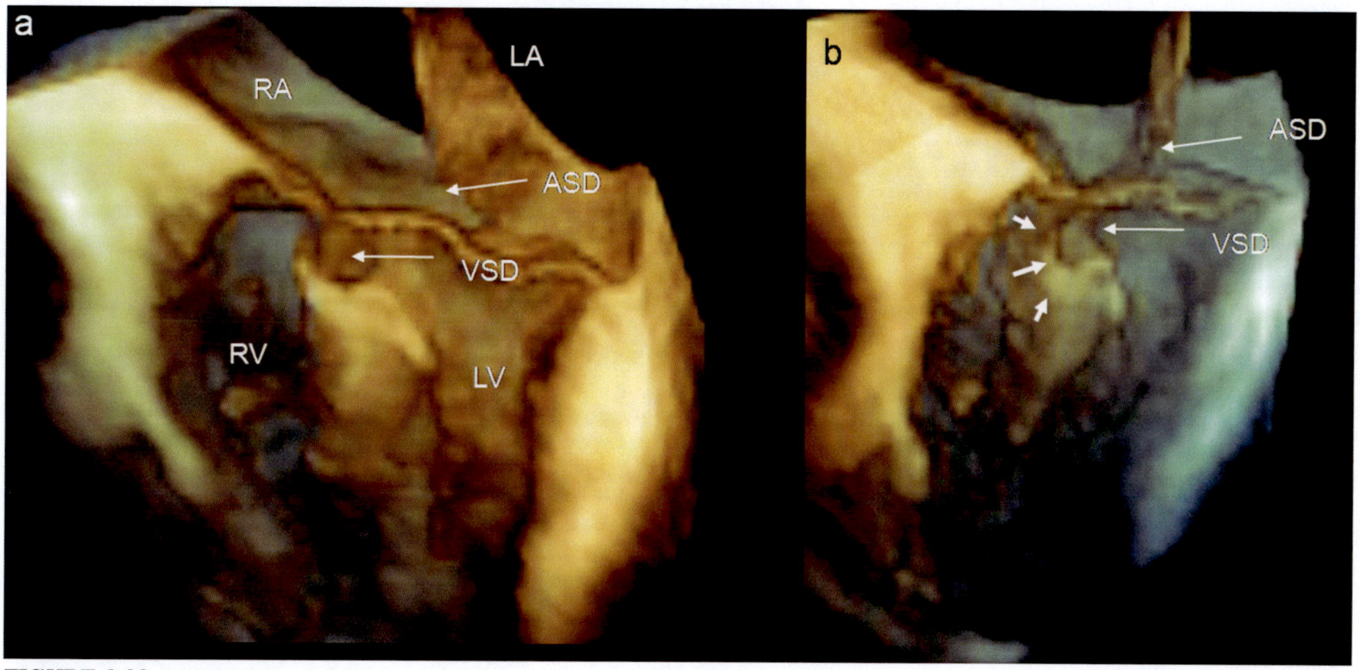

FIGURE 6.29 (a) 3D TEE in full volume modality showing both atrial septum defect (ASD) and ventricular septum defect (VSD) components. (b) Leaflet tissue (*small arrows*) has led to complete closure of the VSD component and to the formation of a pouch-like structure (once called aneurysm of the membranous septum and a frequent cause of spontaneous closure of perimembranous VSD). *Big arrows* point to the atrial and ventricular defects. *RA* right atrium; *LA* left atrium; *RV* right ventricle; *LV* left ventricle.

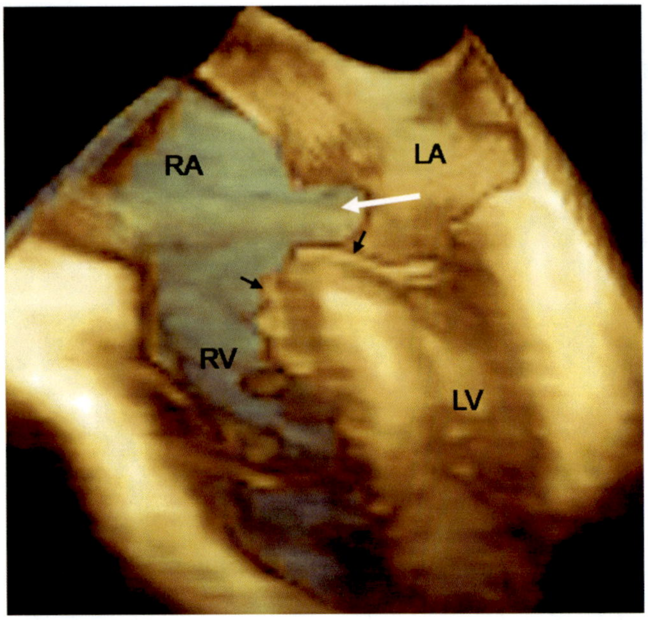

FIGURE 6.30 3D TEE in full volume modality showing the right and left components of the atrioventricular valves at the same level (*small black arrows*). The *white arrow* points to the atrial septal defect. *RA* right atrium; *LA* left atrium; *RV* right ventricle; *LV* left ventricle.

CHAPTER 7

Right and Left Atria

In this chapter, we describe the 3D TEE anatomy of the atria, anatomical variants, and some examples of pathology. The coronary sinus (CS) will be described together with the right atrium, given its anatomical and functional proximity. The atrial septum, which is the medial wall of both atria, because of its anatomical and pathological peculiarities, has been described in Chap. 6.

The continuous and growing development of percutaneous procedures to treat rhythm disturbances has obliged physicians to rediscover the atrial anatomy. A detailed knowledge of the anatomy of the left and right atria and the thoracic veins is essential for the effective application of catheter ablation procedures in atrial fibrillation or flutter. Preprocedural and peri-procedural cardiac imaging may facilitate the identification of anatomic variations, planning of ablation strategy, and has the potential to reduce complications and improve efficacy. In these circumstances, real-time 3D TEE can play a vital role in providing quality images from multiple perspectives.

7.1 THE RIGHT ATRIUM

The right atrium is comprised of a venous component, an appendage, a vestibular portion that leads to the orifice of the tricuspid valve, and a septal component. The superior and inferior caval veins flow into the atrium, forming the venous component, which corresponds to the posterior wall of the right atrium (Figs. 7.1 and 7.2). Inside the right atrium, several relevant structures can be recognized including the crista terminalis, the appendage, the Eustachian valve (EV), the vestibule, and the cavo-tricuspid isthmus (CVTI).

The crista terminalis is a prominent muscular band that separates the smooth wall of the venous component from the rough wall of the atrial appendage (Fig. 7.3). It is a nearly C-shaped band that originates in the antero-medial wall of the right atrium, passes along the anterior border of the superior cavo-atrial junction, sweeps laterally, and descends toward the entrance of the inferior caval vein (Fig. 7.4). It is of variable thickness and width.

The right atrial appendage is triangular in shape and forms a broad junction with the atrial chamber. The appendage protrudes antero-medially from the right atrium (Figs. 7.5 and 7.6).

From the endocardial viewpoint, the wall of the appendage is lined with pectinate muscles (Fig. 7.7). These bundles emerge in branching fashion from the crista terminalis, terminating at the vestibule.

The vestibule is the portion of the atrium immediately proximate to the orifice of the tricuspid valve. Characteristically, it is smooth walled. Its distal margin is marked circumferentially by the hinge line (annulus) of the valvular leaflets (Fig. 7.8).

The EV was described for the first time by the Italian anatomist Bartolomeo Eustachi (born between 1500 and 1513, died 1574). The valve is a crescent-shaped endocardial fold that extends from the anterior margin of the inferior vena cava ostium to the anterior part of the limbus fossa ovalis. Figure 7.9 shows the EV from two different perspectives.

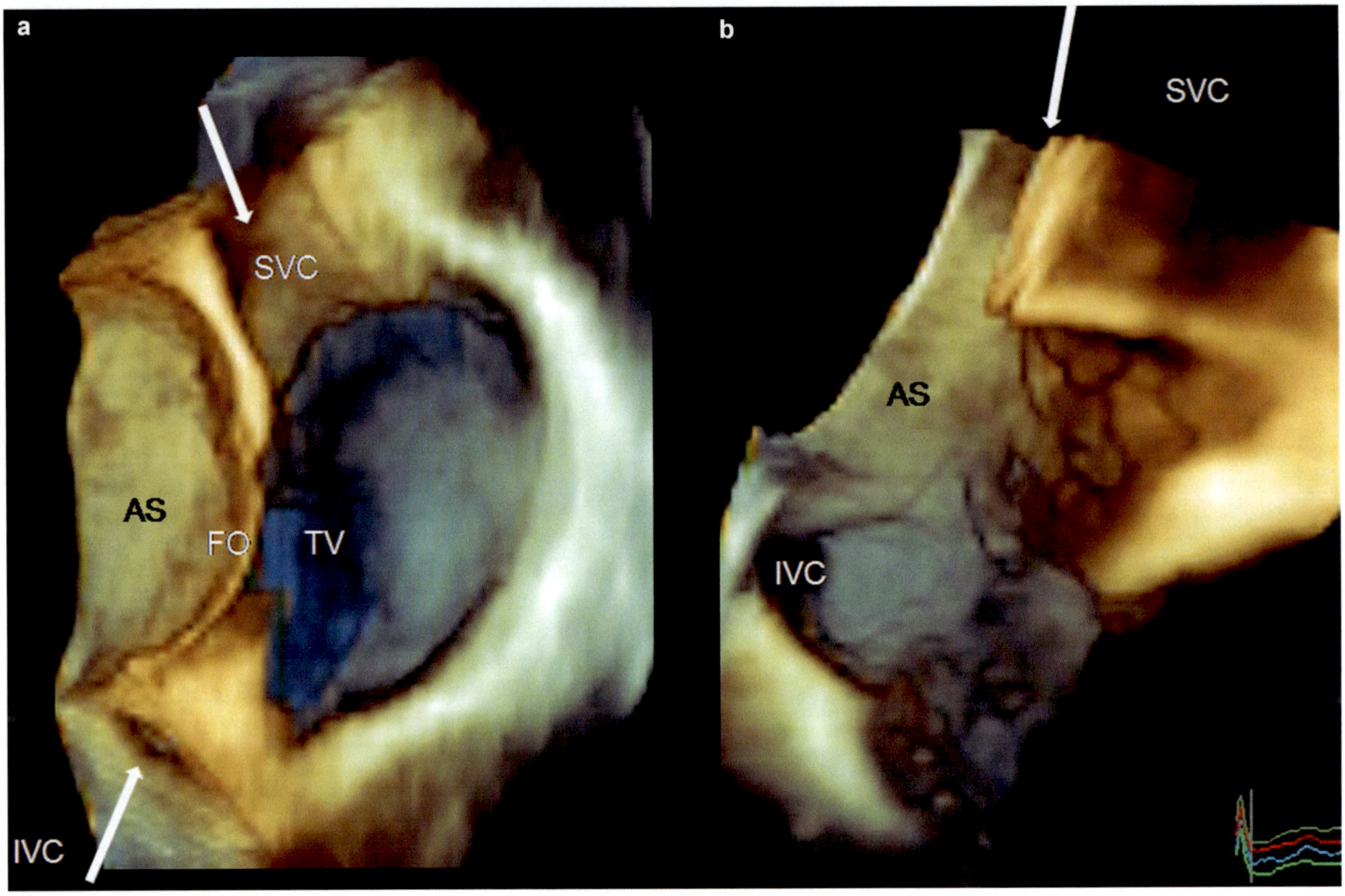

FIGURE 7.1 Real-time 3D TEE images in zoom modality (a, b) showing the entry of the inferior (IVC) and superior (SVC) vena cava into the right atrium (*arrows*). The superior vena cava flow is directed toward the tricuspid orifice (TV), while the inferior vena cava flow is directed toward the fossa ovalis (FO). Because the two caval veins open into the right atrium at different angulations, a single cut cannot show images of both vessels along their longitudinal axes. *AS* atrial septum; *TV* tricuspid valve.

The *CVTI* is bordered anteriorly by the hinge of the tricuspid valve and postero-inferiorly by the right atrial transition to the inferior vena cava. Radiofrequency ablation performed by transecting the CVTI with the ablation line anchored to the tricuspid valve and the inferior vena cava is highly successful in eliminating typical atrial flutter and preventing recurrence. The success of the procedure is highly dependent on the creation of a bidirectional block across the ablation line. Occasionally, despite the ablation, there is continued conduction across the CVTI with recurrence of atrial flutter. Gaps in the ablation lesion due to poor catheter contact have been suggested as reasons for failure. Anatomical variants of CVTI, including sub-Eustachian pouch, encroaching pectinate muscles into the CVTI, or prominent EV might explain these gaps in the ablation line. Three-dimensional TEE might become a useful tool for visualizing normal CVTI as well as its anatomical variants (Figs. 7.10–7.13 and Movie 7.1). In a normal heart, the CVTI is not flat. Usually, a slight recess (a pouch-like depression, named pouch of Keith) can be found inferior to the Eustachian ridge and lateral to the side of the ostium of CS. In some

MOVIE 7.1 The clip shows some anatomical landmarks of the right atrium, such as the Eustachian valve, ostium of the coronary sinus, and the cava-tricuspid isthmus.

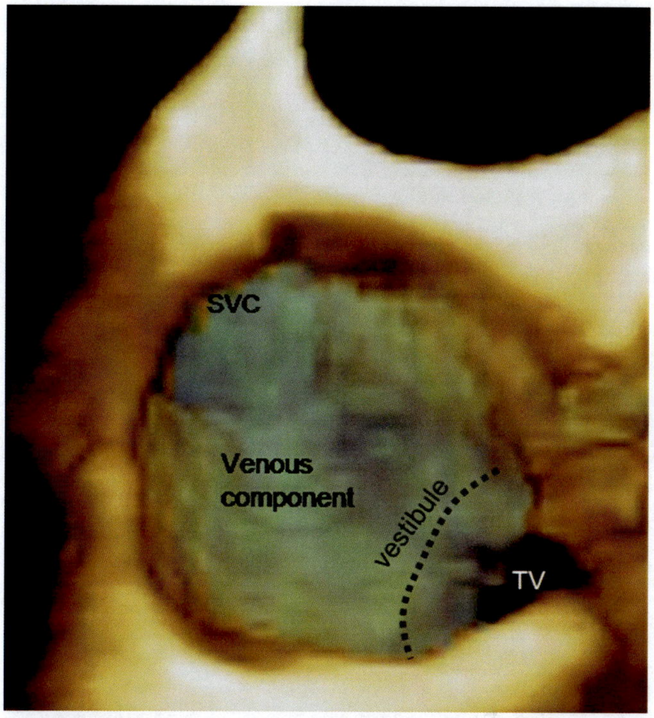

FIGURE 7.2 Real-time 3D TEE image in zoom modality of the right atrium internal cavity obtained after cropping the anterior wall of the right atrium. The figure shows the venous component and the vestibule. The *black dotted line* marks the tricuspid hinge line. *SVC* superior vena cava; *TV*t ricuspidv alve.

patients, the pouch is quite prominent and can cause difficulties with ablation procedure because of a lack of contact of the catheter delivered-energy with the atrial myocardium. In this case, gaps in the ablation line and an inability to create a bidirectional block can occur. For this reason, adequate visualization of the pouch is important. The pouch may be recognized during ablation as a result of an unusual movement of the tip of the catheter or with the right atrial angiography. The sub-Eustachian pouch can also be visualized with 3D TEE, which means that this technique might become useful before and during the ablation procedure (Fig. 7.11). Pectinate muscles may spread out from the crista terminalis and occasionally might cross along the CVTI. This anatomical variation can create difficulties in the ablation procedure (for instance, the catheter might become wedged between two pectinates with inadequate power delivery, or might become unstable between "hills and valleys"). Recognizing this anatomical variant could become important in determining ablation strategy. As shown in Fig. 7.12, real-time 3D TEE can provide images of this anatomical variant.

When an electrode tip catheter is placed in the right ventricle through the femoral vein in patients with a normal EV, proper movements of advancement and clockwise torque will allow the electrode to be correctly placed on

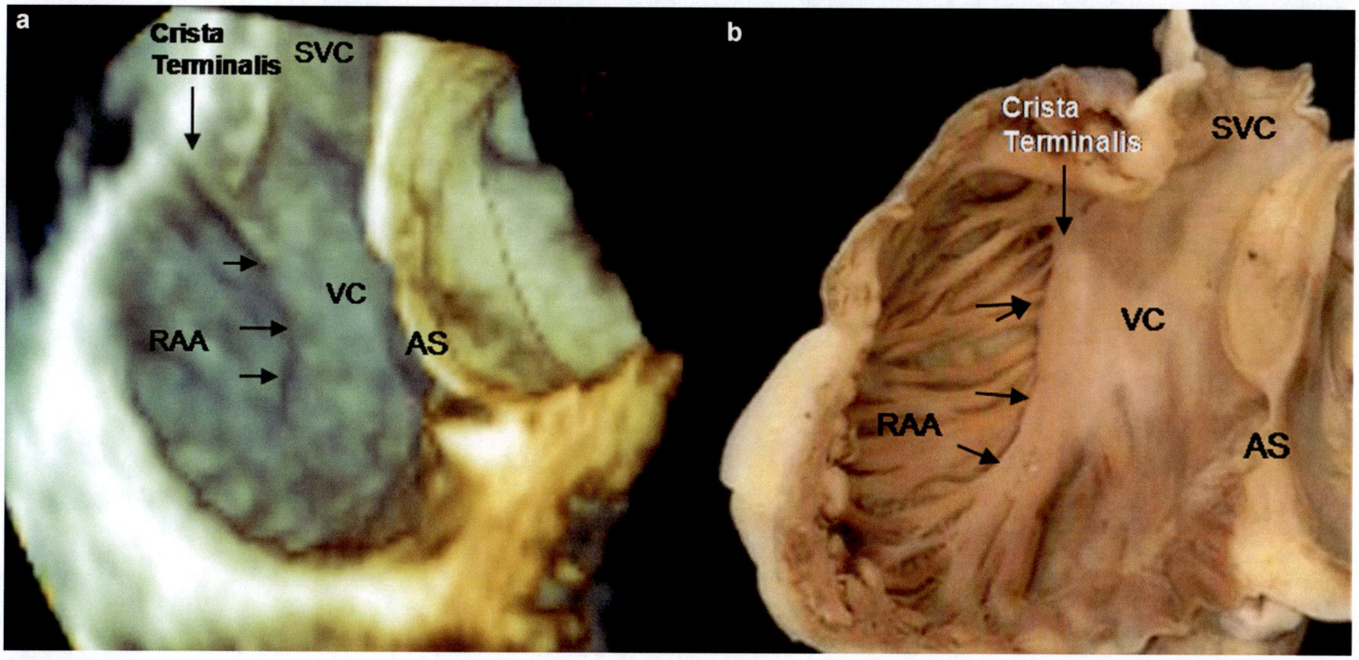

FIGURE 7.3 (a) Real-time 3D TEE image in zoom modality of the right atrium internal cavity showing the crista terminalis and (b) the corresponding anatomic specimen from the same perspective. The crista terminalis forms the boundary between the posteriorly located smooth venous component (VC) and the anterior trabeculated components of the right atrium: the right atrial appendage (RAA). The crista terminalis plays an important role in the genesis of atrial reentry providing an area for conduction block and delay, which leads to initiation, maintenance, and termination of atrial arrhythmia. *SVC* superior vena cava; *AS* atrial septum.

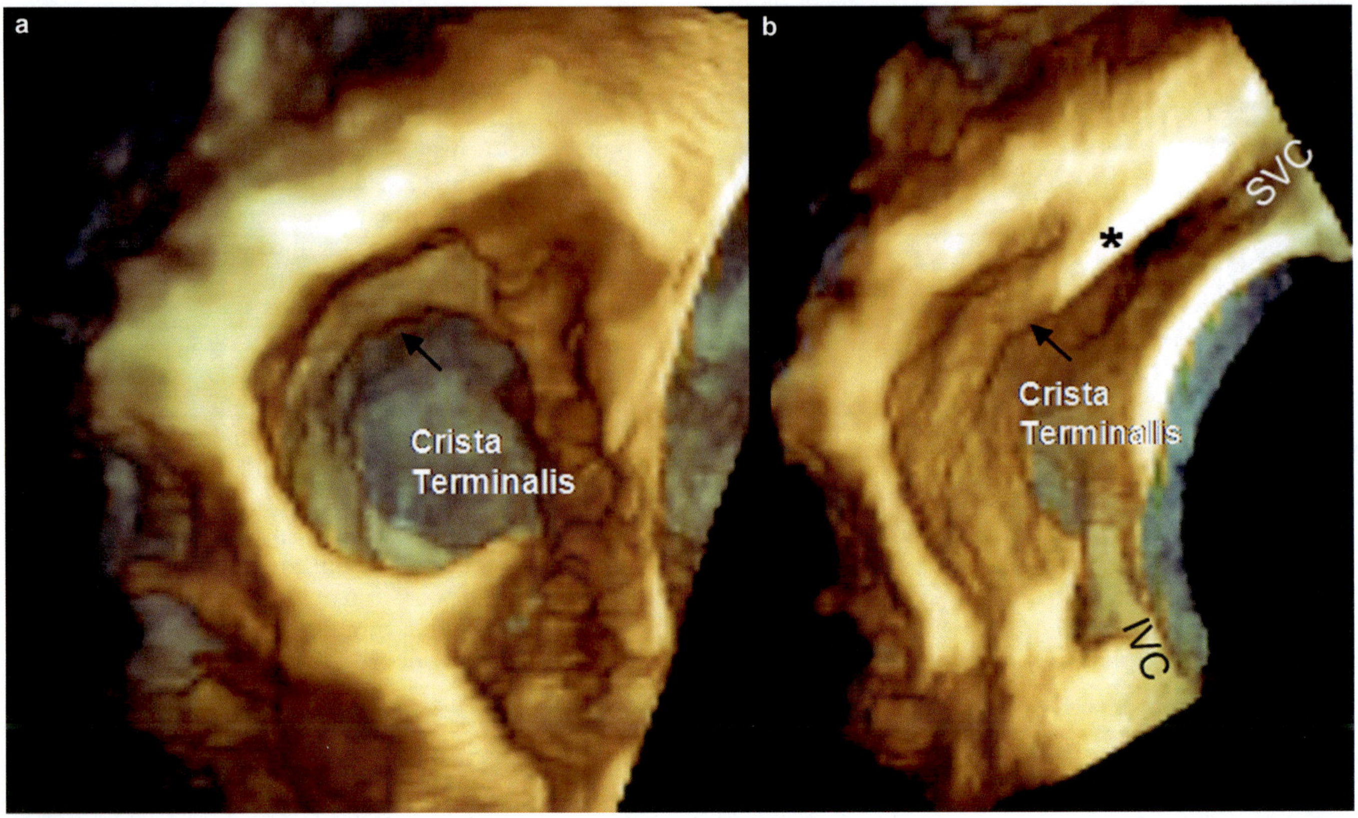

FIGURE 7.4 Real-time 3D TEE images in zoom modality of internal cavity showing the crista terminalis in a view comparable to the right anterior oblique view (a). The crista terminalis has a roughly C-shaped configuration. (b) A deeper cut from the same viewpoint shows the crista terminalis protruding like a bump into the atrial cavity (*asterisk*). *SVC* superior vena cava; *IVC* inferior vena cava.

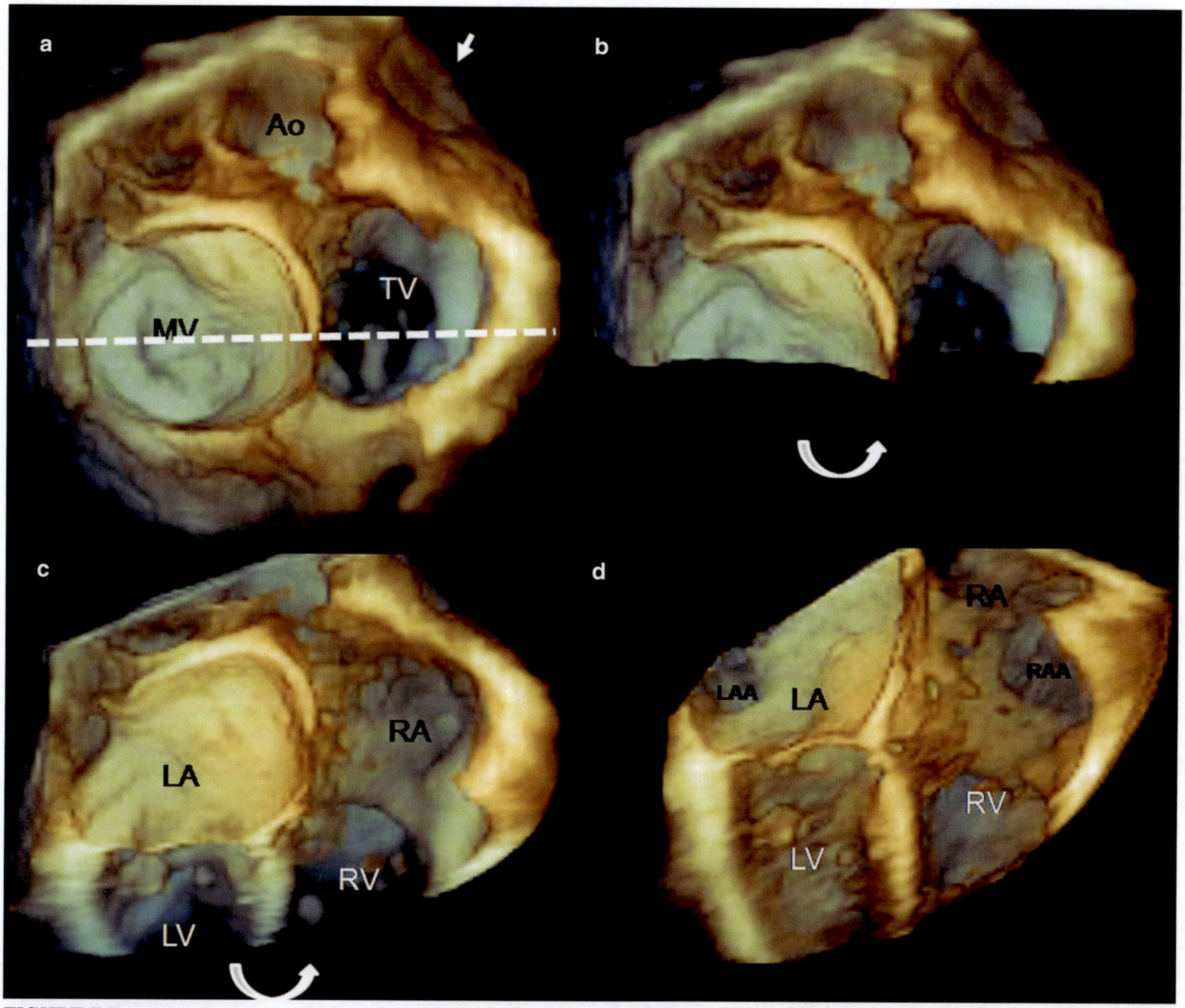

FIGURE 7.5 3D TEE images in full volume modality showing a "four step" approach for visualizing the right atrial appendage (RAA) from a posterior perspective. (a) The base of the heart is visualized from an atrial perspective. An *arrow* points to the RAA. (b) Through a longitudinal cut, (*dotted line*) the posterior half of the heart is "electronically" removed. (c, d) The anterior half of the heart is rotated to obtain a longitudinal view. The internal surfaces of the anterior walls of the four cavities seen from a posterior perspective are then imaged. In particular, the opening of the left atrial appendage (LAA) and right atrial appendage (RAA) into the corresponding atrial chambers are well depicted. *MV* mitral valve; *TV* tricuspid valve; *Ao* aorta; *LA* left atrium; *RA* right atrium; *LV* left ventricle; *RV* right ventricle.

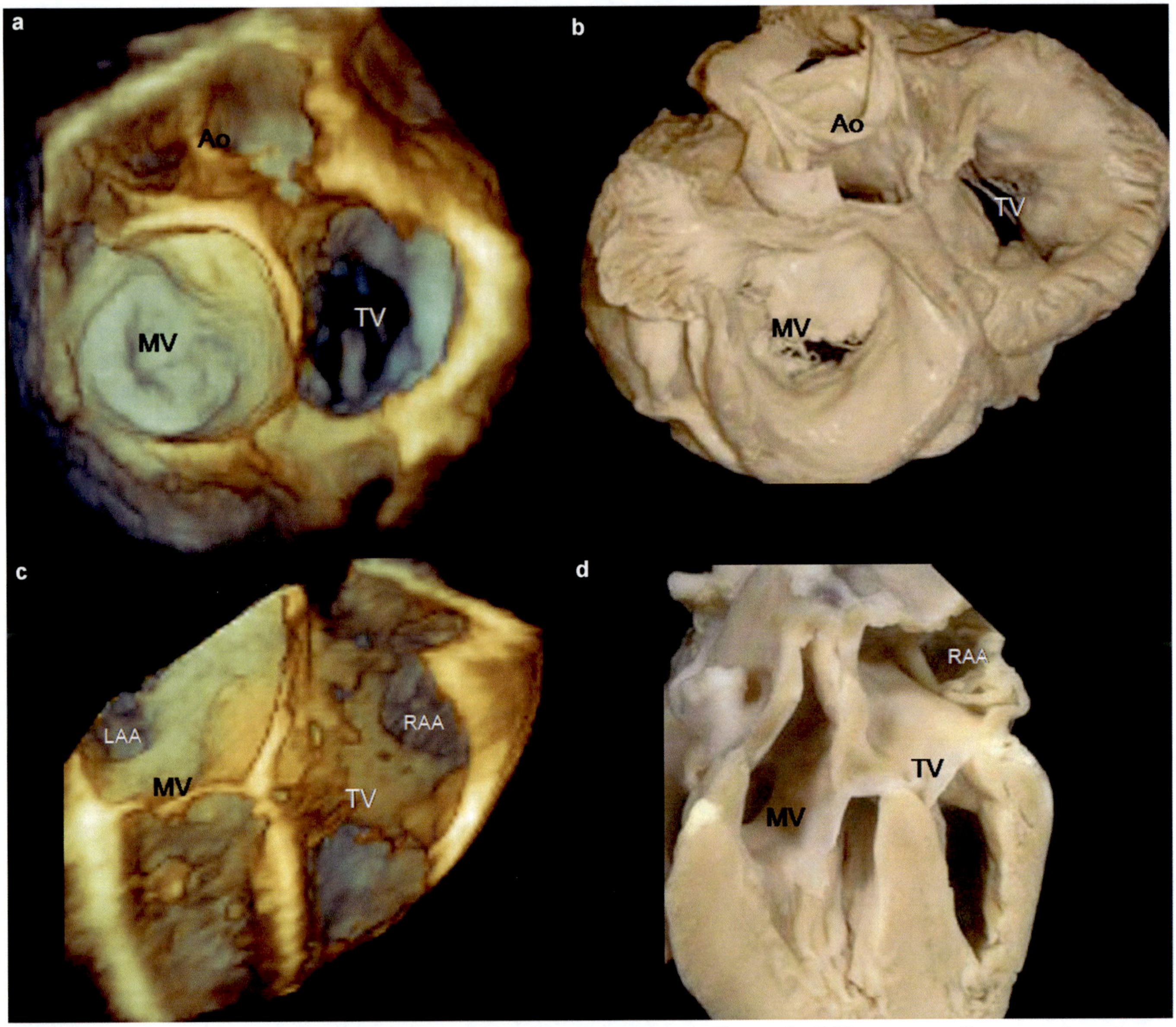

FIGURE 7.6 (a, c) 3D TEE images in full volume modality. The same images as in Fig. 7.5. (b, d) The corresponding anatomic specimens. *MV* mitral valve; *TV* tricuspid valve; *Ao* aorta; *LAA* left atrial appendage; *RAA* right atrial appendage.

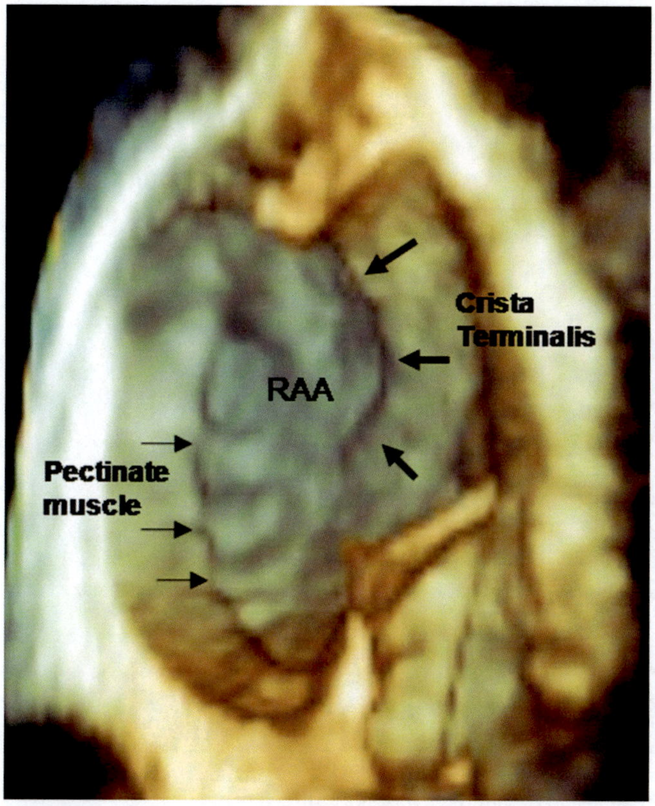

FIGURE 7.7 Real-time 3D TEE images in zoom modality of the right atrium internal cavity. The view is from a posterior/rightward perspective. The figure shows the right atrial appendage (RAA). *Bold arrows* indicate the crista terminalis. *Thin arrows* indicate the pectinatem uscles.

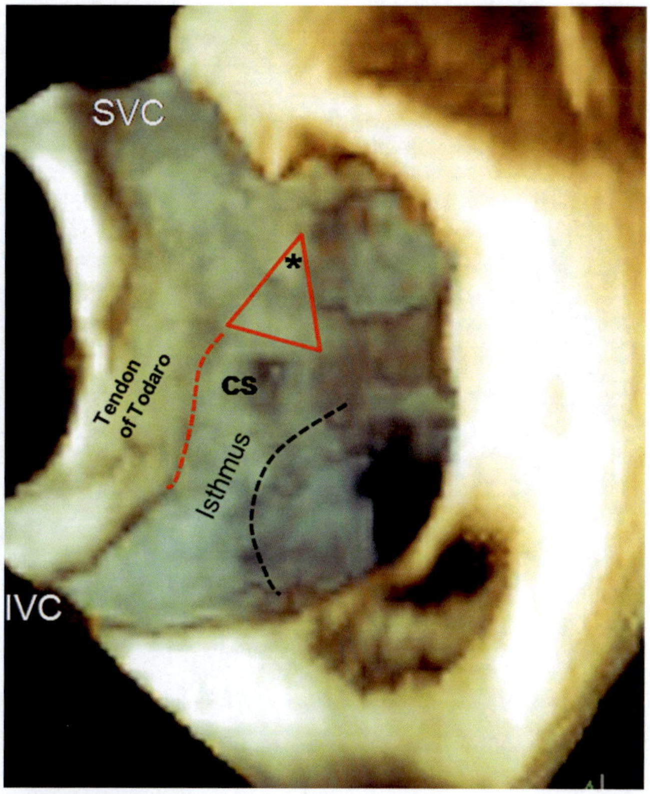

FIGURE 7.8 Real-time 3D TEE image in zoom modality of the right atrium internal cavity, showing the vestibule and cavo-tricupid isthmus. The isthmus is recognized by electrophysiologists as the region of slow conduction that is ablated to interrupt the circuit of common atrial flutter. Above the ostium of coronary sinus is the triangle of Koch (*red triangle*) with the atrio-ventricular node towards its apex (*asterisk*). A thin fibrous cord known as the Todaro tendon (*dotted red line*) runs within the musculature of the sinus septum, from the insertion of the Eustachian valve (not visible) to the central fibrous body. The *black dotted line* marks the tricuspid hinge line. *SVC* superior vena cava; *IVC* inferior vena cava; *CS* coronary sinus.

the CVTI. In patients with prominent EV, the crest of the ridge acts as a fulcrum and when the same clockwise torque is applied on the catheter, the tip may move in an unanticipated direction. The use of an appropriate guiding sheath will often solve the problem. In Fig. 7.13, a prominent EV is imaged by using real-time 3D TEE.

7.1.1 3D TEE Examples of Right Atrial Pathology

Right atrial thrombi are usually related to the presence of central venous catheters. Quite rarely, thrombi can be seen spontaneously even if the patient has atrial fibrillation. The most plausible reason is that, in contrast to the left atrial appendage (LAA), the right atrial appendage has a broad junction with the right atrium preventing a favorable milieu for thrombi formation. Occasionally, however, a thrombus can be detected in the right atrium. Figure 7.14 shows a thrombus in the right atrium with both 2D and real-time 3D TEE.

7.2. THE CORONARY SINUS

In the normal heart, the CS is a wide venous channel of about 2–3 cm in length often located proximally to the atrio-ventricular groove and usually running along the inferior wall of the left atrium, or in the atrio-ventricular groove ending in the right atrium. The CS can be visualized by real-time 3D TEE from many perspectives (Figs. 7.15–7.19).

7.2.1 Example of Coronary Sinus Anomaly

A relatively frequent anomaly of CS is coronary sinus dilatation. One of the most common causes of an abnormal dilatation of the CS is a persistent left superior vena cava (PLSVC). The anomaly is estimated to be present in

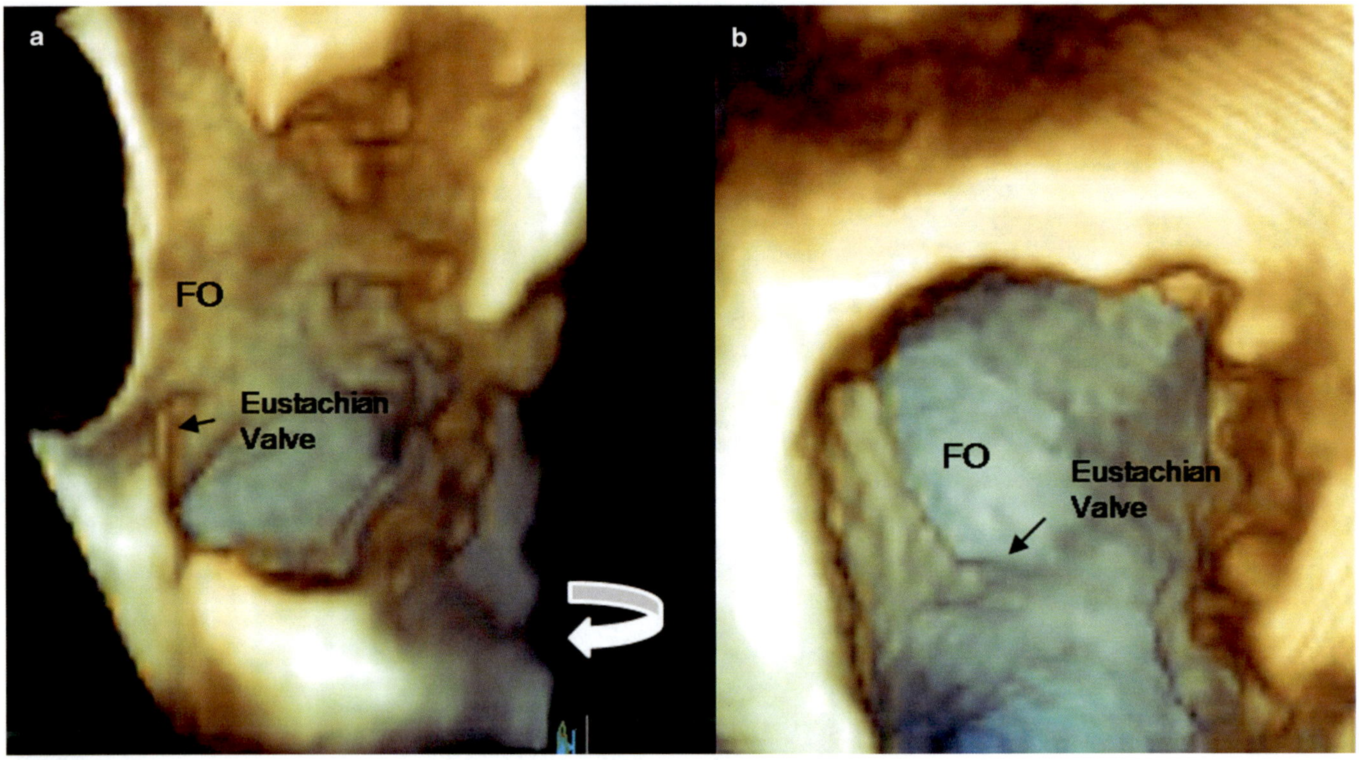

FIGURE 7.9 Real-time 3D TEE images in zoom modality show the Eustachian valve from lateral (a) (*black thin arrow*) perspective and (b) "en face" (*black arrow*). The *curved white arrow* indicates the rotation of the image to obtain the perspective shown.

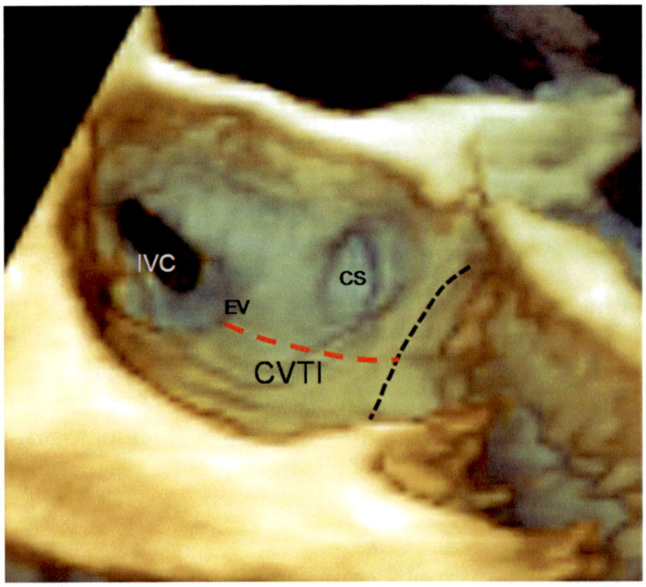

FIGURE 7.10 Real-time 3D TEE showing the cavo-tricuspid isthmus (CVTI) bordered by the inferior vena cava (IVC) postero-inferiorly and the hinge of the tricuspid valve anteriorly (*black dotted lines*). The *red dotted line* indicates the ablation path. *EV* Eustachian valve; *CS* coronary sinus.

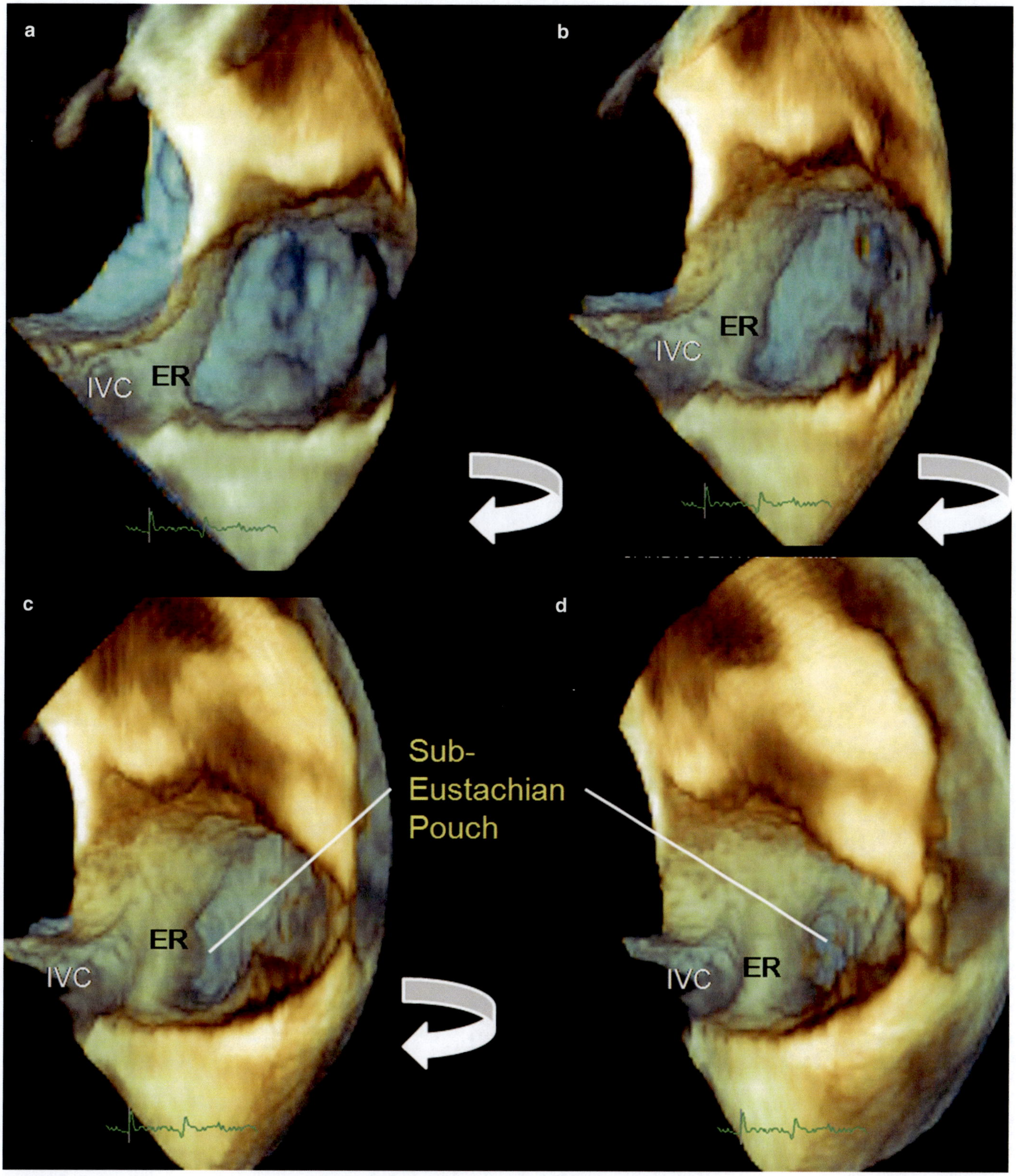

FIGURE 7.11 (a) Real-time 3D TEE in zoom modality showing the inferior vena cava (IVC) and a prominent Eustachian ridge (ER). (b–d) With a right-to-left rotation (*curved arrows*) a sub-Eustachian pouch is then imaged.

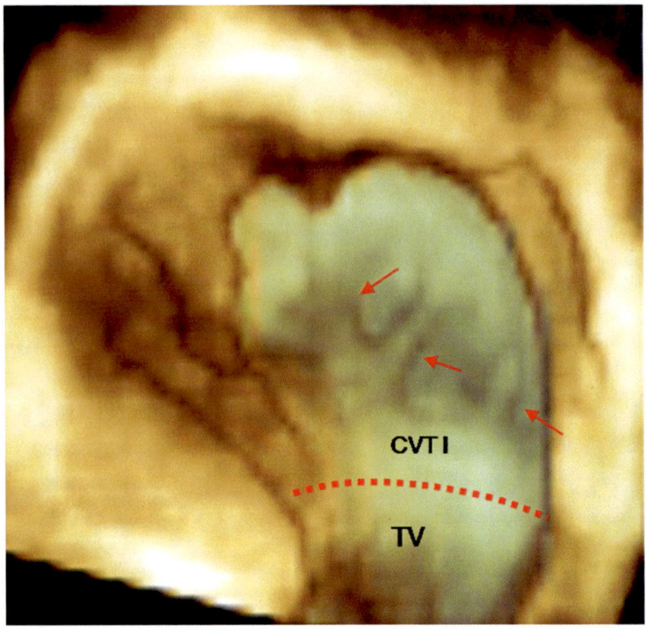

FIGURE 7.12 Real-time 3D TEE showing pectinate muscles (*red arrows*) encroaching the cavo-tricuspid isthmus (CVTI). The *dotted red line* indicates the hinge of the tricuspid valve (TV).

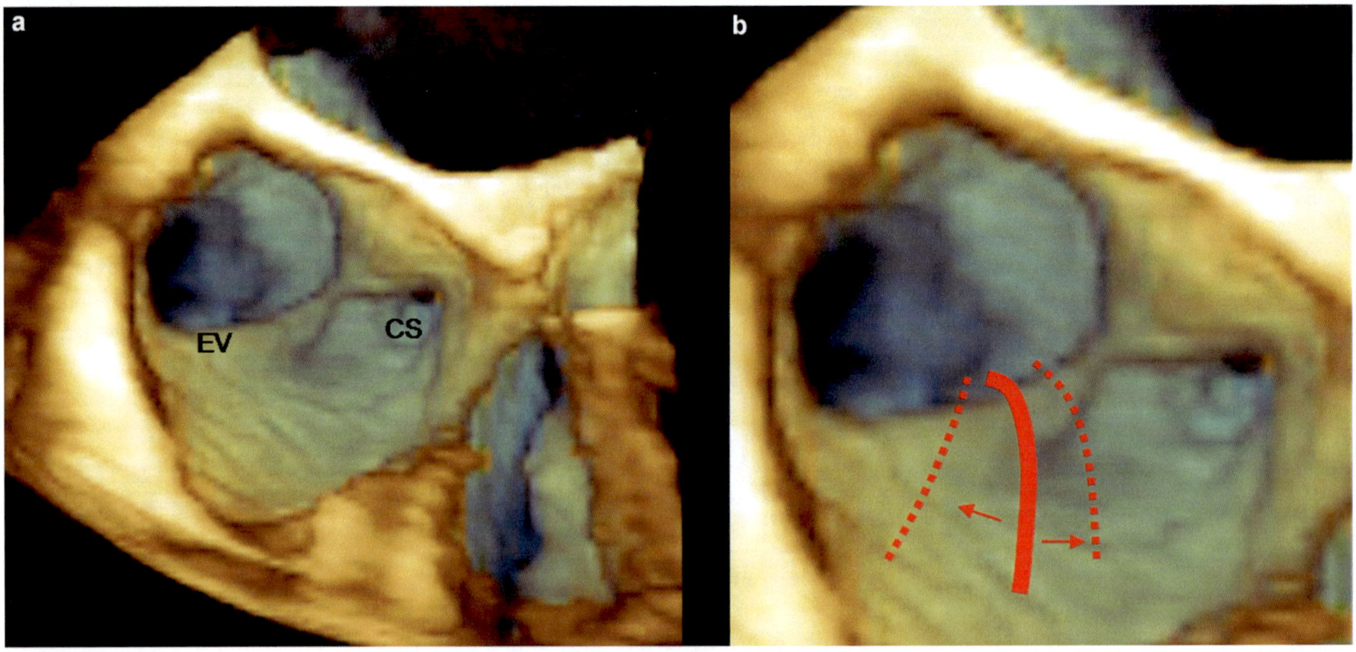

FIGURE 7.13 (a) RT 3D TEE showing a prominent Eustachian valve (EV). In this case, the crest of the ridge acts as a fulcrum and becomes the only point of contact. (b) When a torque is applied, the tip of the catheter may move in an unanticipated direction. *CS* coronary sinus.

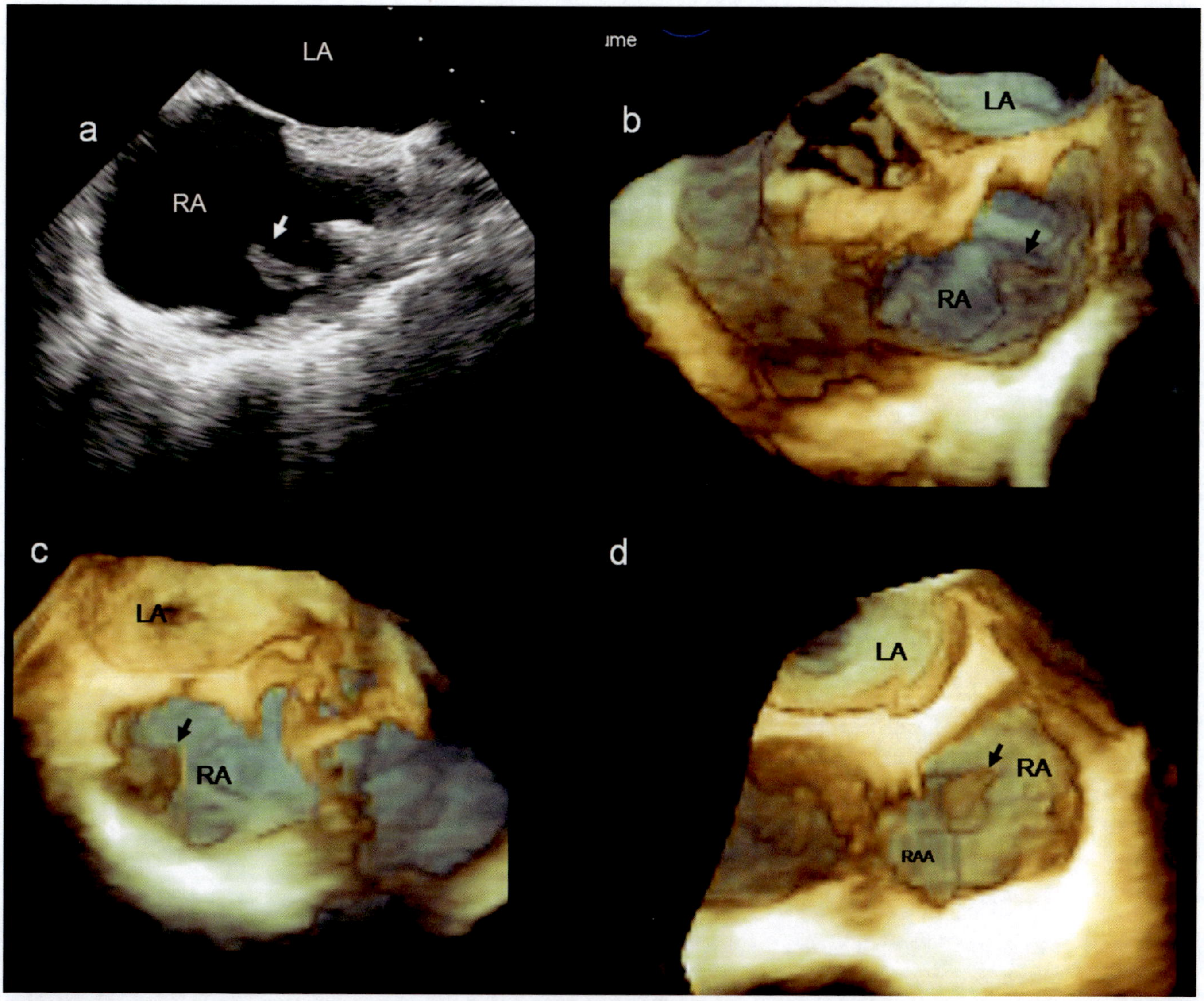

FIGURE 7.14 (a) 2D TEE image of a right atrial thrombus (*arrow*). (b–d) Real-time 3D TEE images from different perspectives of a right atrial thrombus (*arrow*). *LA* left atrium; *RA* right atrium; *RAA* right atrium appendage.

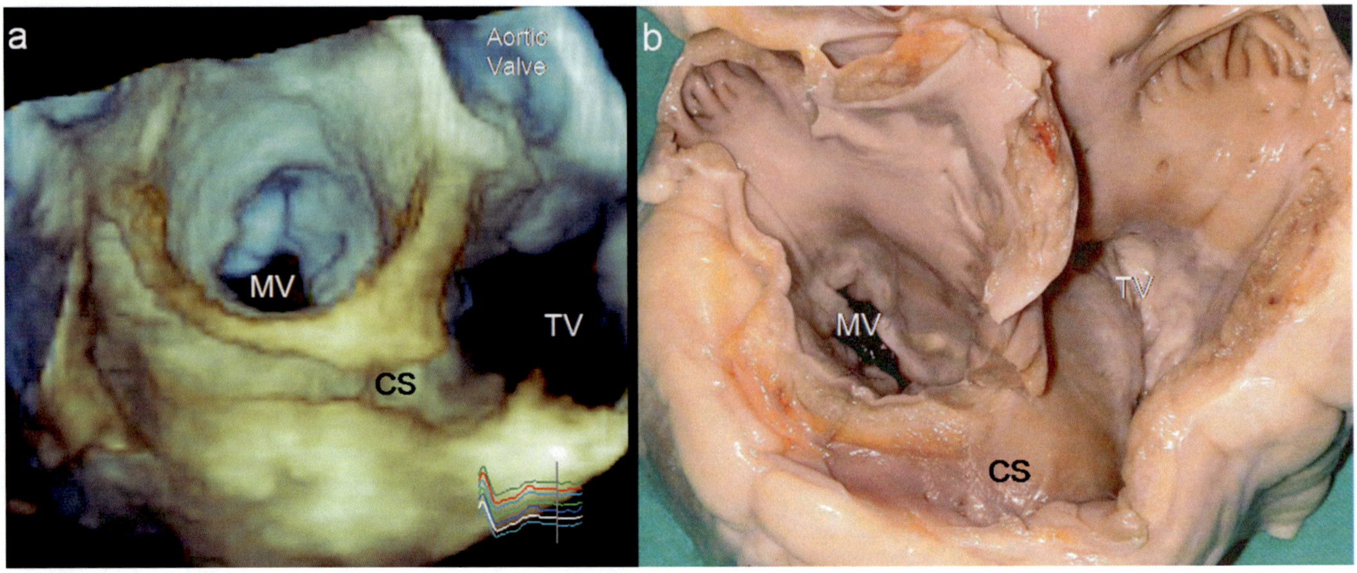

FIGURE 7.15 (a) Real-time 3D TEE in zoom modality showing the mitral valve (MV) and the coronary sinus (CS) and (b) the corresponding anatomical specimen. Viewed from above with a slight upward angulation, the coronary sinus describes a gentle curve in the left inferior coronary sulcus and opens in the right atrium between the inlet of the inferior vena cava and the tricuspid orifice at the inferior border of the Koch triangle. *TV*t ricuspidv alve.

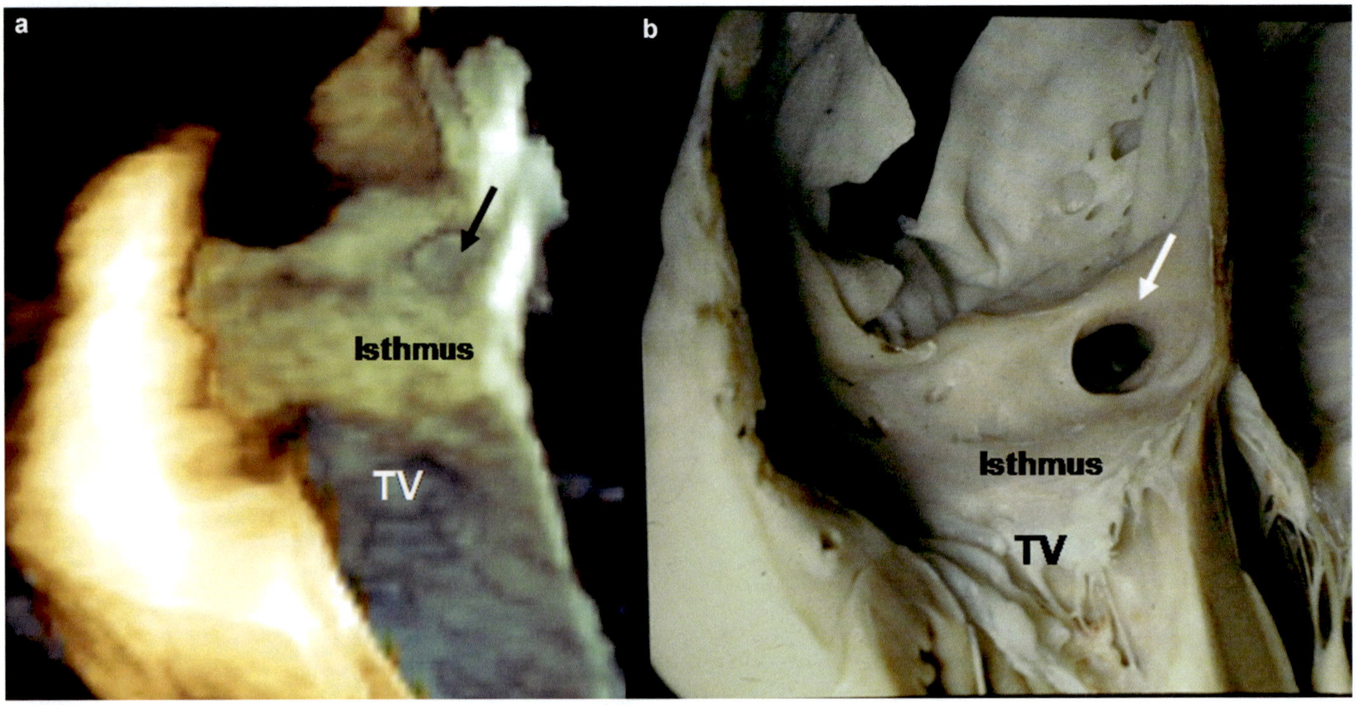

FIGURE 7.16 (a) 3D TEE in full volume modality after cropping the antero-lateral part of the volume data set, showing the tricuspid valve (TV) and the ostium of coronary sinus (*arrow*).(b)T he corresponding anatomical specimen.

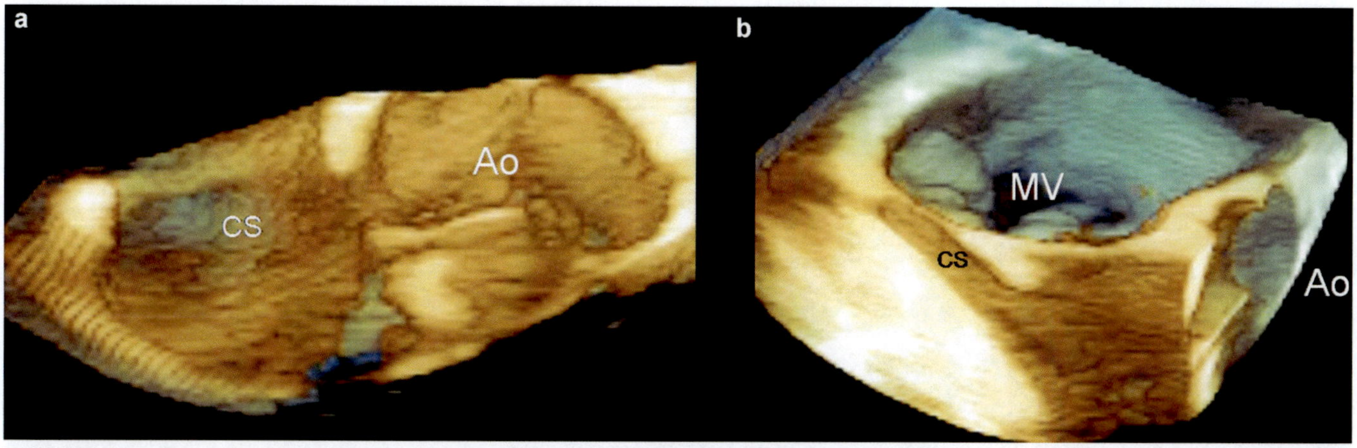

FIGURE 7.17 (a) Real-time 3D TEE in zoom modality showing the ostium of the coronary sinus (CS) "en face." (b) The same volume data set after cropping longitudinally the venous channel. The spatial relationship with the aortic valve (Ao) and the mitral valve (MV) can be seen.

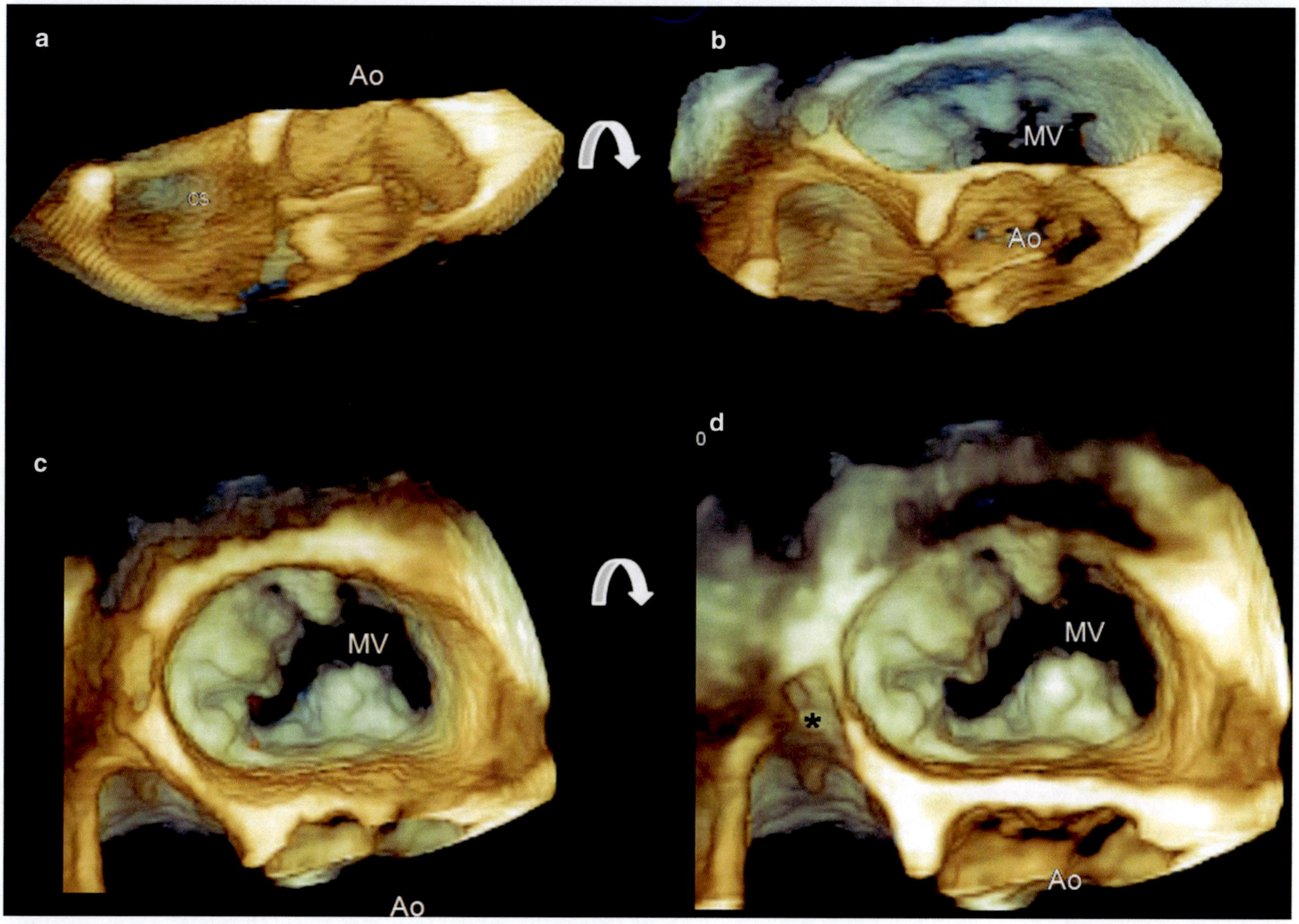

FIGURE 7.18 (a) Real-time 3D TEE in zoom modality showing the ostium of the coronary sinus. The next panels show the same image with progressive downward angulation. (b) The mitral valve (MV) appears in the image (c, d) from an atrial perspective. (d) The *asterisk* marks the floor of the coronary sinus imaged after cropping the roof. *Ao* aorta.

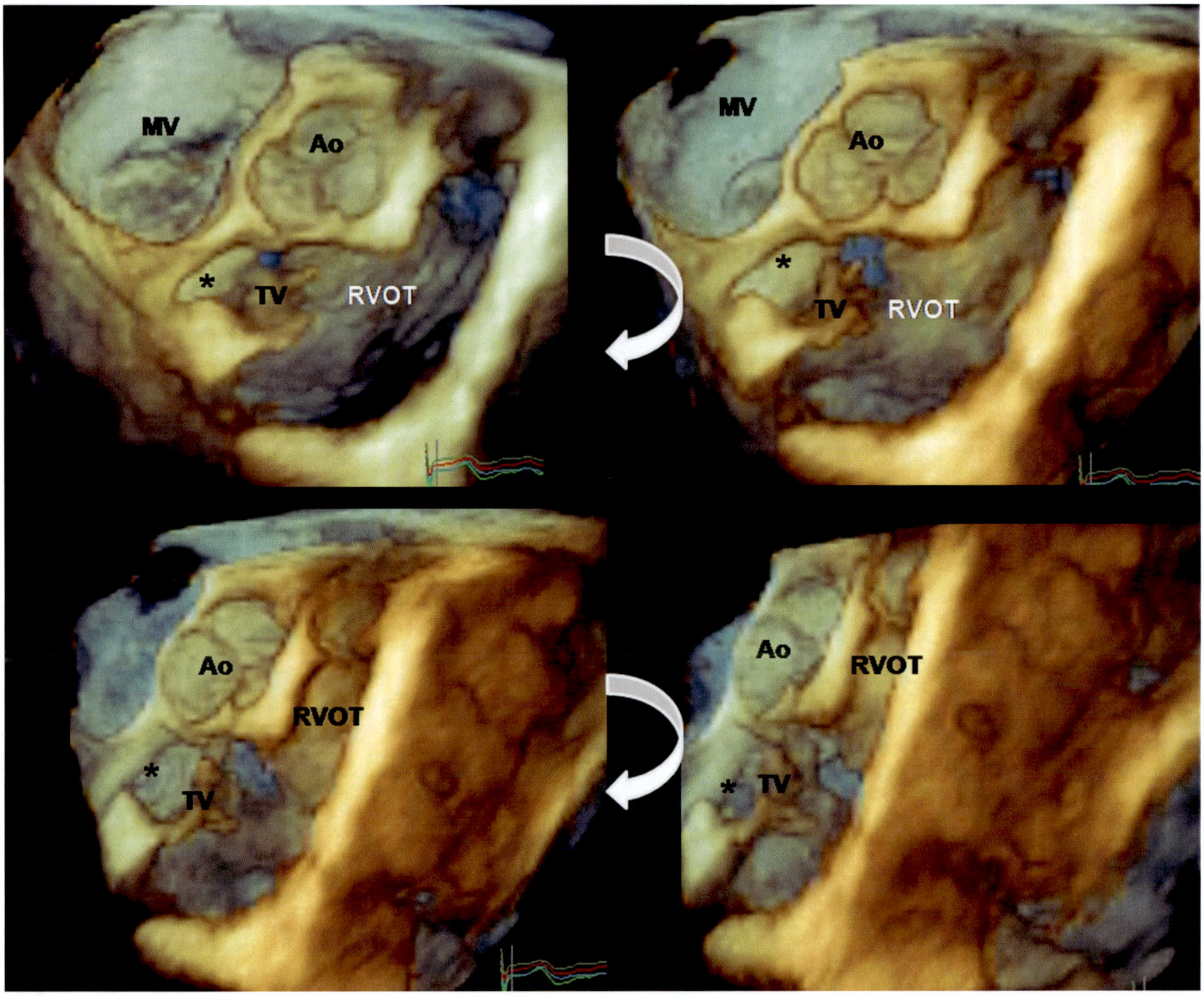

FIGURE7.19 3D TEE in full volume modality, after cropping the anterior wall of the right ventricle. The relationships between the ostium of coronary sinus (*asterisk*) and the surrounding structures such as aorta (Ao), tricuspid valve (TV), mitral valve (MV), and right ventricle outflowt ract(RVOT)c anb ed isplayed.

0.3–0.5% of the general population and in 2–4% of patients with other congenital heart defects. In early embryonic development, the venous blood in the upper part of the body drains into the right atrium via the left and right anterior cardinal veins. After approximately 8 weeks of gestation, the left brachiocephalic vein develops as a bridge between the left and right cardinal veins. Later on, most of the left-sided cardinal system below this bridge disappears, leaving only the CS and a remnant of the left cardinal vein known as the ligament of Marshall. Simple failure of obliteration of the left anterior cardinal vein results in the PLSVC. PLSVC most commonly drains into the CS leading to its dilatation. Real-time 3D TEE can image the entire abnormally dilated CS, although the entry of PLSVC is not usually visualized since most of its course is outside of the pyramidal volume data set. Figure 7.20 shows a dilated CS due to PLSVC (Movie 7.2).

In the same case, the ostium of a large posterior vein is also imaged in Fig. 7.21.

MOVIE7.2 An example of dilated coronary sinus due to persistent superior vena cava.

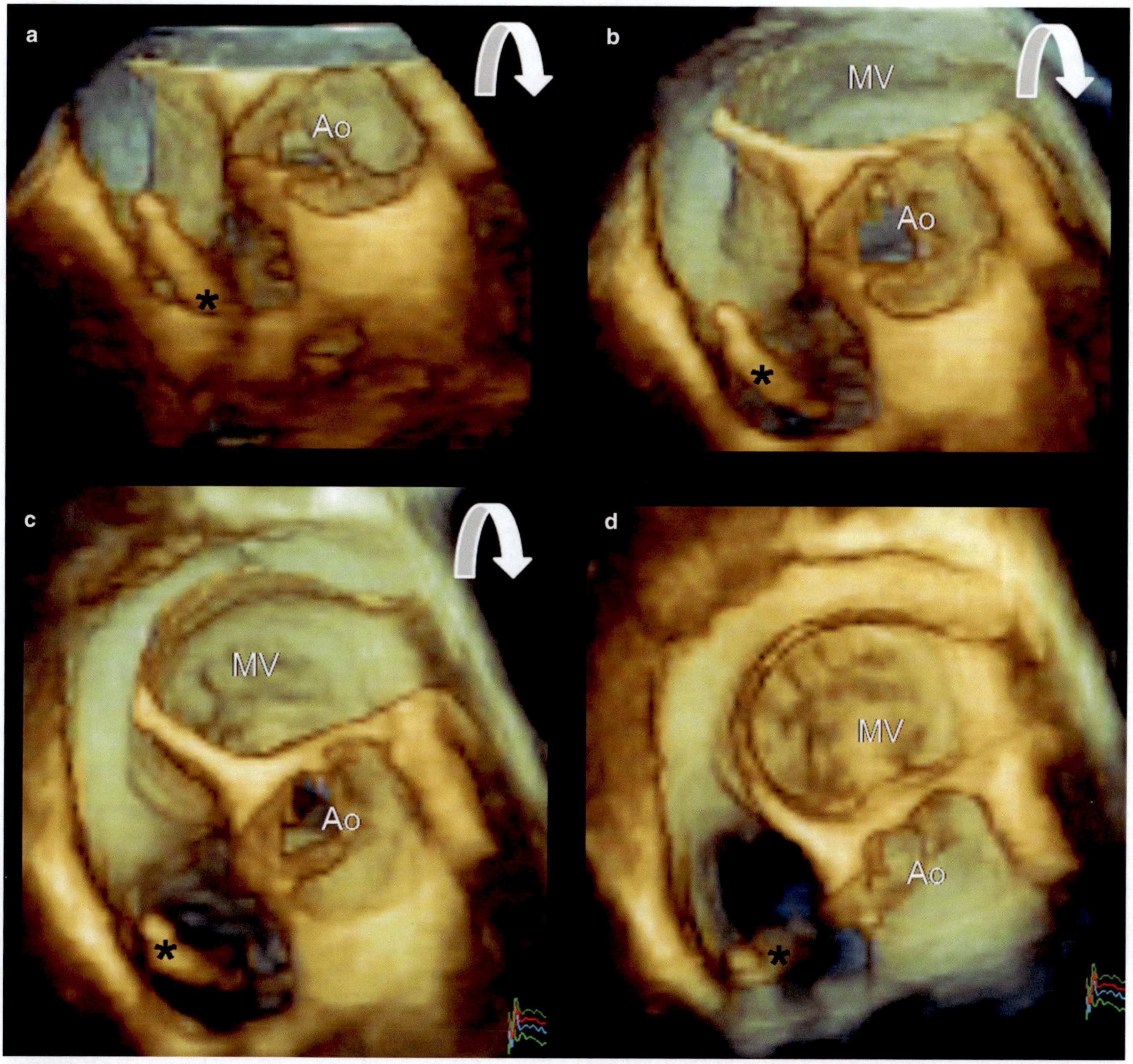

FIGURE 7.20 3D TEE in full volume modality (a-d) showing a large dilated coronary sinus caused by persistent left superior vena cava. The *asterisk* marks a catheter passing through the right atrium. By rotating up-down the volume set data (*curved arrows*), the entire semicircular course of the coronary sinus is revealed. *MV* mitral valve; *Ao* aorta.

7.3 THE LEFT ATRIUM

The left atrium is the most posteriorly situated cardiac structure. Consequently, its posterior wall is adjacent to the course of the esophagus, separated only by the pericardium. Like the right atrium, the left atrium consists of three components: the appendage, the vestibule, and the venous component. The left atrium is a predominantly smooth wall-shaped cavity, because unlike the right atrium, there are no anatomical markers and its trabeculated appendage is rather smaller than the rest of the atrium. The vestibule of the left atrium surrounds circularly the outlet part of the left atrium which leads to the mitral valve (Fig. 7.22).

The LAA is a frequent target of 2D TEE examination. The ability of 2D TEE to detect thrombi in the LAA (in the clinical setting of atrial fibrillation) made this technique a useful tool prior to the use of procedures such as electrical

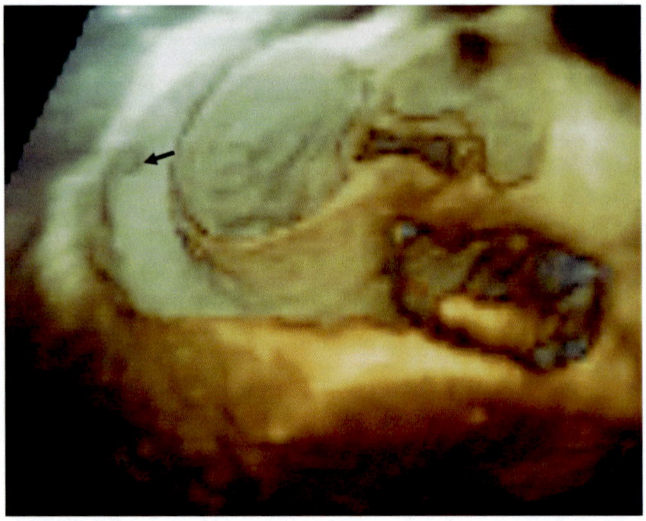

FIGURE 7.21 3D TEE in full volume modality of the same case as shown in Fig. 7.20. A slight change in orientation shows a round vascular ostium (*arrow*) that is presumably a large posterior vein (middlec ardiacv ein).

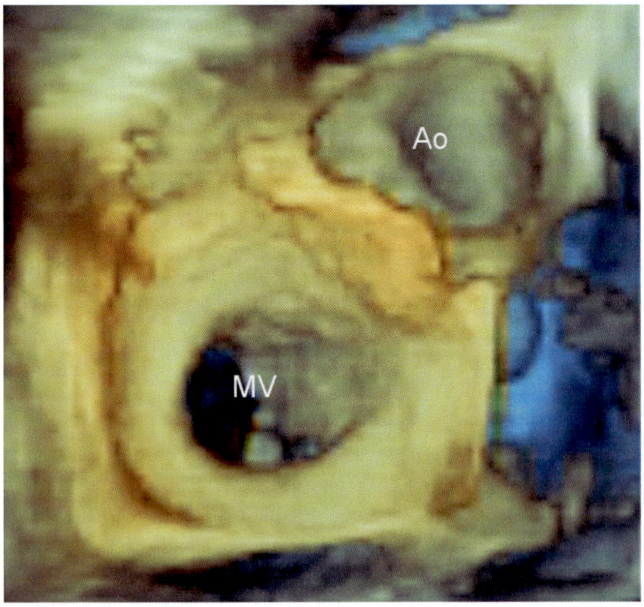

FIGURE 7.22 3D TEE in full volume modality showing the smooth-walled vestibule surrounding the mitral valve (MV). *Ao* aorta.

cardioversion and ablation. From an anatomical point of view, LAA is probably the most variable structure of the heart. It may be tubular, curved or hook-shaped with one, two, or more lobes that spread in different directions. Because of this complex and variable anatomy, it is likely that 3D TEE will enhance the ability of TEE to explore the internal structure of the LAA. Although there is no evidence yet available, it is also likely that this technique will improve the ability of TEE to distinguish small thrombi, hidden in small or very peripheral lobes, from pectinate muscles. Figure 7.23 shows 3D TEE of LAA imaged from different perspectives (Movie 7.3).

MOVIE 7.3 The left atrial appendage imaged from left atrial perspective.

Figures 7.24 and 7.25 show the ability of real-time 3D TEE to image fine anatomical details.

A smooth ridge separates the entrance of the appendage from the ostium of the upper left pulmonary vein (Fig. 7.26). This ridge might have a bulbous tip and can be mistaken for a pedunculated mass arising from the lateral wall of the left atrium. From an atrial perspective, when both ostia of the LAA and upper left pulmonary vein are imaged "en face," the ridge is easily recognized as a prominent structure dividing the two ostia (see also the paragraph on pulmonary veins).

Figure 7.27 shows the spatial relationship between the mitral valve and the LAA.

Pulmonary veins Anatomical details of the pulmonary veins, especially at the point of venous insertions into the left atrium, have become clinically important owing to the use of catheter ablation in treating patients with atrial fibrillation. The pulmonary veins and veno-atrial junctions are considered to have an important role in initiating and maintaining atrial fibrillation. Current commonly used ablation strategies aim to isolate the veins from the left atrium.

Pulmonary veins originate from a capillary network on the walls of the airsacs, where they are continuous with the capillary ramifications of the pulmonary artery. Joining together, they form one vessel for each lung lobule. These vessels merge into a single vein for each lobe; three for the right, and two for the left lung. The vein from the middle lobe of the right lung usually unites with that from the upper lobe. The most common pattern is to have two veins from the hilum of each lung. They open separately into the posterior part of the left atrium. Visualization of all four pulmonary veins with 2D transesophageal echocardiography has been described. Similarly, 3D TEE visualizes all four pulmonary veins by using two different angulations for the right and left veins. Figure 7.28 shows both left pulmonary veins and their relationship with the LAA.

The left upper pulmonary vein (LUPV) is imaged easily with real-time 3D TEE. With 2D TEE, the vein is viewed to the right of the LAA separated by a ridge-like projection in the left atrium. With real-time 3D TEE, new perspectives can be achieved. One of the easiest to obtain

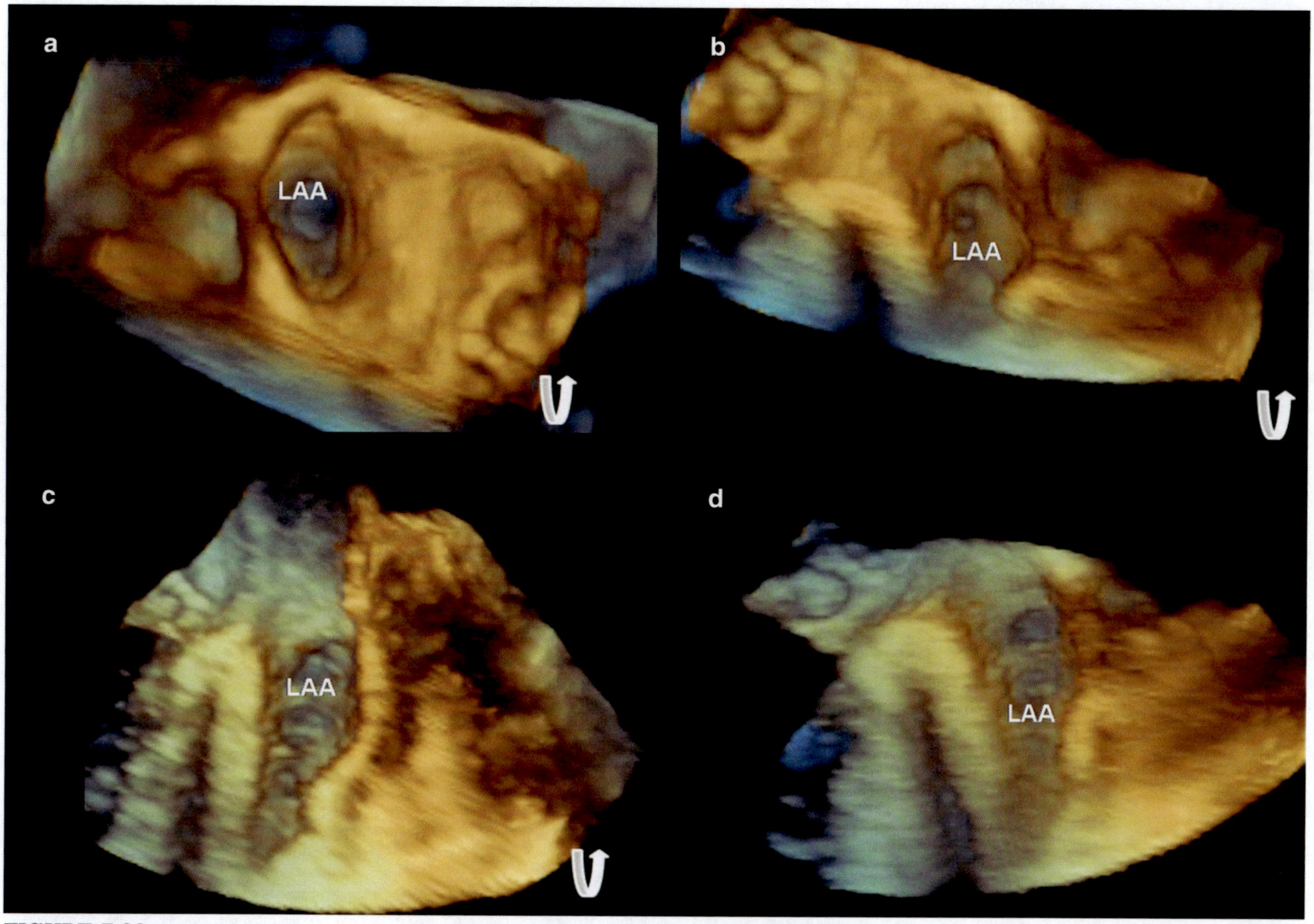

FIGURE 7.23 Real-time 3D TEE of the left atrial appendage (LAA) in zoom modality. In the four panels, the image is progressively up-angulated (*curved arrows*) to show the LAA from different perspectives: (a) an overhead image of the LAA, (c) an image from the left antero-lateral perspective, (b) an intermediate view between the overhead perspective and the left antero-lateral perspective, (d) an upward angulation oft hei mages eeni n(c).

is the "en face" perspective showing the ostium of the LUPV from above. A ridge separates the vein from the LAA(Fig. 7.29a ndM ovie 7.4).

Not uncommonly, in both the overhead (Fig. 7.30) and lateral perspectives (Fig. 7.31), the last run of branches into the LUPV can be recognized.

A standardized procedure, similar to that in 2D TEE, is required for imaging with 3D image of both left pulmonary veins in a single projection (Fig. 7.32). With 3D TEE one can perform rotation and cutting of 3D images in any direction, without losing the spatial relationship between structures, provides an "en face" view of the orifice of both veins (Fig. 7.33 See also movie 7.5).

As in the case of the left pulmonary veins, we can also create an image of both right pulmonary veins in one shot (Fig. 7.34). Figure 7.35 shows a progressive rotation of 3D images to provide an "en face" view of the orifices of both veins. The right pulmonary veins are located adjacent to the plane of the atrial septum and pass immediately behind the superior vena cava. The relationship between the right upper pulmonary veins and superior vena cava can be seen in Fig. 7.36.

MOVIE 7.4 The left atrial appendage and left upper pulmonary vein separated by a ridge-like projection in the left atrium seen from the left atrial perspective.

MOVIE7.5 The left upper and lower pulmonary veins viewed from above.

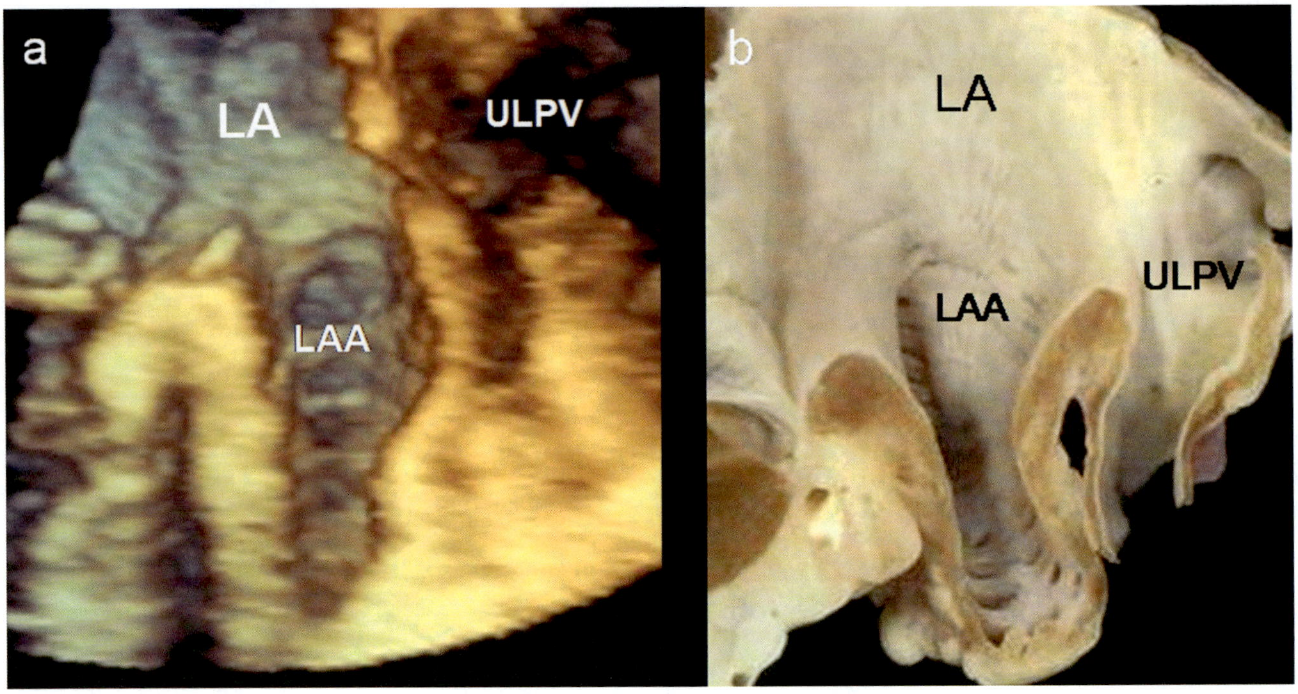

FIGURE 7.24 (a) Real-time 3D TEE of the left atrial appendage in zoom modality and (b) the corresponding anatomical specimen taken from a similar perspective. *LAA* left atrial appendage; *LA* left atrium; *ULPV* upper left pulmonary vein.

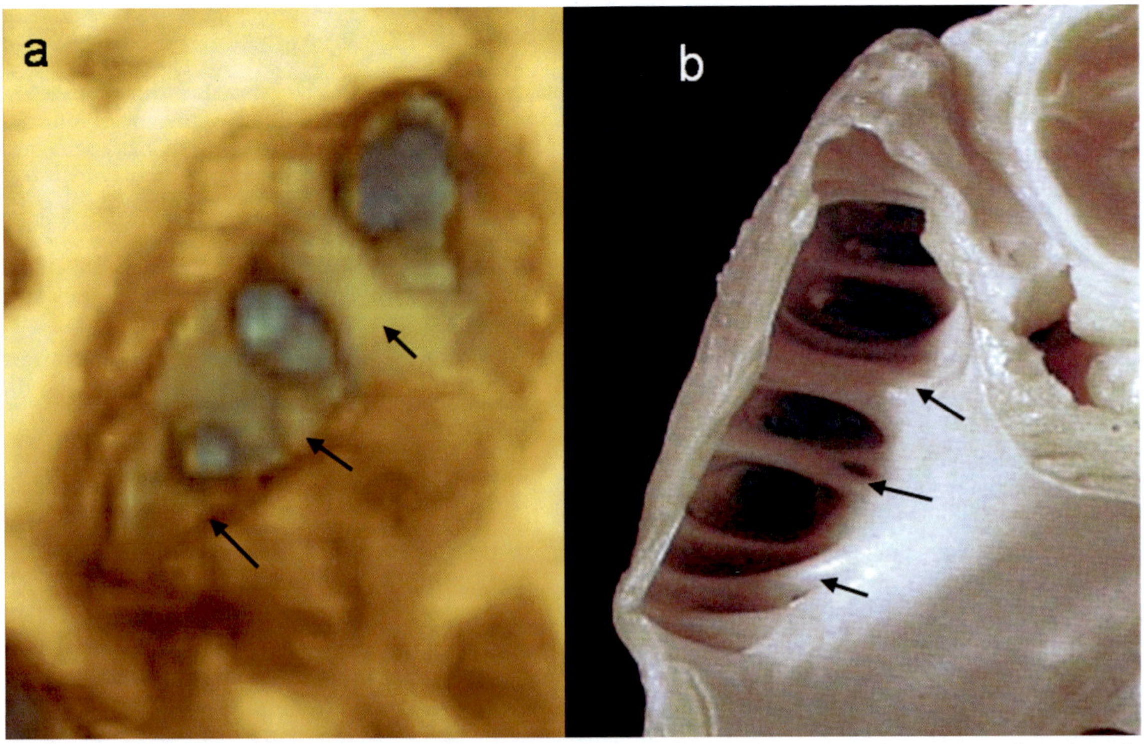

FIGURE 7.25 (a) Real-time 3D TEE of the left atrial appendage in zoom modality and (b) the corresponding anatomical specimen from an overhead perspective so as to reveal an image "en face" of lobes and pectinate muscles (*arrows*). The pectinate muscles appear as fine ridges lining the lumen of the appendage.

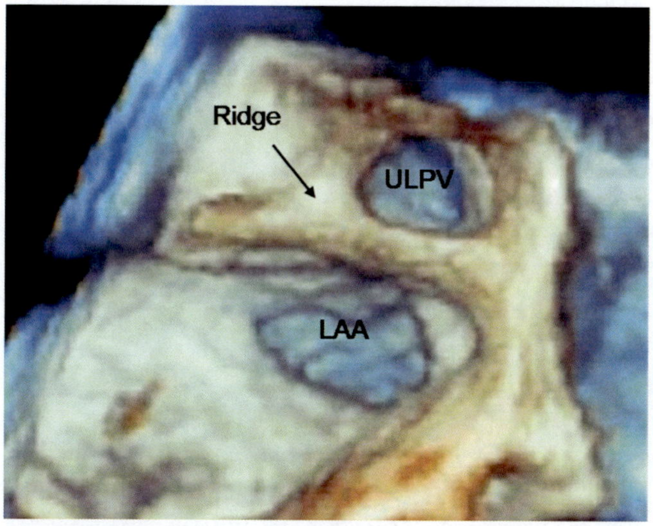

FIGURE 7.26 Real-time 3D TEE in zoom modality showing both ostia of the left atrial appendage (LAA) and the left upper pulmonaryv ein(LUPV)d ividedb yt her idge.

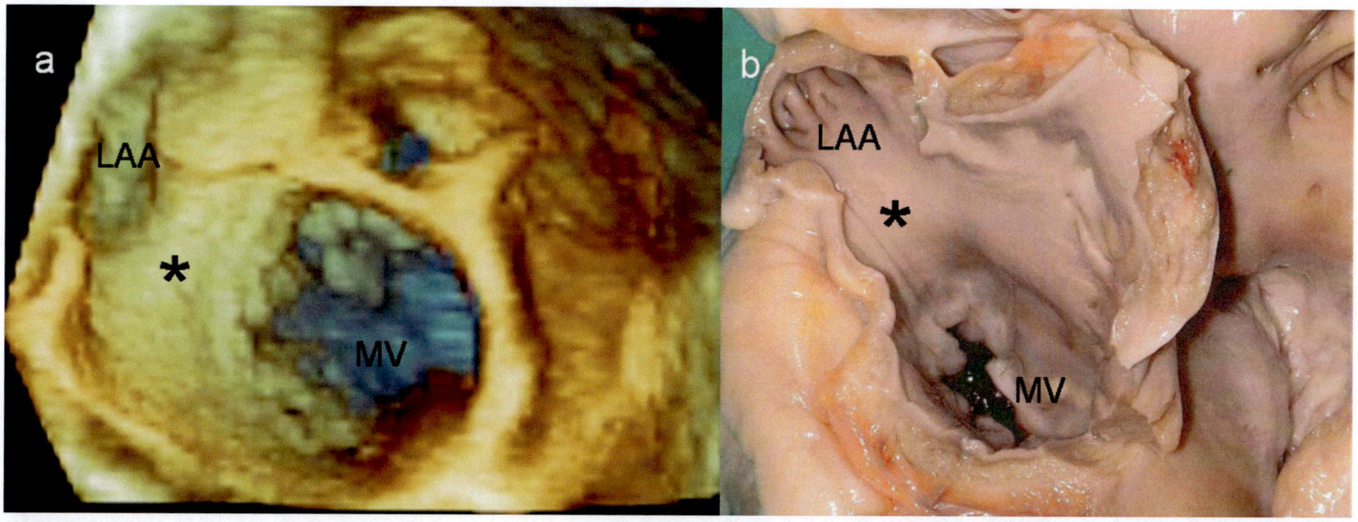

FIGURE 7.27 (a) Real-time 3D TEE in zoom modality from a slightly angulated atrial perspective showing the mitral valve (MV) and the left atrial appendage (LAA) and (b) the corresponding anatomical specimen. The *asterisk* marks the smooth atrial wall between the two structures.

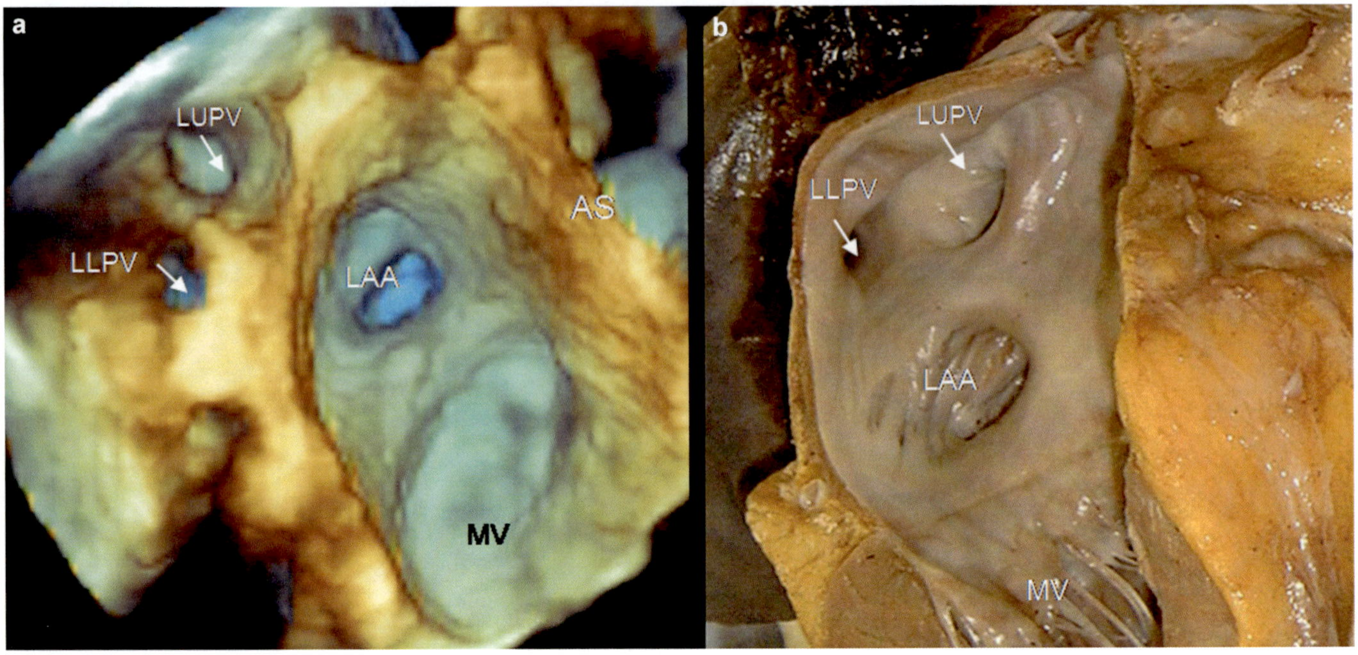

FIGURE 7.28 (a) Real-time 3D TEE showing both pulmonary veins and (b) the corresponding anatomical specimen. *LUPV* left upper pulmonary vein; *LLPV* Left lower pulmonary vein; *LAA* left atrial appendage; *MV* mitral valve; *AS* atrial septum.

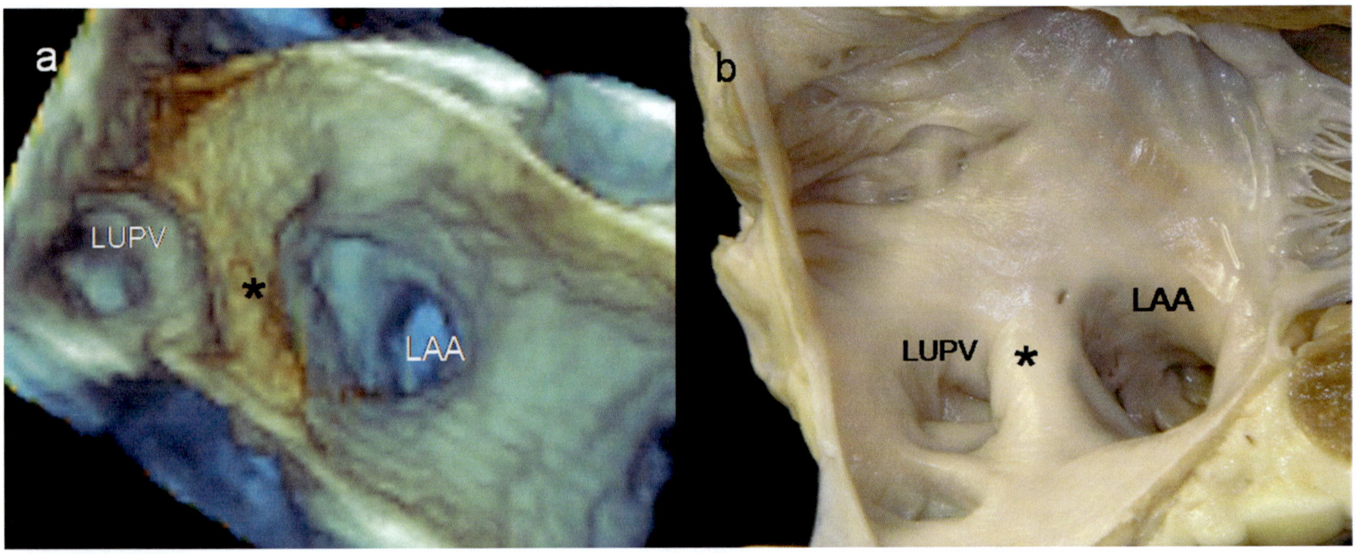

FIGURE 7.29 (a) Real-time 3D TEE in zoom modality showing the left atrial appendage (LAA) and left upper pulmonary vein (LUPV) from an overhead perspective. (b) A similar anatomical perspective. The *asterisk* marks the "ridge" between the ostium of the LAA and the LUPV.

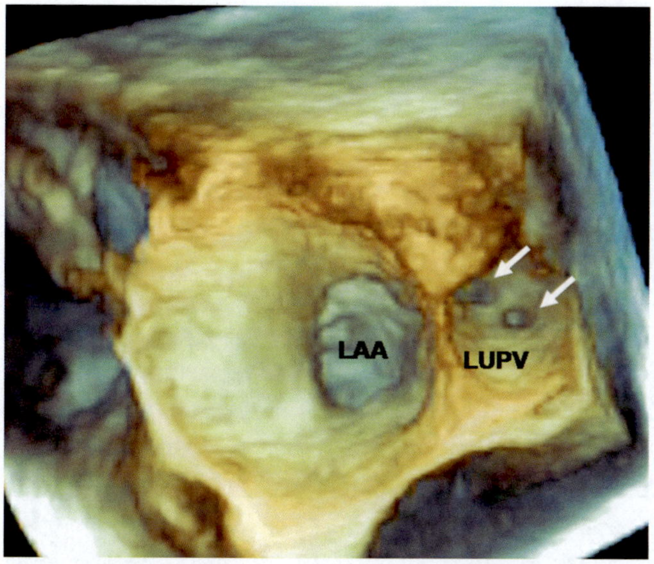

FIGURE 7.30 Real-time 3D TEE in zoom modality showing the left atrial appendage (LAA) and the left upper pulmonary vein (LUPV) from an overhead perspective. The confluence of two secondary branches into the LUPV can be seen (*arrows*). *LAA* left atrial appendage.

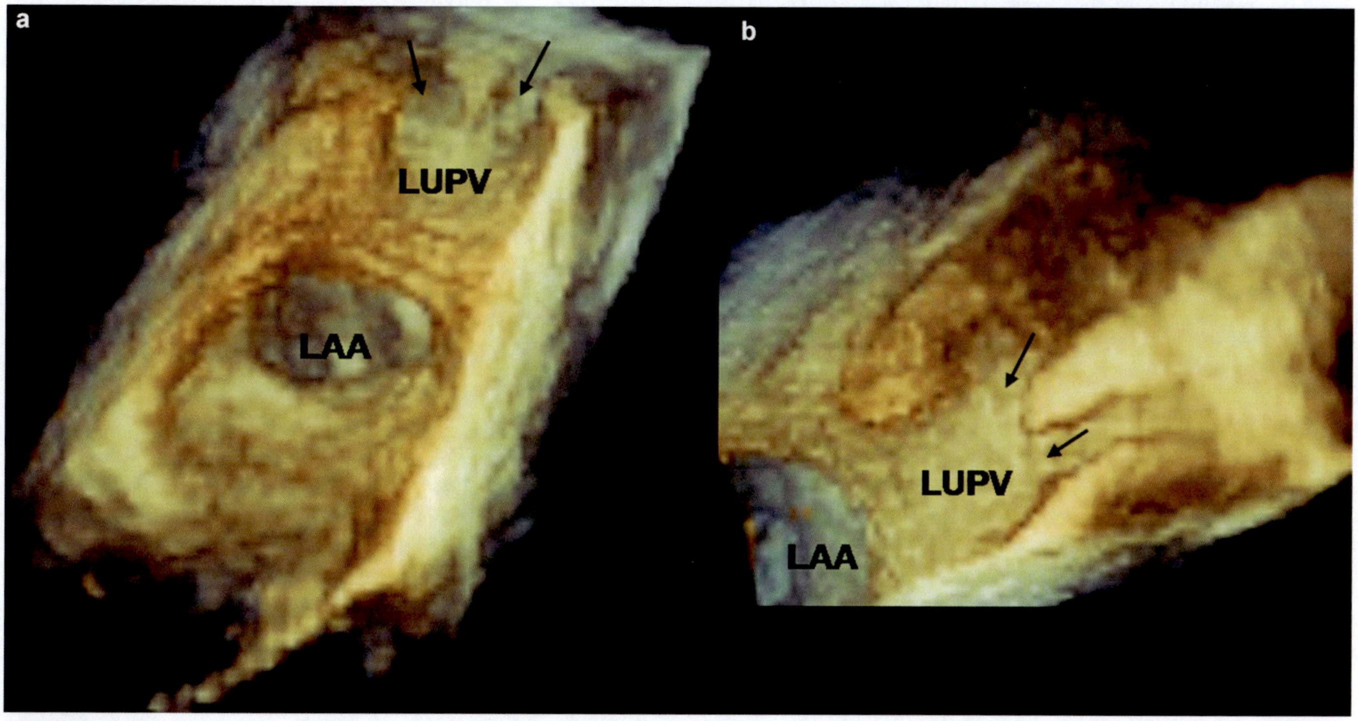

FIGURE 7.31 (a) Real-time 3D TEE in zoom modality showing the left atrial appendage (LAA) and the left upper pulmonary vein (LUPV) from an overhead perspective. (b) A lateral left-hand perspective after cropping the LUPV longitudinally. The *arrows* indicate the confluence ofb ranchesi ntot heL UPV.

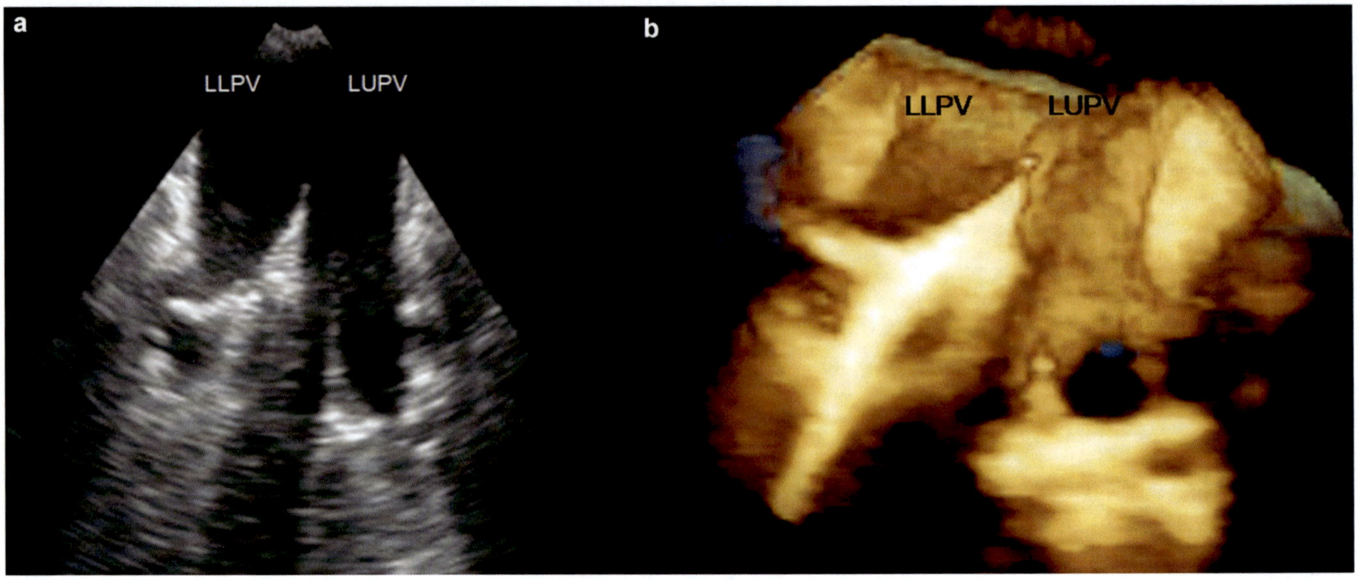

FIGURE 7.32 (a) 2D TEE and (b) real-time 3D TEE in zoom modality showing the left upper (LUPV) and the left lower (LLPV) pulmonary veins in the same longitudinal cut. Images in 2D TEE are obtained after having set the transducer at 100–120° and rotating the shaft to the patient's left side. Once 2D images of both veins have been obtained, live or zoom modality can display their 3D images. With 2D images the veins are better defined. The reason is that the third dimension makes the wall of veins somewhat less clear in 3D images than in 2D images.

Theoretically, with real-time 3D TEE we should be able to visualize all four pulmonary veins in one shot. However, the right and left pairs of veins are widely separated, and they lie very close to the transducer. At this transducer distance, the pyramidal beam is too narrow to visualize the entire roof of the left atrium including the pulmonary veins. Figure 7.37 shows a composite image of the four veins.

Not infrequently, there are variations such as a common vein on one side (Figs. 7.38 and 7.39) or bilaterally where the upper and lower veins combine before entering the atrium. There may also be accessory veins.

Quantitative accurate measurements of the pulmonary veins' ostia can be obtained by tracing the contour of the ostia as seen "en face" (Fig. 7.40).

7.3.1 Examples of Left Atrial Pathology

Thrombi may form anywhere in the right and left cardiac cavities. The LAA, however, with its complex pouch-like shape and presence of multiple lobes is by far the most vulnerable area. Any condition leading to blood stasis in the left atrium predisposes to thrombus formation in the LAA. Real-time 3D TEE appears to be an excellent tool for creating images of this structure of complex geometry and for detecting thrombi. The diagnosis of a thrombus with 2D TEE is based on the recognition of a mass with a characteristic texture (different shades of gray in comparison to the surrounding structures) often associated with spontaneous echo contrast. With real-time 3D TEE, shades of gray or variation of colors give us mostly the perception of depth rather than that of texture. As a result, a thrombus is detected as a mass with a texture similar to that of the surrounding structures which are located in the same z-plane Fig. (7.41). The advantages of real-time 3D TEE is that the shape of the thrombus is better defined and that the thrombus can be seen from any perspective (Figs. 7.42). 2D sections derived from 3D data can display some of the texture (Movies 7.6 and 7.7).

Atrial myxomas are the most common primary heart tumors accounting for 40–50% of all cardiac tumors. Approximately, 90% are solitary and pedunculated, and 75–85% occur in the left atrial cavity. Up to 25% of cases are found in the right atrium. Myxomas are polypoid, round, or oval. They are gelatinous with a smooth or lobulated surface and are usually white, yellowish, or brown. The most common point of attachment is at the border of the fossa ovalis in the left atrium, although myxomas can also originate from the posterior atrial wall, the anterior atrial wall, or the atrial appendage. The mobility of the tumor depends

MOVIES 7.6 and 7.7 Show a thrombus in left atrial appendage from two different perspectives.

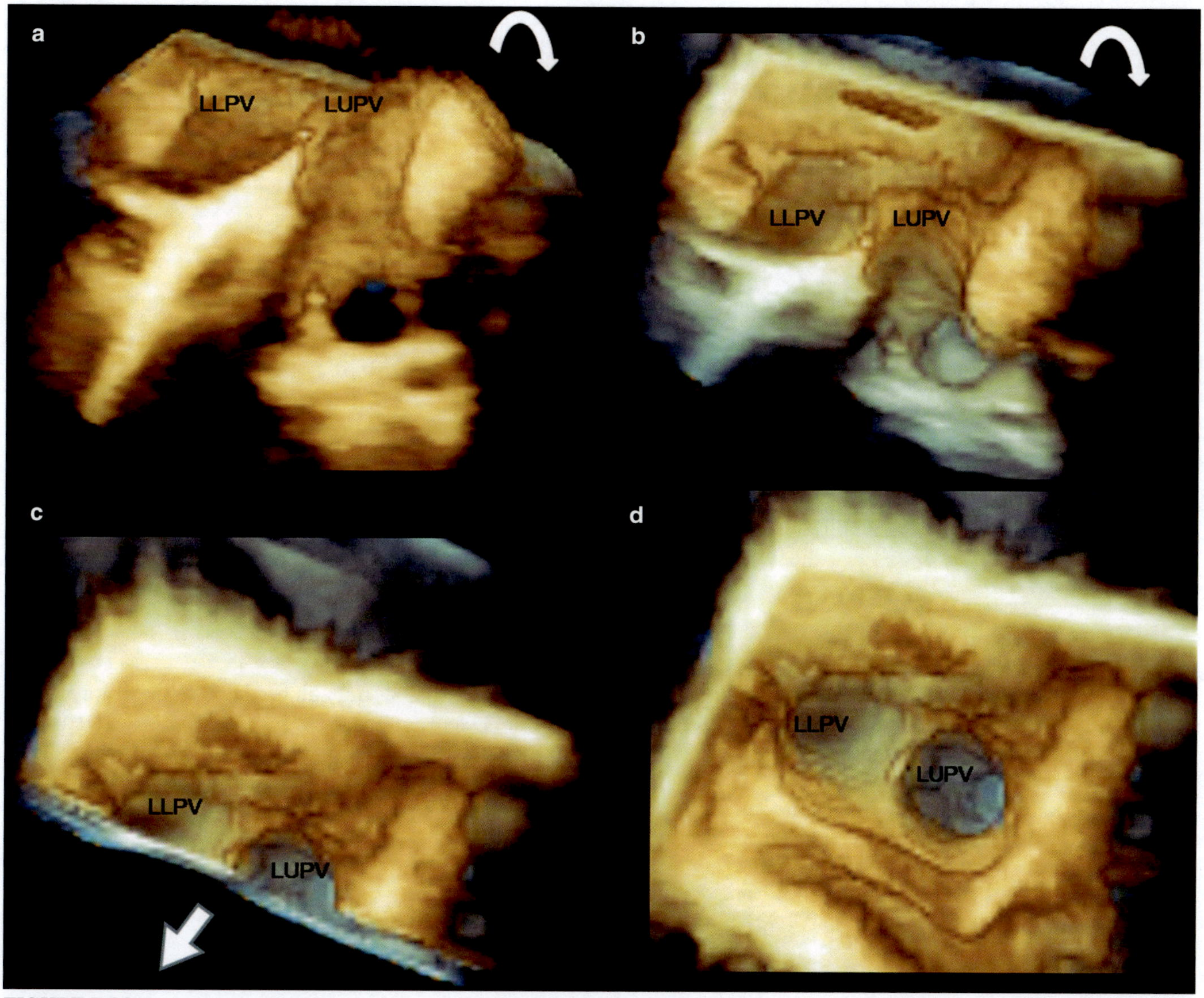

FIGURE 7.33 (a) Real-time 3D TEE in zoom modality showing a longitudinal cut of the left upper (LUPV) and the left lower (LLPV) pulmonary veins. (b-d) The rotations (*curved arrows*) and expansion of the image (*straight arrow*) lead to a progressive disclosure of the orifices ofb othv einsi n “enf ace”p erspective.

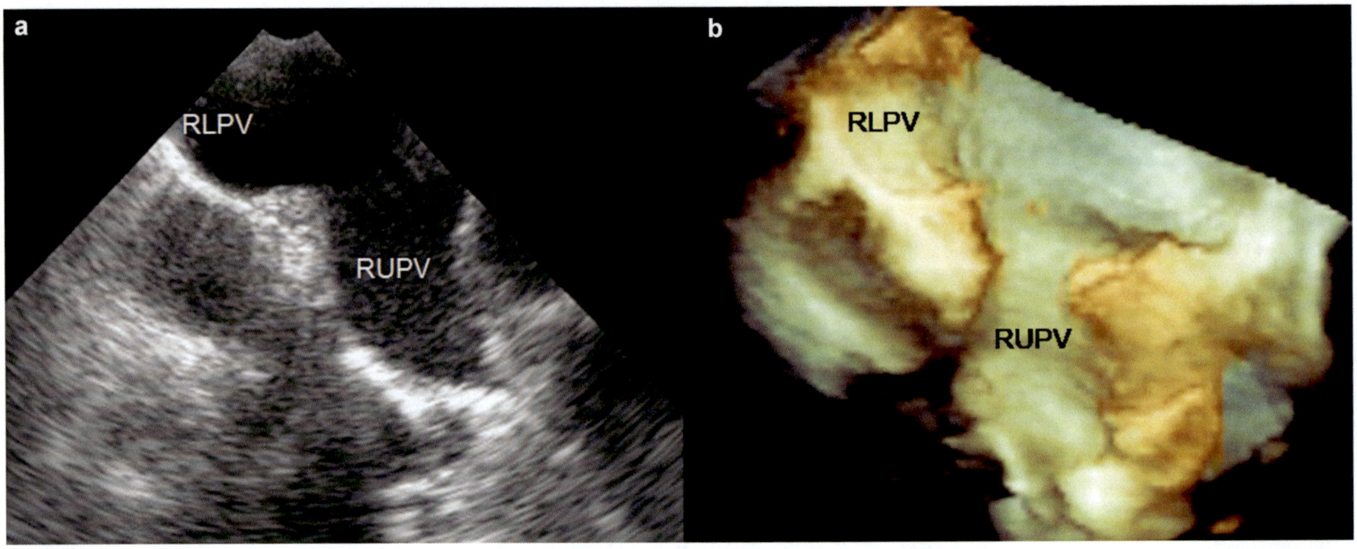

FIGURE 7.34 (a) 2D TEE and (b) real-time 3D TEE in zoom modality showing the right upper (RUPV) and the right lower (RLPV) pulmonary veins in the same longitudinal cut. Images on 2D TEE are obtained after having set the transducer at 60–80° and rotating the shaft to the patient's right-hand side. Once again, the 2D image appears clearer.

upon the extent of its attachment to the interatrial septum and the length of the stalk. Symptoms are produced by mechanical interference with cardiac function or embolization. Being intravascular and friable, myxomas account for most cases of tumor embolism. Embolism occurs in about 30–40% of patients. The site of the embolism is dependent upon the location (left or right atrium) and the presence of an intracardiac shunt. Two-dimensional echocardiography is the diagnostic procedure of choice (Fig. 7.43).

RT 3D TEE does not add further relevant information with the exception of a more precise location in respect of the atrial cavity and an "overall view" (Fig. 7.44 and Movie 7.8). Once diagnosed, atrial myxoma must be surgically removed.

MOVIE 7.8 The clip shows a large left atrial myxoma attached to anterior atrial wall viewed from above.

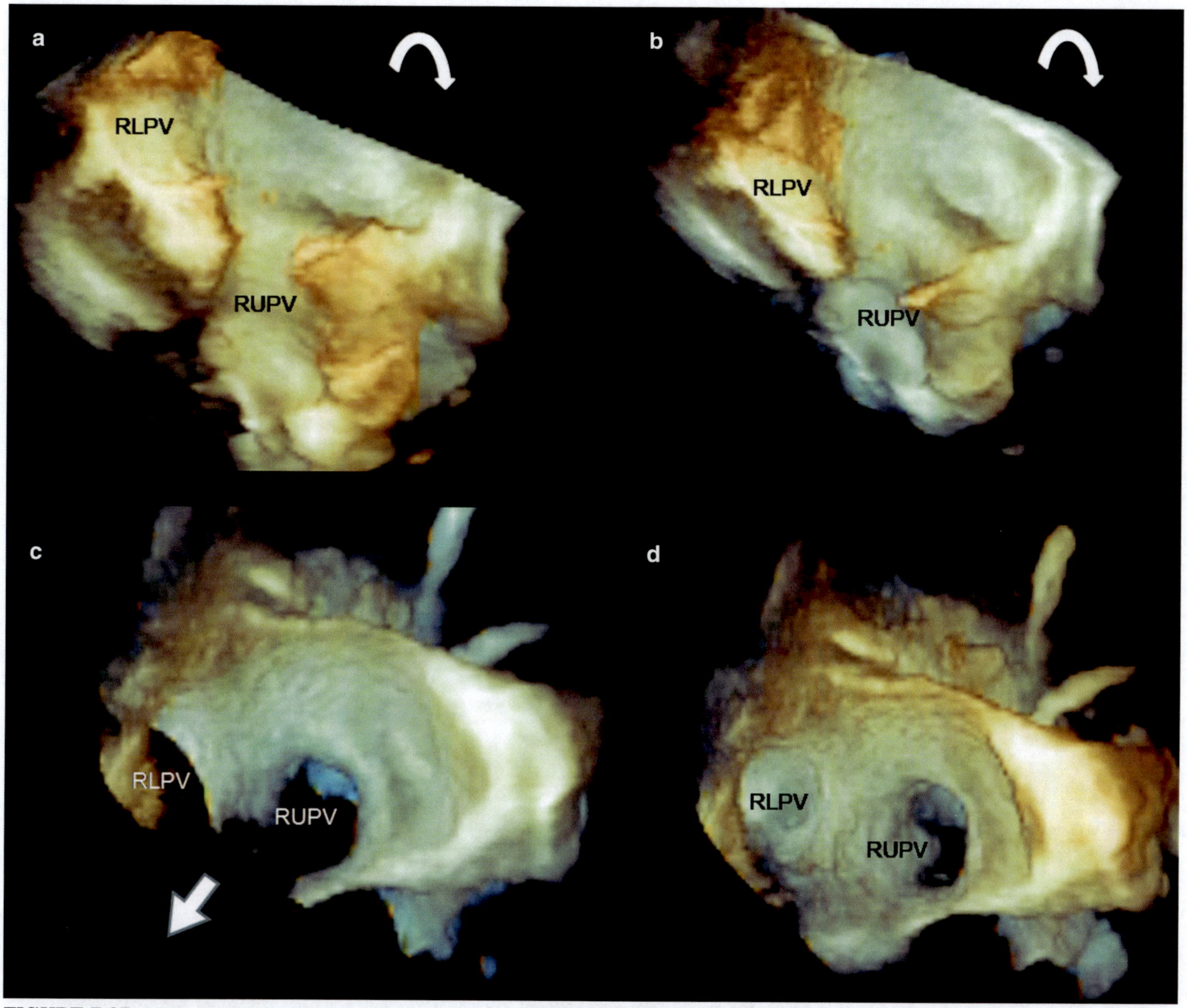

FIGURE 7.35 (a) Real-time 3D TEE in zoom modality showing a longitudinal cut of the right upper (RUPV) and the right lower (RLPV) pulmonary veins. (b-d) Progressive rotations (*curved arrows*) and the expansion of the image (*straight arrow*) lead to the progressive appearance of the orificeo fb othv einsi n "enf ace" perspective.

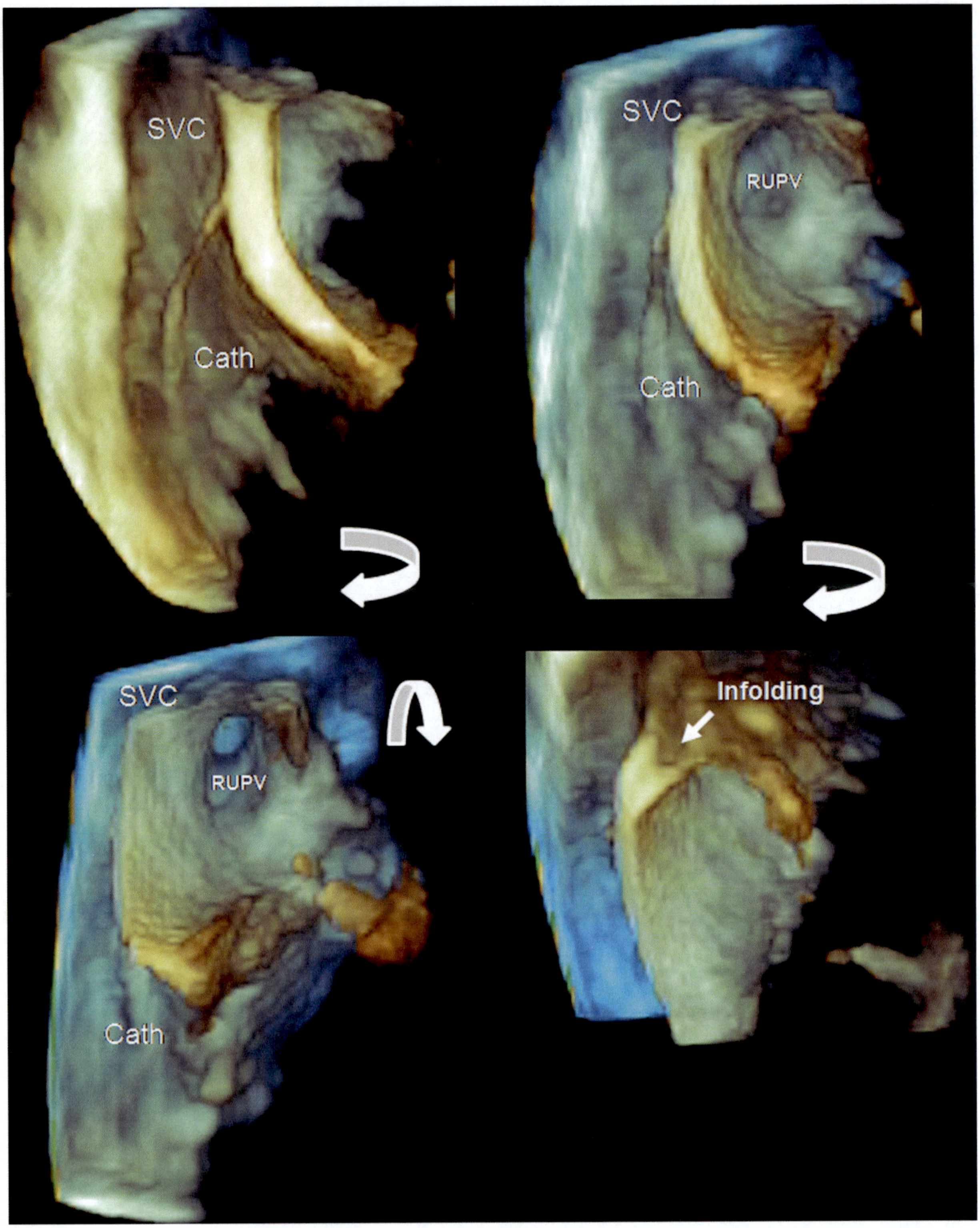

FIGURE 7.36 Real-time 3D TEE in zoom modality showing the relationship between the superior vena cava (SVC) and right upper pulmonary vein (RUPV). A long axis view of the SVC imaged in a patient undergoing cavo-tricuspid isthmus ablation for a typical atrial flutter. By a progressive counterclockwise rotation of the image (*curved arrows*) the right upper pulmonary vein is revealed. An up-down angulation (*curved arrow*) shows the enfolding (*small straight arrow*) forming the *septum secundum* which separates the SVC from the RUPV. *Cath* catheter.

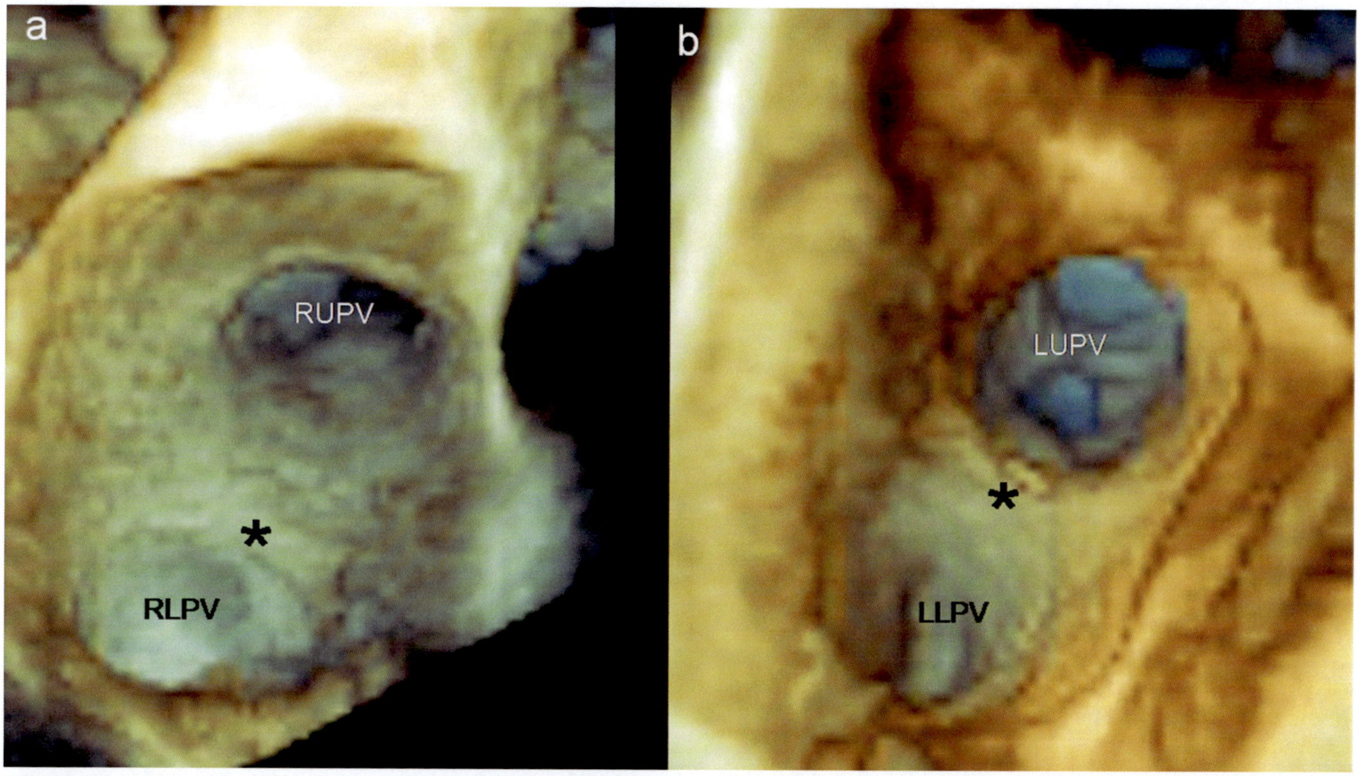

FIGURE 7.37 Real-time 3D TEE in zoom modality showing both pairs of pulmonary veins (a, b). The *asterisks* mark the carina (or ridge) between the orifices of upper and lower veins. The narrow pyramidal beam does not allow all four pulmonary veins to be included in one image (see text). *RUPV* right upper pulmonary vein; *RLPV* right lower pulmonary vein; *LUPV* left upper pulmonary vein; *LLPV* left lower pulmonaryv ein.

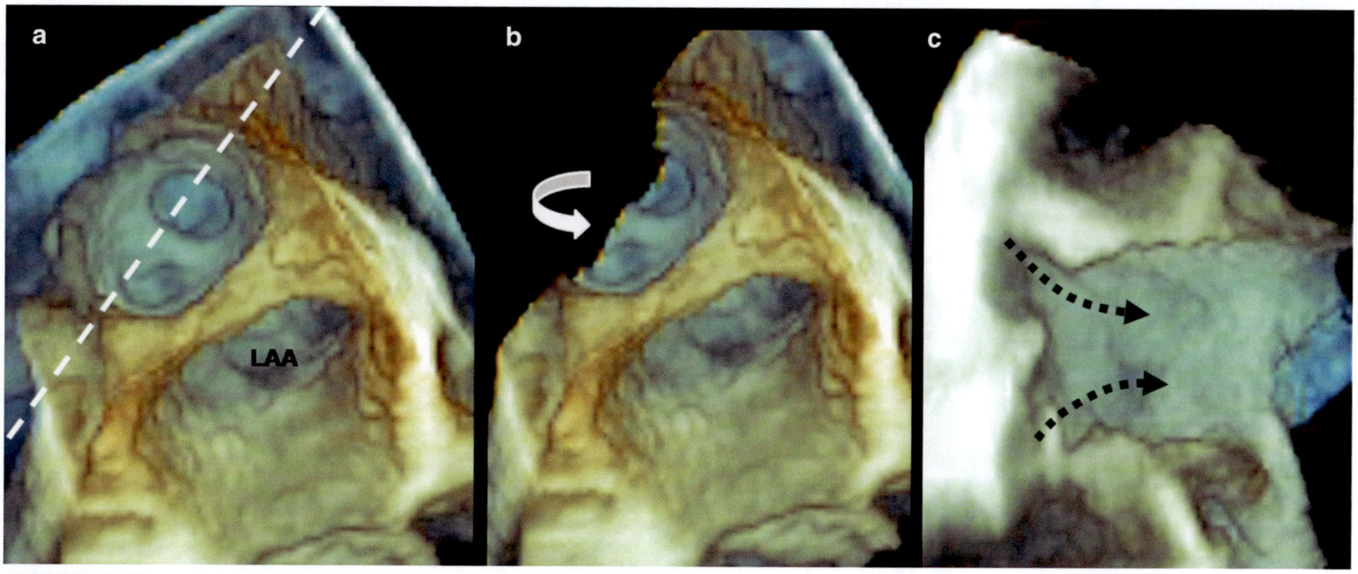

FIGURE 7.38 Real-time 3D TEE in zoom modality showing a common left vein ostium opening in the left atrial cavity. (a) The vein is seen "en face" with the *dotted line* marking the cutting plane. (b) The *curved arrow* indicates the rotation of the image to show in (c) the common vein from its long axis viewpoint. The *black dotted arrows* indicate the confluence of two veins. *LAA* left atrial appendage.

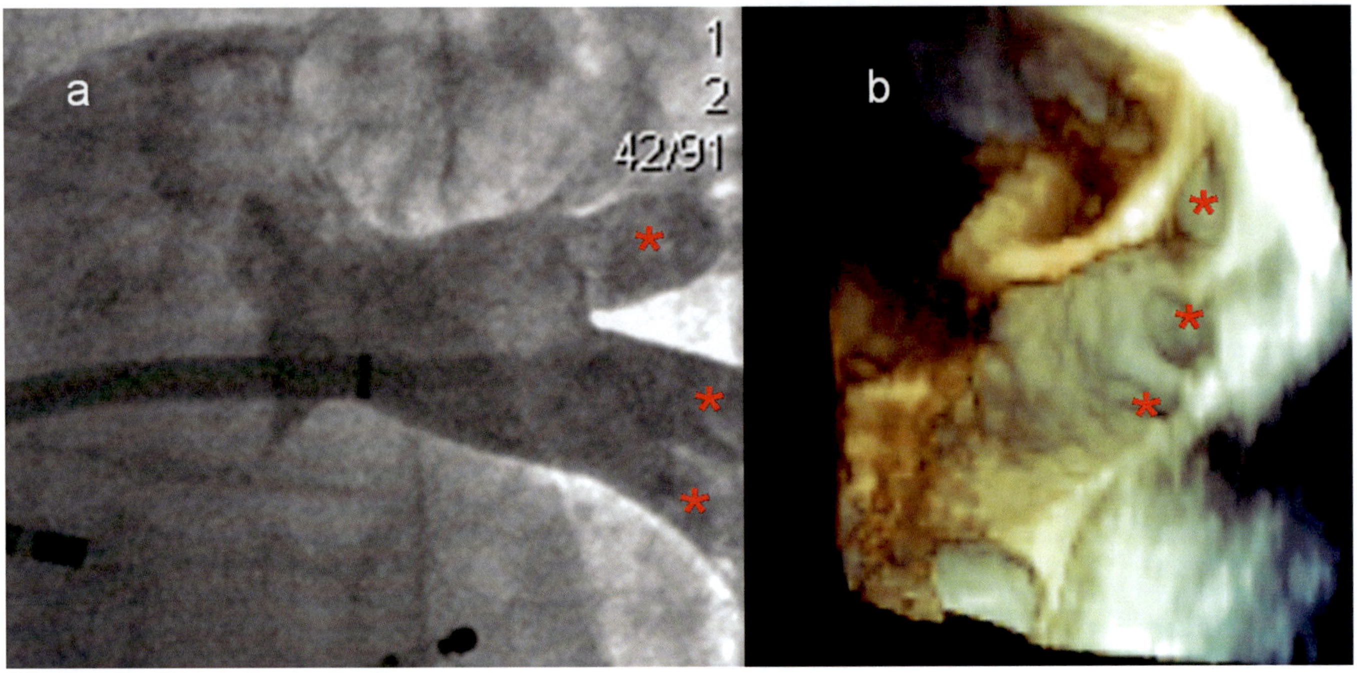

FIGURE 7.39 (a) Angiographic and (b) RT 3D TEE images of the single pulmonary vein shown in Fig. 7.38. The vein is formed by the confluence of three branches (indicated by *asterisks*).

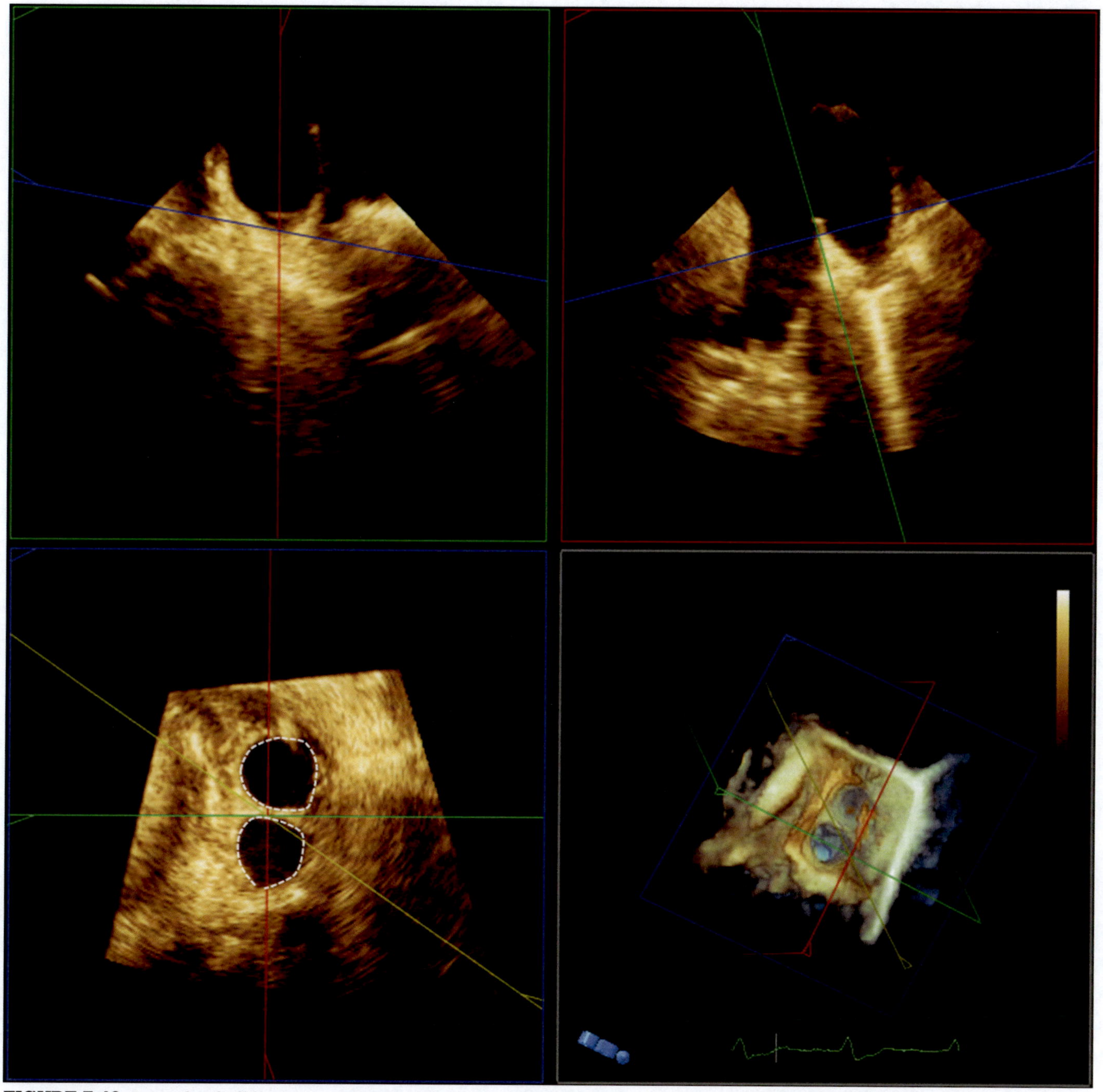

FIGURE 7.40 Example of off-line measurements of the ostia of the left pulmonary veins using a dedicated software.

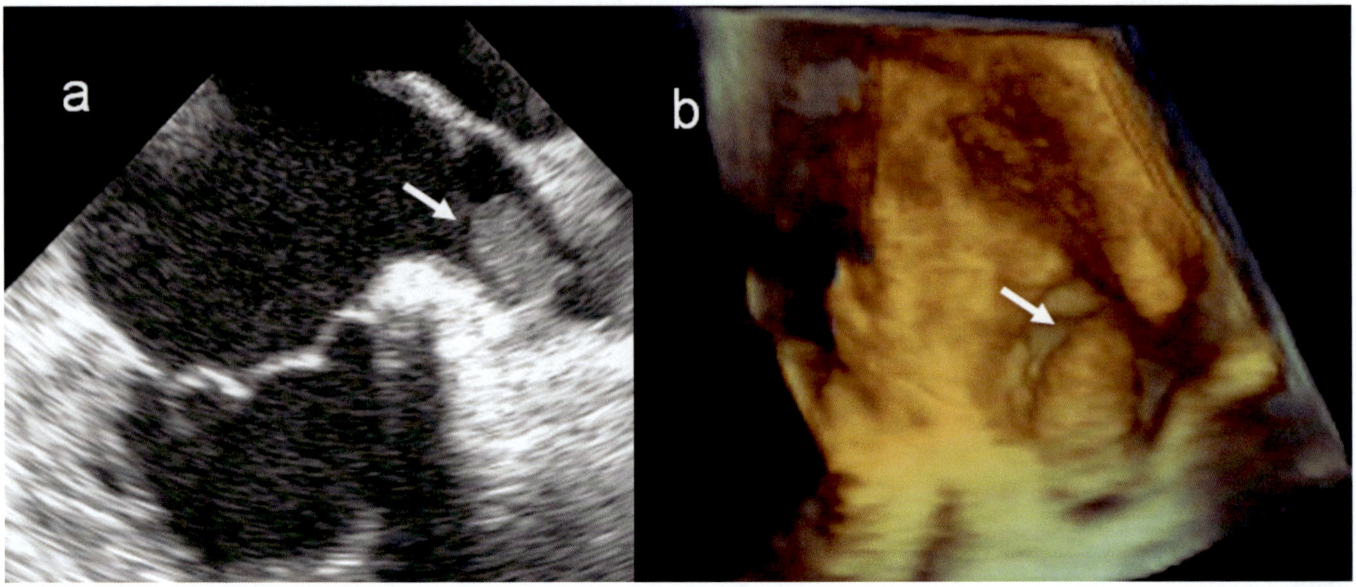

FIGURE 7.41 (a) 2D TEE and (b) real-time 3D TEE showing a large thrombus in the left atrial appendage (*arrow*). While the different texture helps in the recognition of the mass as a thrombus in the 2D image, in real-time 3D TEE projections, the variations of color are helpful to characterize better the shape of the mass and its position on the z-plane rather than its texture. In 3D images, the texture of the thrombus is similar to the wall of the appendage.

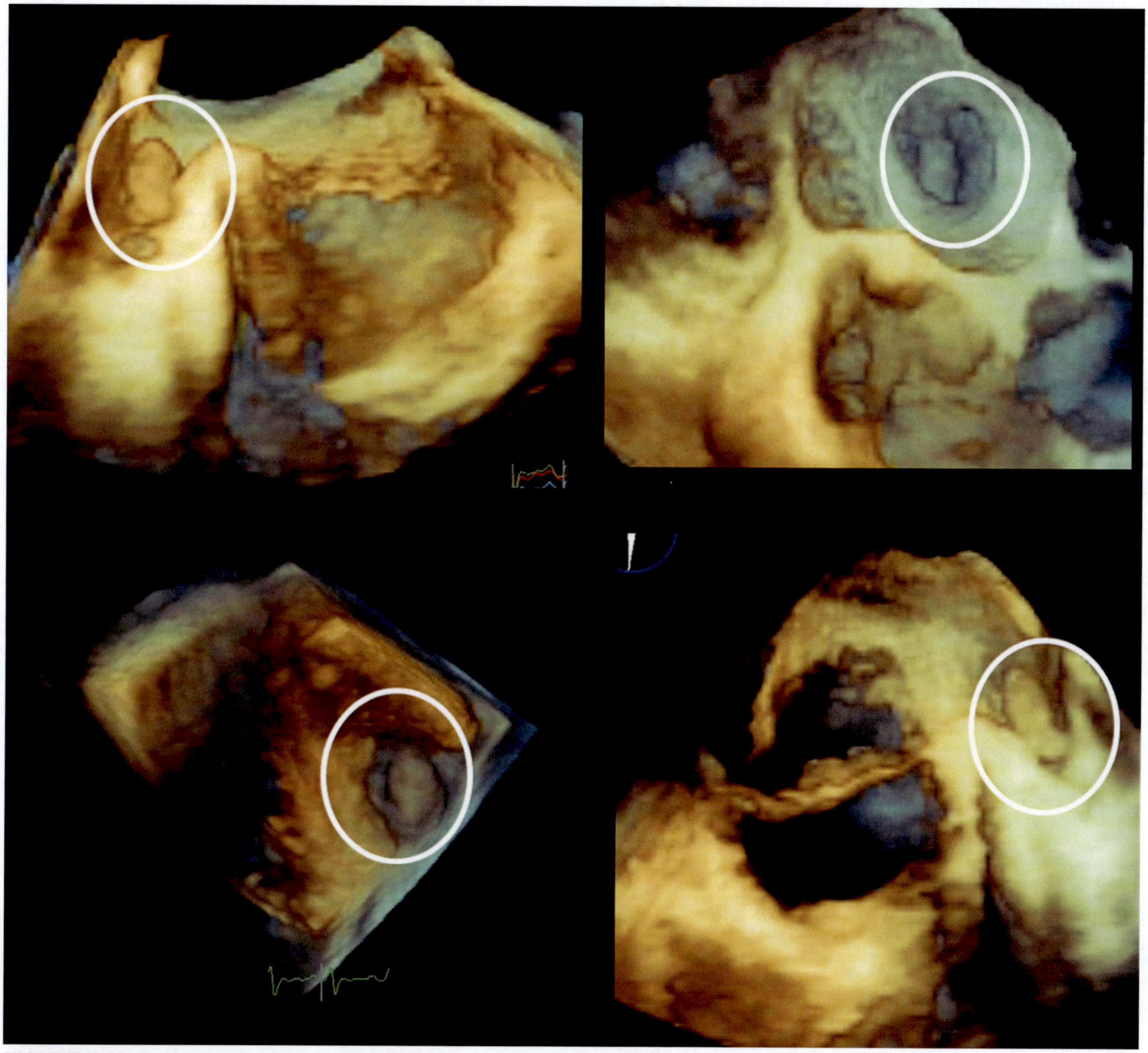

FIGURE 7.42 3D TEE in full volume modality displaying a thrombus from different perspectives (*circle*).

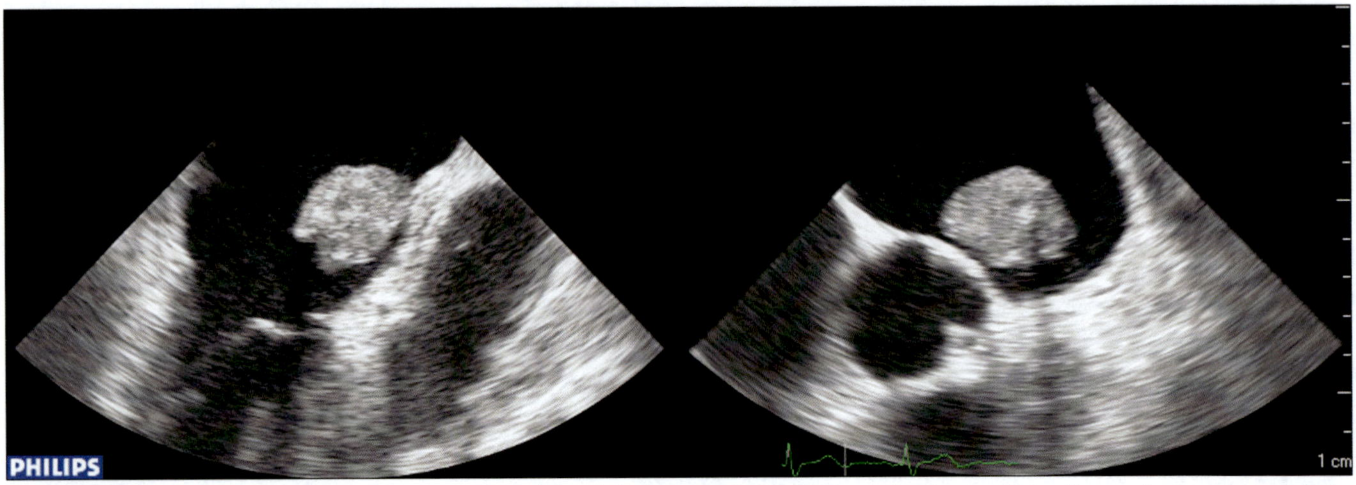

FIGURE 7.43 Conventional 2D TEE showing a classic left atrial myxoma. The 2D TEE examination is still the diagnostic procedure of choice for the diagnosis and for characterization of the size, shape, site and texture of the tumor.

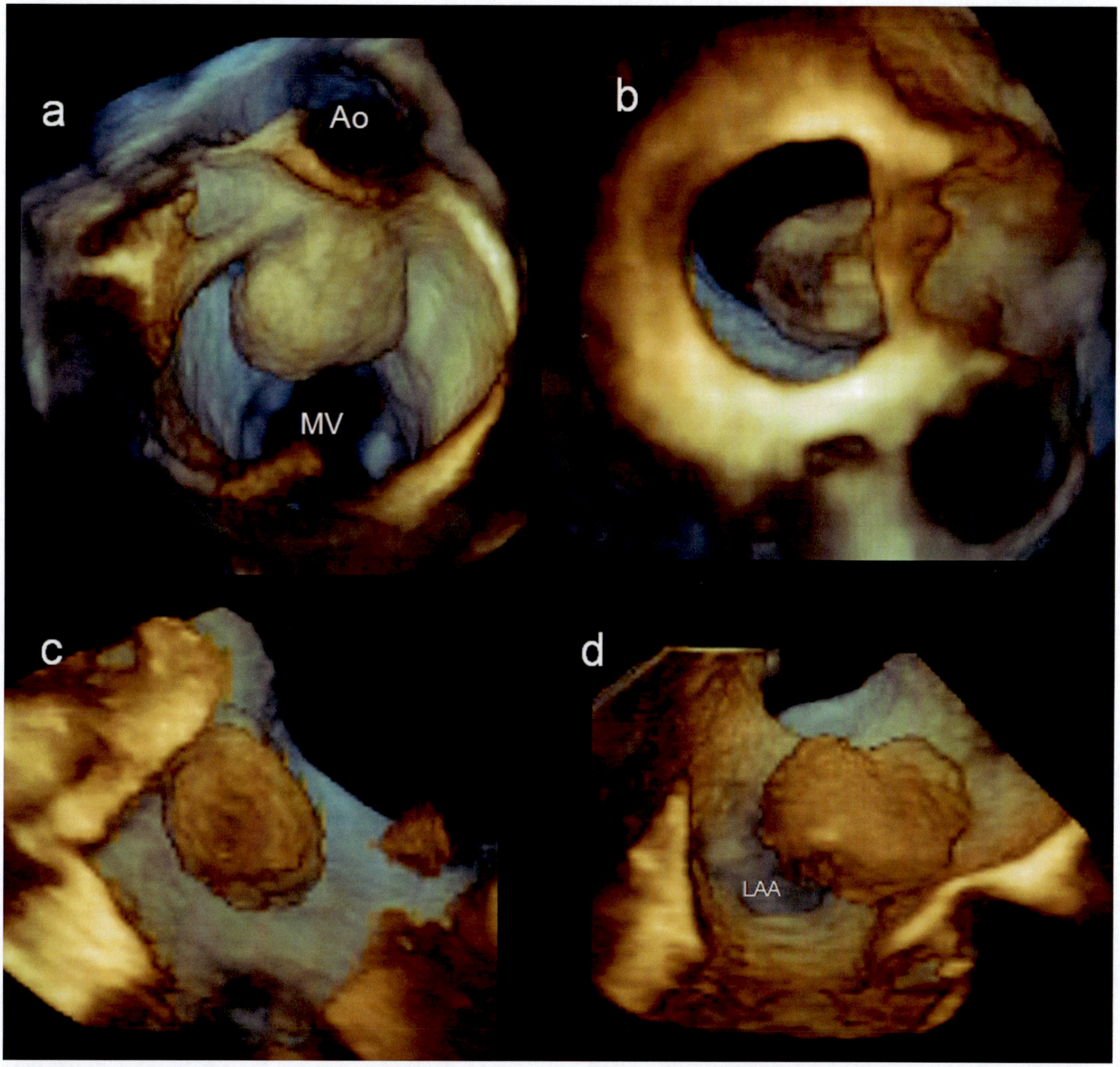

FIGURE 7.44 RT 3D TEE in zoom modality showing the atrial myxoma in the same patient as in Fig. 7.43. The myxoma can be seen from different perspectives: (a) above, (b) below, (c) antero-lateral and (d) posteromedial. With its vision of "overall view," RT 3D TEE offers a better understanding of the relationship with the surrounding structures, such as the aorta (Ao), and the left atrial appendage (LAA). *MV* mitral valve.

CHAPTER8

TheR ight Ventricle

The right ventricle is the most anteriorly situated cardiac chamber, lying directly behind the sternum. It "wraps around" the left ventricle (Fig. 8.1). The internal appearance of the right ventricle is typical. The shape of the cavity can be imaged as an open "V" with a wide muscular separation between the tricuspid and the pulmonic valves(Fig. 8.2).

The right ventricle can be divided into three portions: the inlet, the apical, and the outlet components (Fig. 8.3). The most constant characteristic feature of the right ventricle is the presence of coarse apical trabeculations in contrast to the fine trabeculations found in the left ventricle (Fig. 8.4). From the transgastric TEE view, the apex of the right ventricle is closer to the transducer than from the midesophagus, and even the finest trabeculations can sometimesbea ppreciated (Fig. 8.5).

The right ventricle is characterized by the presence of other structures such as the crista supraventricularis, the trabecula septomarginalis, and the moderator band.

The *crista supraventricularis* is the prominent muscular structure that separates the inlet (tricuspid valve) from the outlet (pulmonic valve) (Fig. 8.6).

The trabecula septomarginalis is a Y-shaped muscle band that appears like a column holding the ventriculo-infundibular fold in its arms (Figs. 8.7 and 8.8). The posterior arm points toward the tricuspid valve and the membranous septum. Usually, but not always, the body of the Y adheres to the septum, and in cross-sectional imaging, it can appear as a bump on the septum. When abnormally formed or hypertrophied, it can serve to divide the ventricular cavity into two chambers. The body of the trabecula septomarginalis ends near the apex, splitting into several smaller muscle bundles. One of these usually takes a characteristic course crossing the right ventricular cavity. This branch has been named the moderator band because it was thought, wrongly, to limit the diastolic expansion of the chamber (Fig. 8.9).

The moderator band extends toward the anterior wall and joins the base of the anterior papillary muscle (Figs. 8.10 and 8.11).

The outlet portion of the right ventricle consists of the infundibulum, a circumferential muscular structure that supports the leaflets of the pulmonic valve (Figs. 8.12 and 8.13).

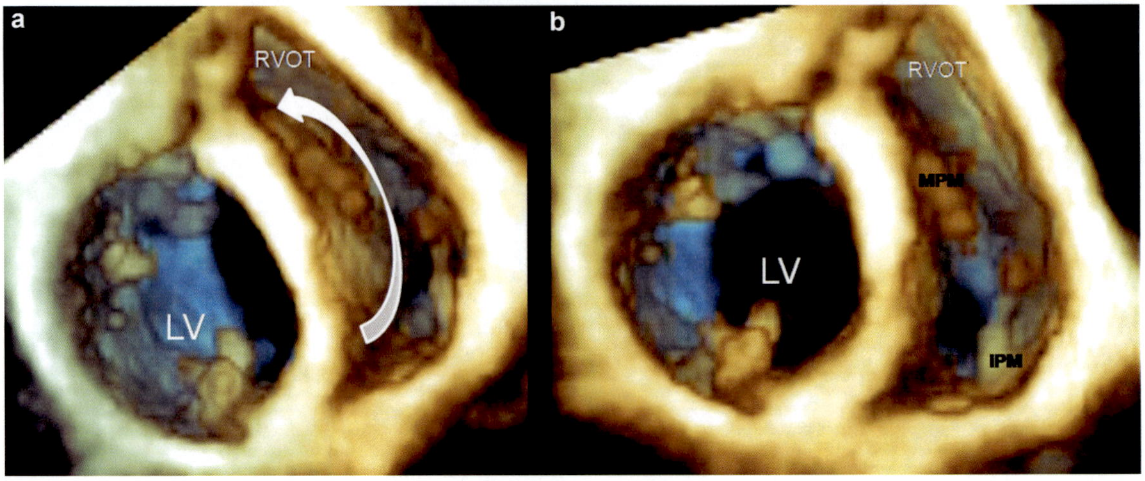

FIGURE 8.1 3D TEE images in full volume modality after cropping the ventricles along a midventricular transverse plane at two different levels. Views from the atrial perspective shows the right ventricle wrapping around (*curved arrow*) the left ventricle (LV). The inferior (IPM) and medial (MPM) papillary muscles can be imaged. *RVOT* right ventricle outflow tract.

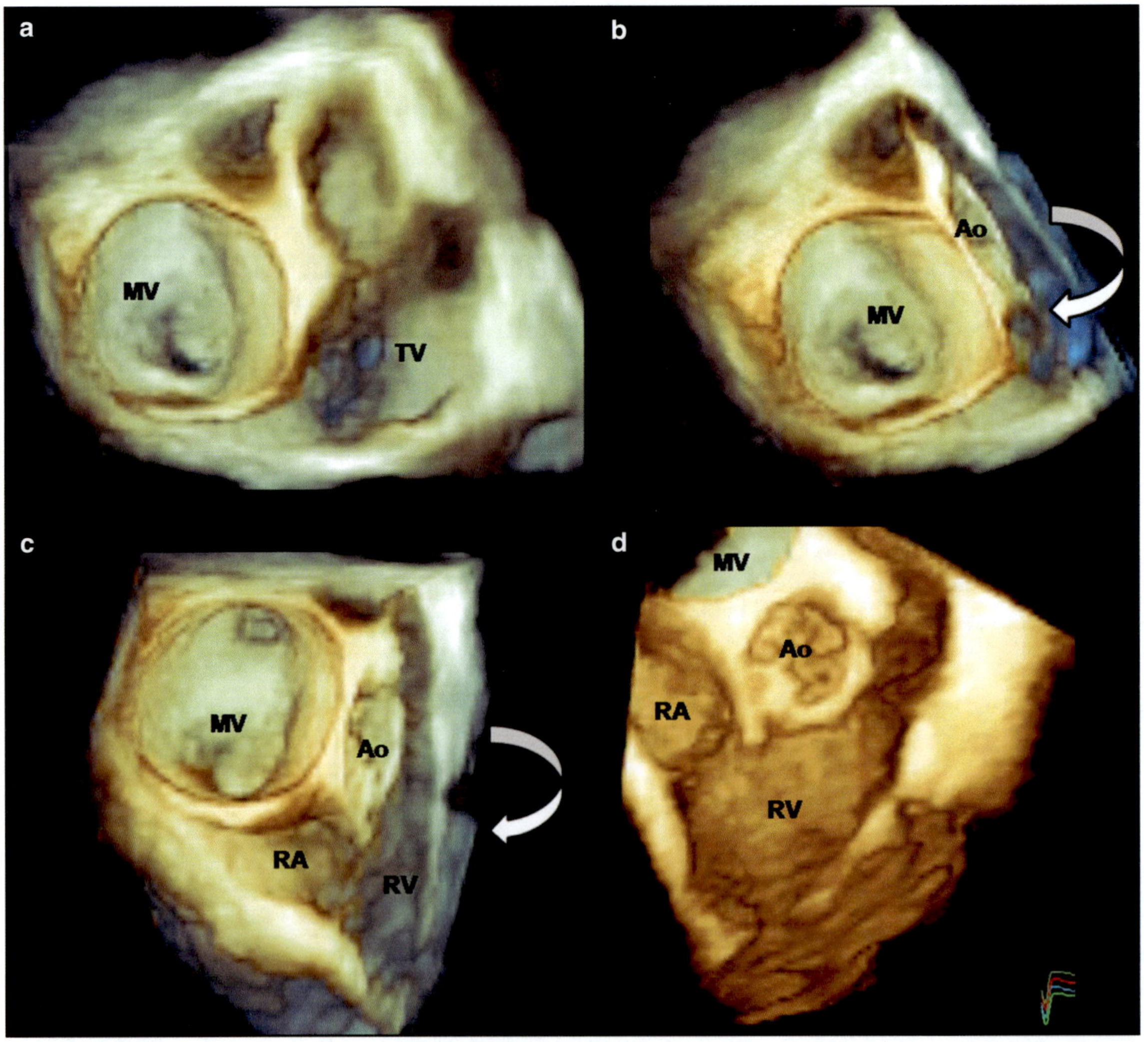

FIGURE 8.2 3D TEE in full volume modality. A four step approach to visualize the right ventricle: (a) the base of the heart is seen from the atrial perspective; (b) an oblique cut plane is made in the antero-lateral right ventricular wall; *curved arrows* in (b, c) indicate the direction of the progressive rotations leading to the image in (d). *MV* mitral valve; *TV* tricuspid valve; *Ao* aorta; *RA* right atrium; *RV* right ventricle.

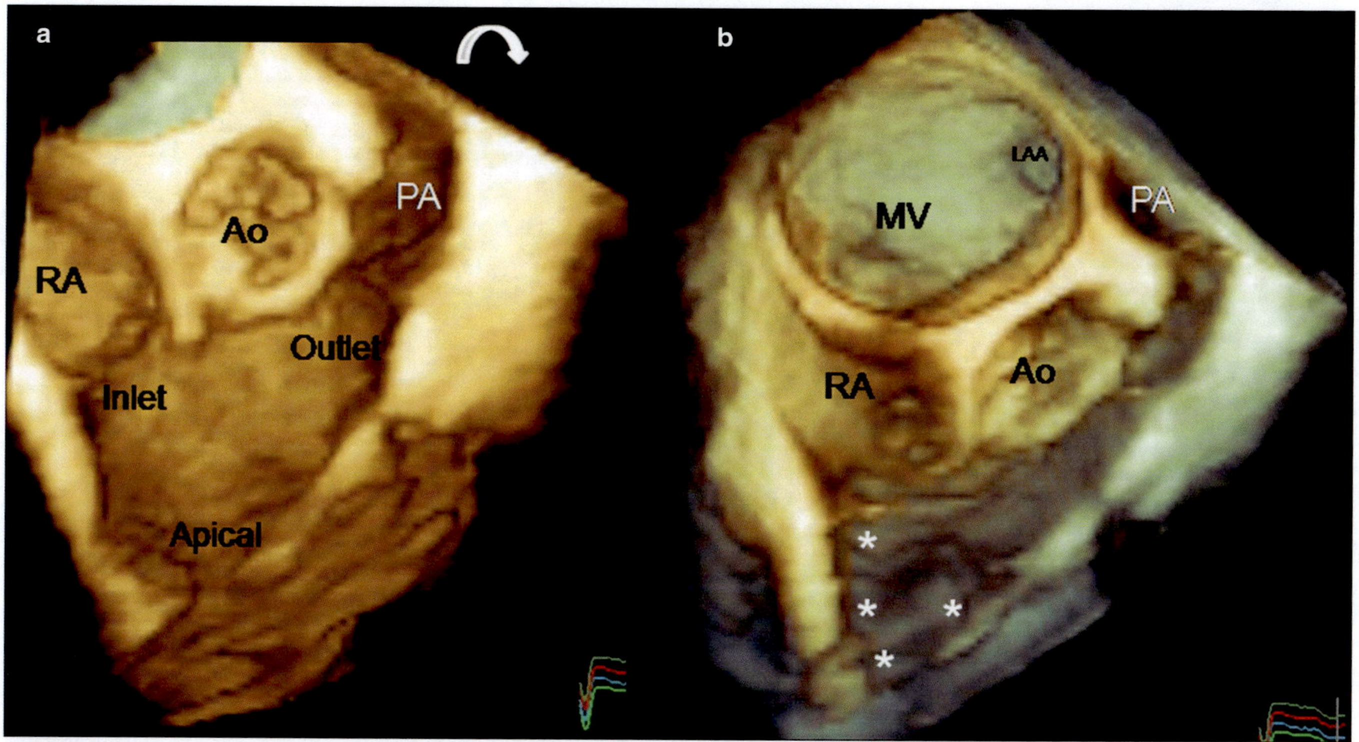

FIGURE 8.3 3D TEE image in full volume modality after cropping the antero-lateral wall of the right ventricle (see Fig. 8.2) showing (a) the "en face" septal surface of the right ventricle. Based on their location, the three portions can be distinguished: the inlet, the apical, and the outlet component; (b) a slight angulation enables the visualization of the coarse trabeculations typical of the right cavity (*asterisks*). The fine balance of gain (in order to separate structures from the noise) and the distance of the apex from the transducer do not allow precise imaging of the trabeculations. *Ao* aorta; *RA* right atrium; *PA* pulmonary artery; *MV* mitral valve; *LAA* left atrial appendage.

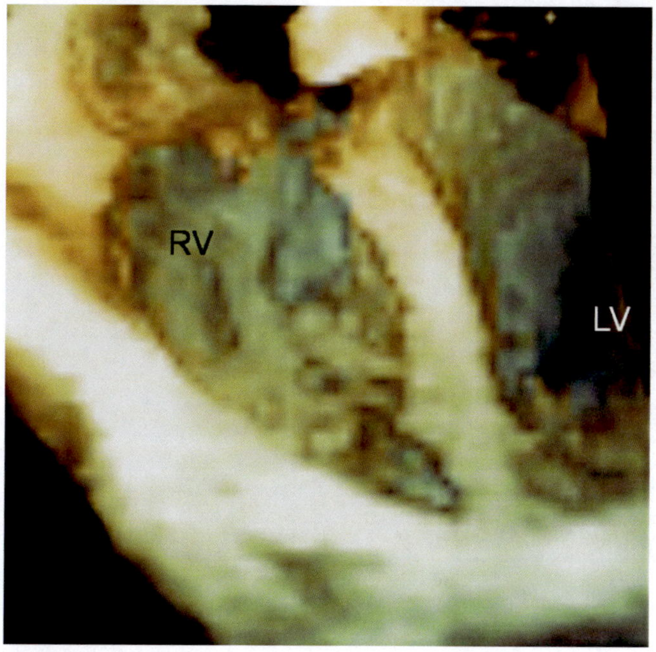

FIGURE 8.4 3D TEE image in full volume modality after cropping the left lateral margin of the heart. From this perspective, the trabeculations are clearly visible. *RV* right ventricle; *LV* left ventricle.

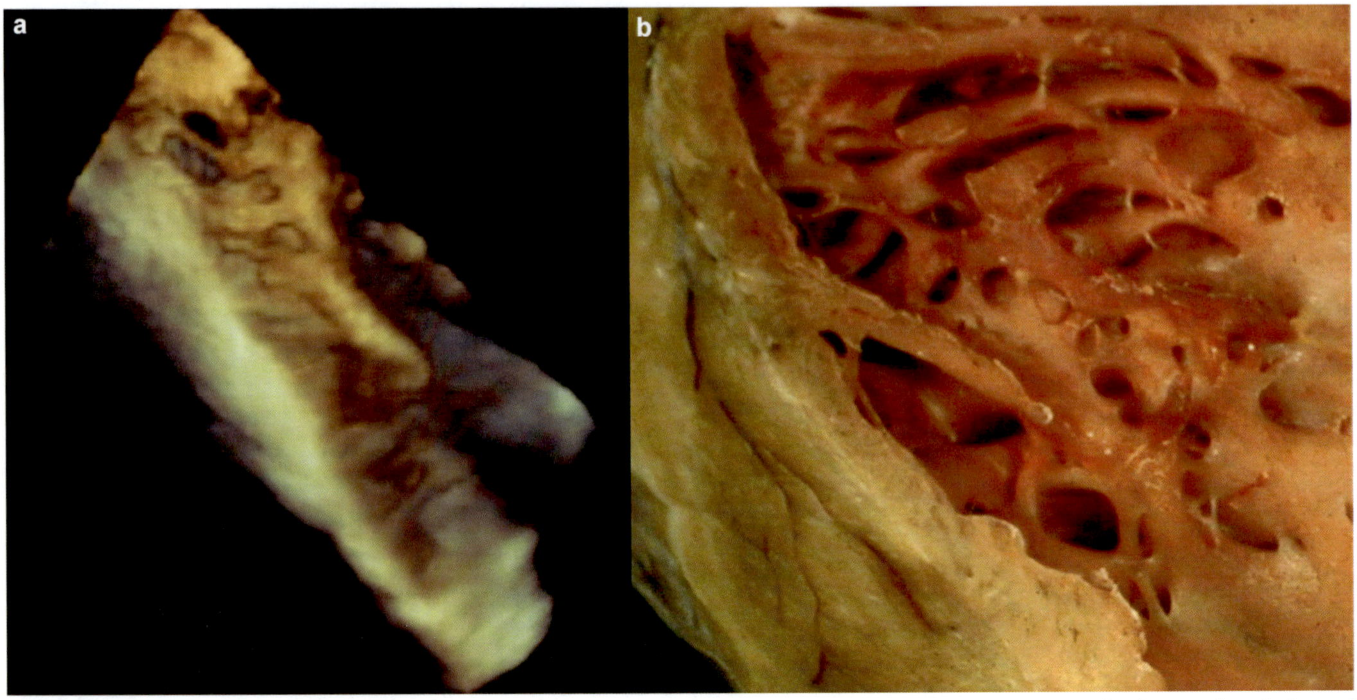

FIGURE 8.5 (a) Real-time 3D TEE image in live modality from the transgastric longitudinal view showing even the finest trabeculations of the right ventricle; (b) a corresponding anatomical specimen.

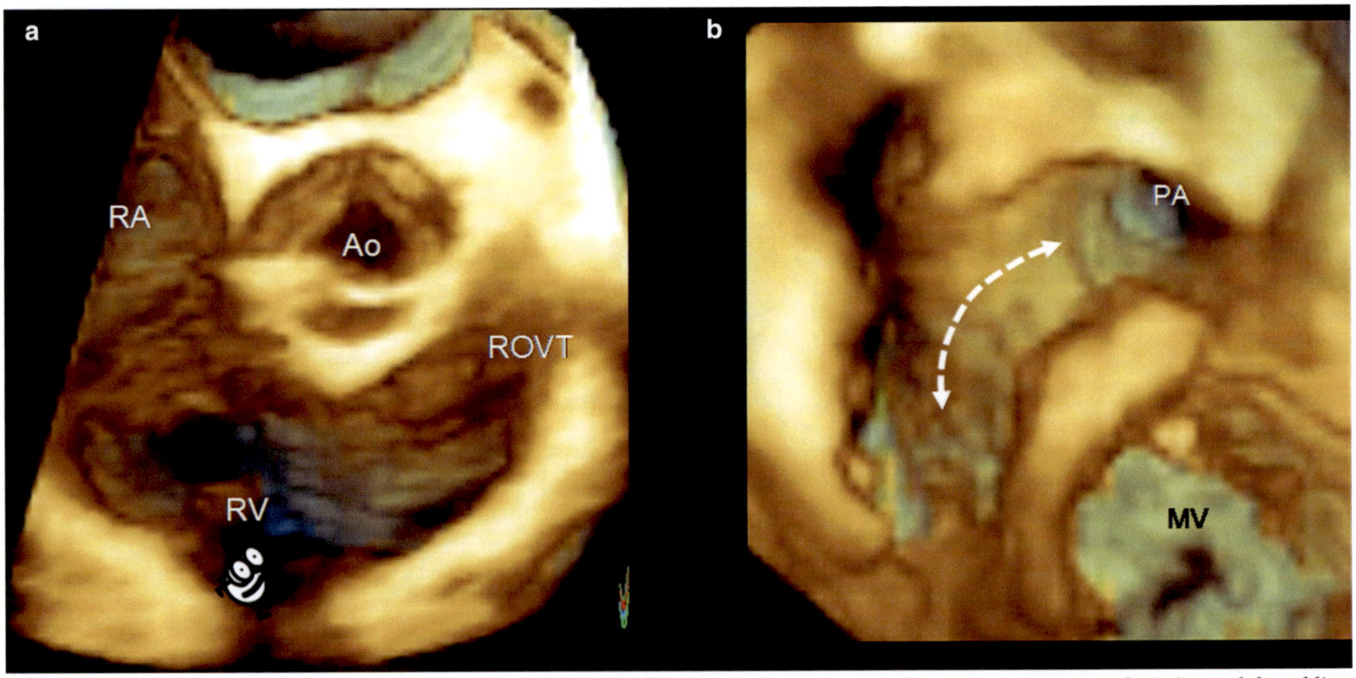

FIGURE 8.6 (a) 3D TEE images as viewed from the RV apex (a), displaying the crista (b). The crista supraventricularis (*curved dotted line; see also chap.2*) *RA* right atrium; *Ao* aorta; *RVOT* right ventricular outflow tract; *RV* right ventricle; *MV* mitral valve; *PA* pulmonary artery.

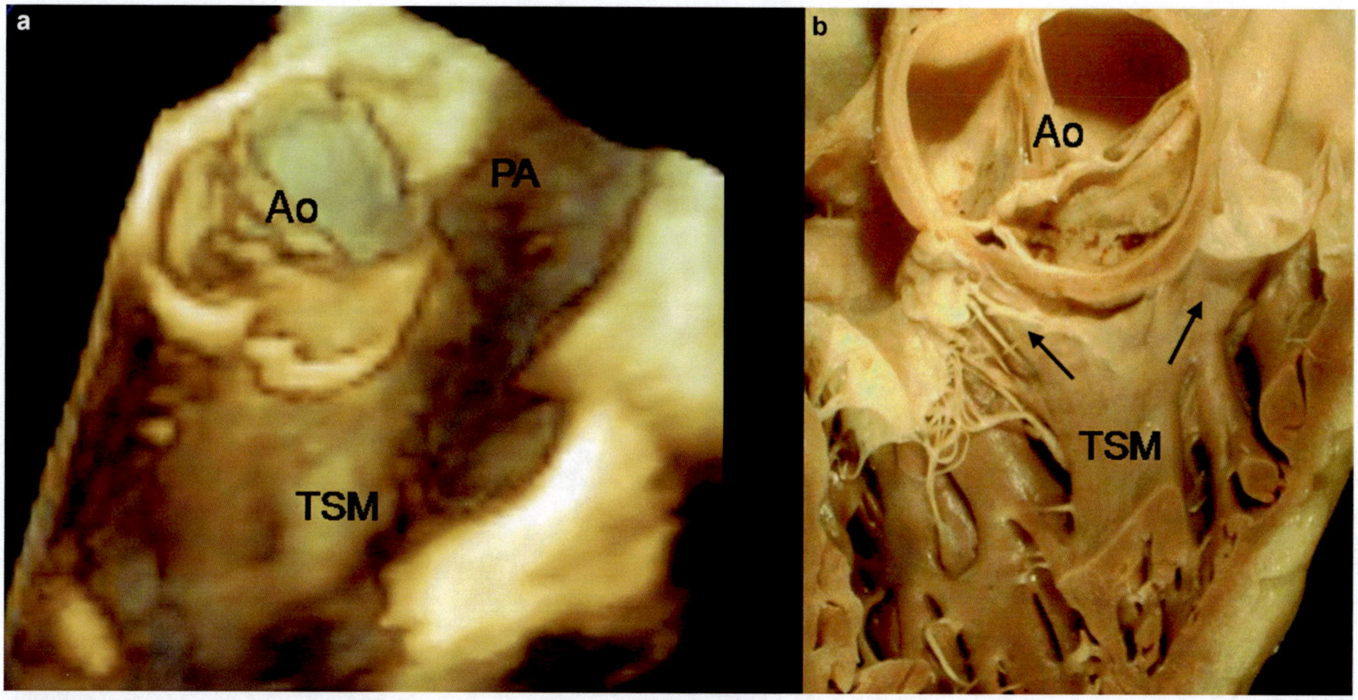

FIGURE 8.7 (a) 3D TEE image in full volume modality. The trabecula septomarginalis (TMS) may appear after cropping the anterior wall of the right ventricle. However, in most cases the trabecula is not distinguishable; (b) a corresponding anatomical specimen. The "arms" (*arrows*) of the TMS are better seen in the specimen than in the 3D RT TEE images. *PA* pulmonary artery; *Ao* aorta.

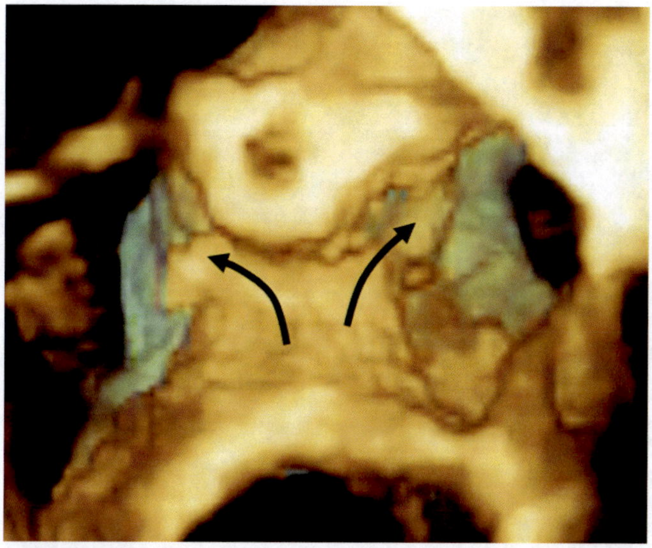

FIGURE 8.8 3D TEE image in full volume modality after cropping most of the anterior wall of the right ventricle. The trabecula septomarginalis and its arms (*curved arrows*)c an be appreciated.

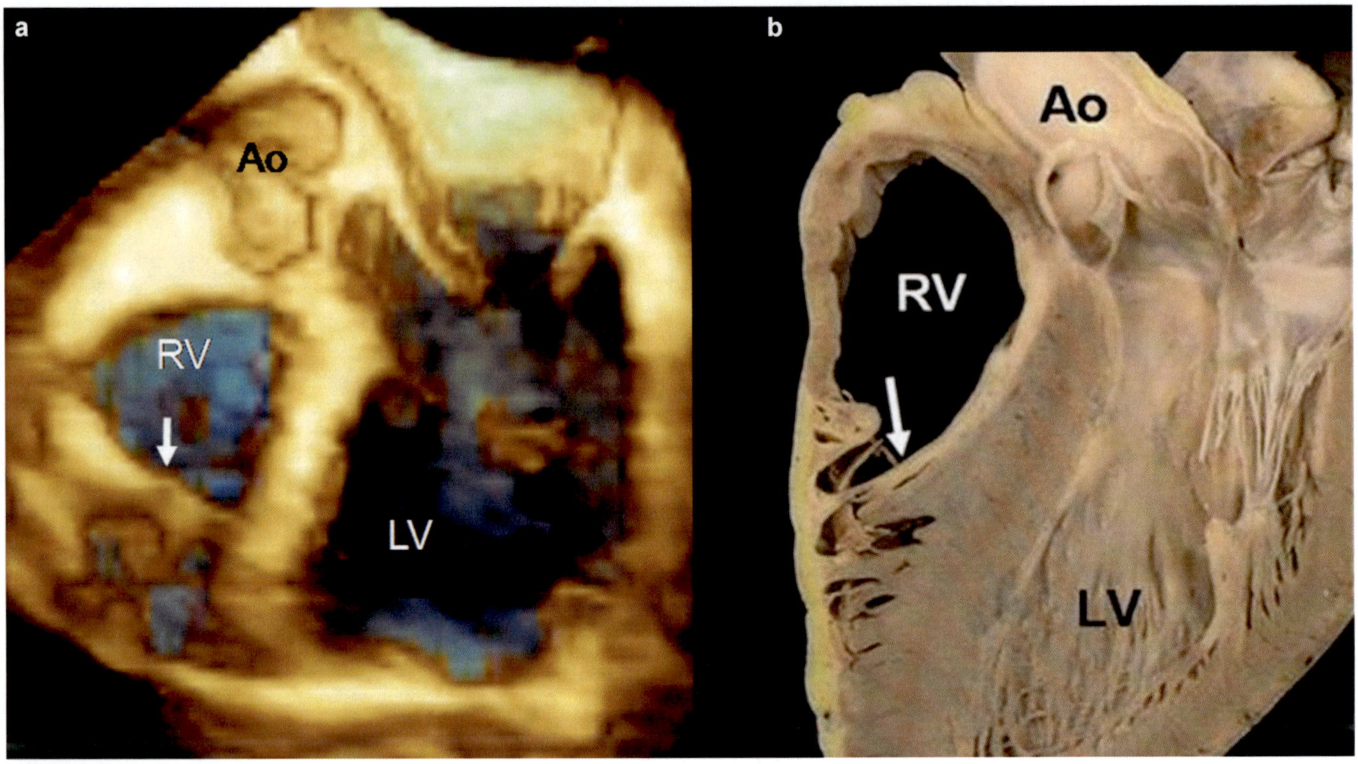

FIGURE 8.9 (a) 3D TEE image in full volume modality after properly cropping the volume data set to obtain an image of the moderator band (*arrow*) and (b) the corresponding anatomical specimen. *Ao* aorta; *RV* right ventricle; *LV* left ventricle.

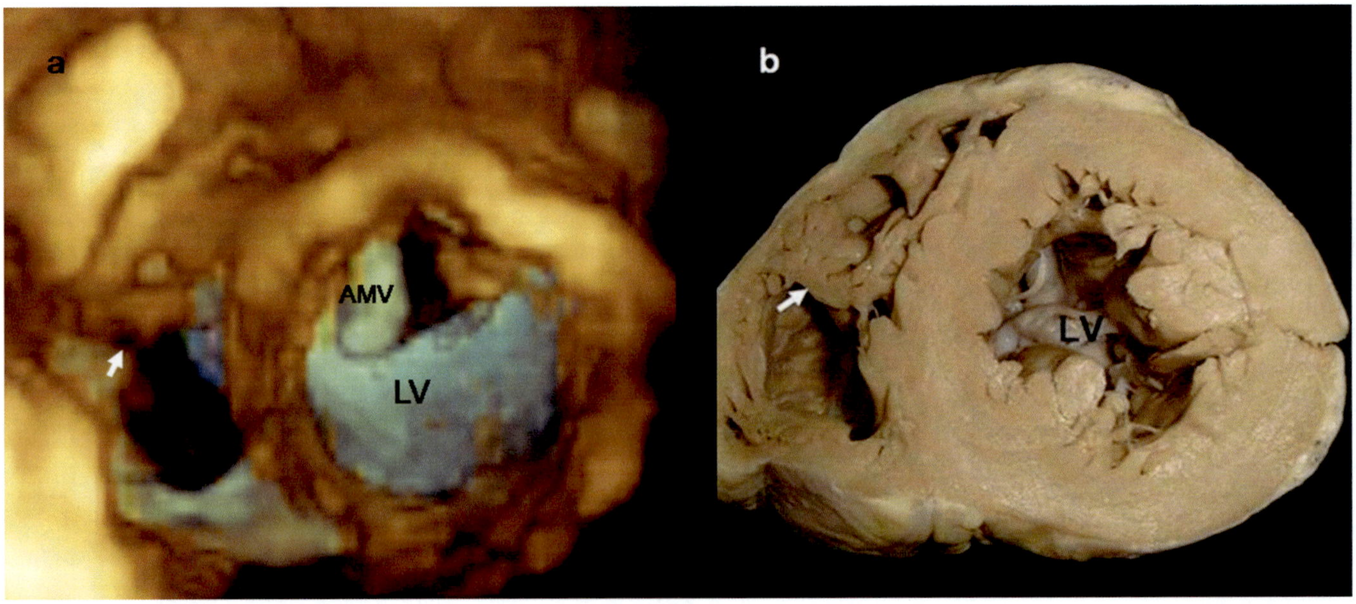

FIGURE 8.10 (a) 3D TEE image in full volume modality after cropping transversally the volume data set and (b) the corresponding anatomical specimen showing the moderator band (*arrow*) from a left ventricular perspective. The anterior mitral leaflet (AML) in its opening position can also be imaged inside the left ventricle (LV).

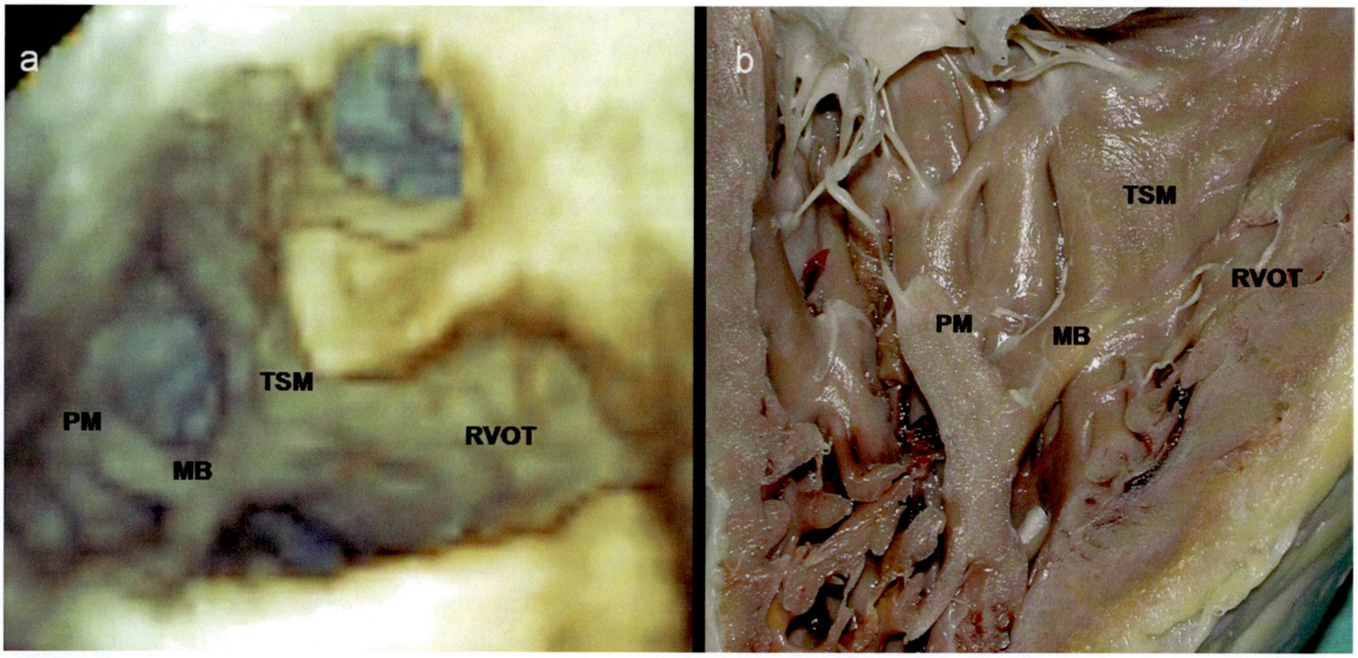

FIGURE 8.11 (a) 3D TEE image in full volume modality and (b) the corresponding anatomical specimen showing the trabecula septomarginalis (TSM) and the moderator band (MB) crossing the right ventricular cavity and joining the anterior papillary muscle (PM). *RVOT* right ventricle outflowt ract.

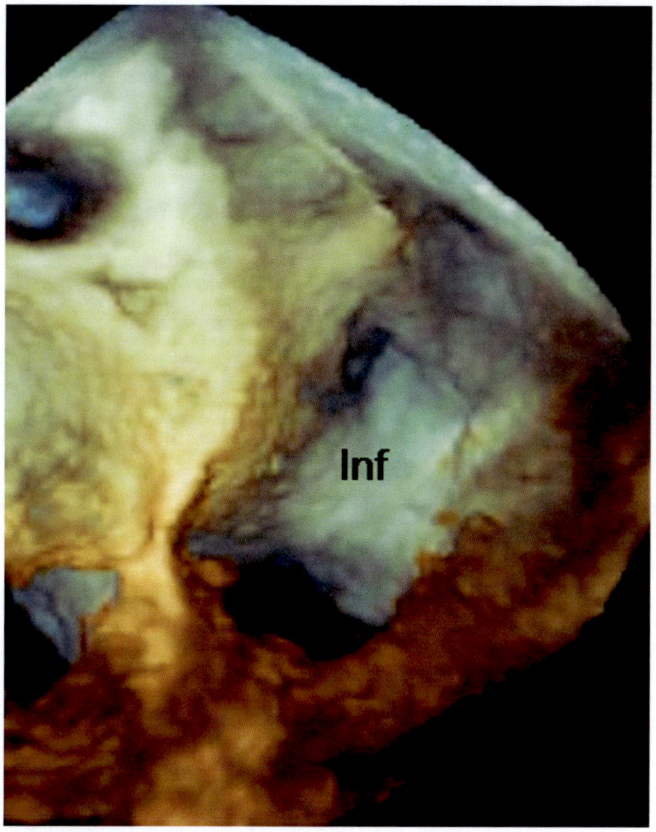

FIGURE 8.12 Real-time 3D TEE image in zoom modality showing the internal surface of the infundibulum (Inf) from an anterolateralp erspective.

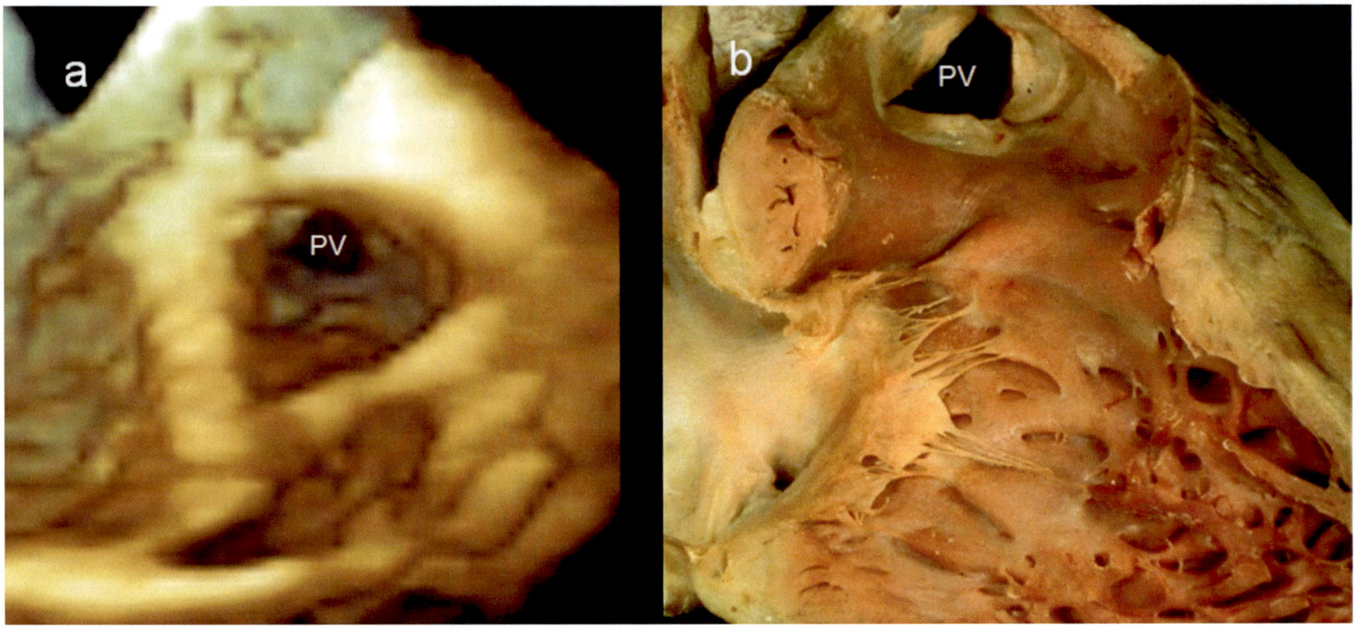

FIGURE 8.13 (a) 3D TEE image of the infundibulum from a right ventricular perspective showing the infundibulum and the pulmonic valve (PV) in opening position; (b) an anatomical specimen from a similar perspective.

CHAPTER9

TheL eft Ventricle

The left ventricle forms the apex and the lower part of the left heart border. It is shaped like a cone (ellipsoid of revolution) with its long axis directed from the apex to the base. Real-time 3D TEE may depict the internal configuration of the ventricle by properly cutting the left ventricle through longitudinal planes. Sections parallel to the ventricular long axis reveal the ellipsoid geometry (Fig. 9.1), while short axis cross-sections, perpendicular to long axis, reveal a roughly circular geometry (Fig. 9.2). The endocardial surface is irregular compared to the epicardial surface owing to the presence of two groups of papillary muscles and trabeculations. Papillary muscles are left ventricular muscular protuberances that anchor the valvular chords to the left ventricular wall. The two groups are located beneath the commissures, occupying antero-lateral and postero-medial positions (Fig. 9.3). Papillary muscles are conceptualized as being directly continuous with the solid portion of the heart wall, the compact myocardium. But tomographic imaging has consistently shown that the bases of the papillary muscles are not solid. Instead, they are composed of muscular continuations from the trabeculations that line the ventricularc avity(Fi g.9. 4).

Like the right ventricle, the left ventricle possesses an inlet, an apical trabecular component, and an outlet. The inlet component contains the mitral valve and extends from the atrio-ventricular junction to the attachment of the papillary muscles (Fig. 9.5).

The apical trabecular portion is the most characteristic feature of the morphological left ventricle and contains fine trabeculations. As for papillary muscles, the distance between the transducer and the left ventricle does not permit consistently good images of the left ventricular trabeculations to be obtained from mid esophagus. In some cases, they can be appreciated from a transgastric viewpoint (Fig. 9.6).

The outlet component of the left ventricle supports the aortic valve and consists of both muscular and fibrous

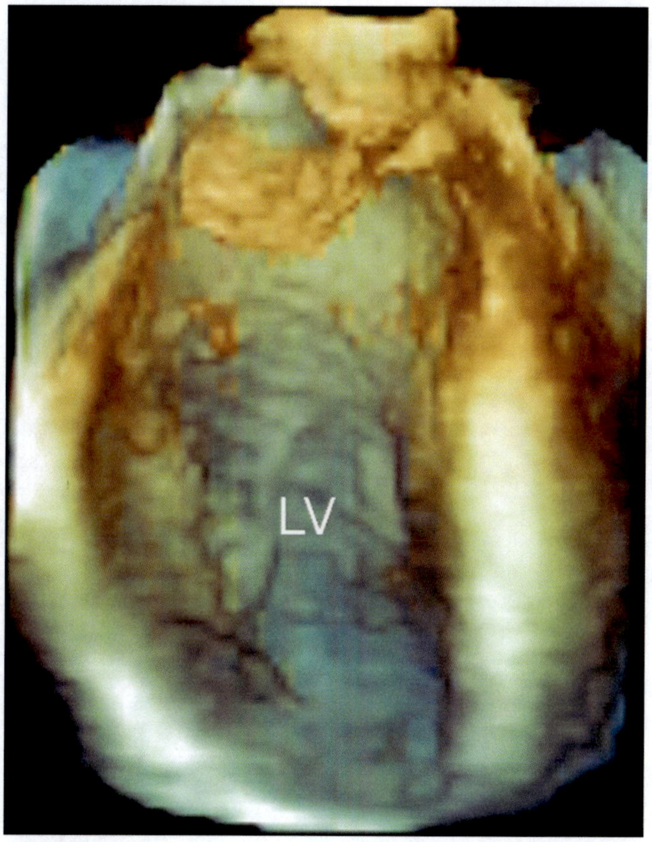

FIGURE 9.1 3D TEE in full volume modality. A longitudinal cut shows the ellipsoid shape of the left ventricle (LV) cavity.

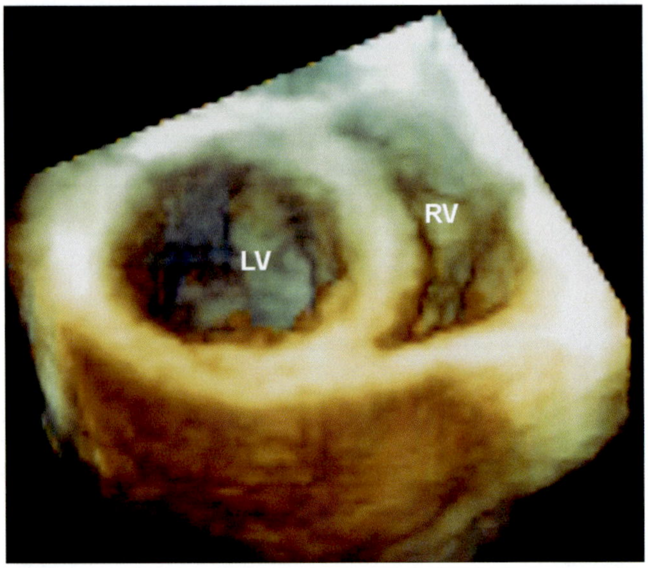

FIGURE 9.2 3D TEE in full volume modality. A transversal cut reveals the circular geometry of the left ventricle (LV) cavity. *RV* right ventricle.

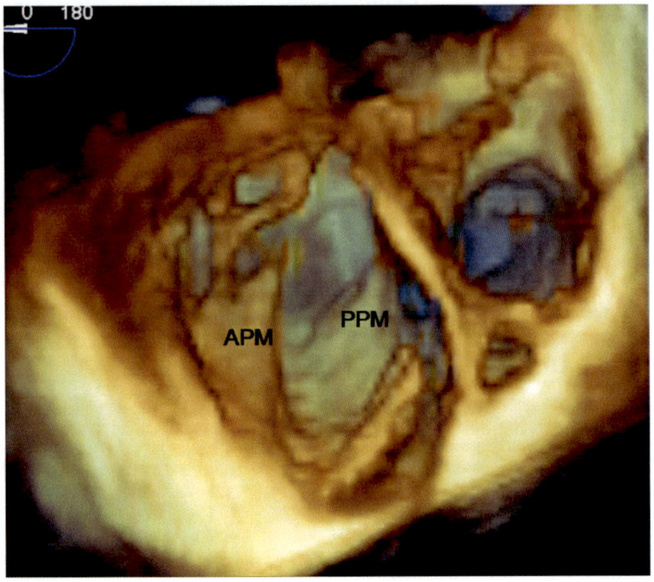

FIGURE 9.3 3D TEE in full volume modality. After properly cropping the lateral wall of the left ventricle, the antero-lateral (APM) and postero-medial (PPM) papillary muscles are displayed.

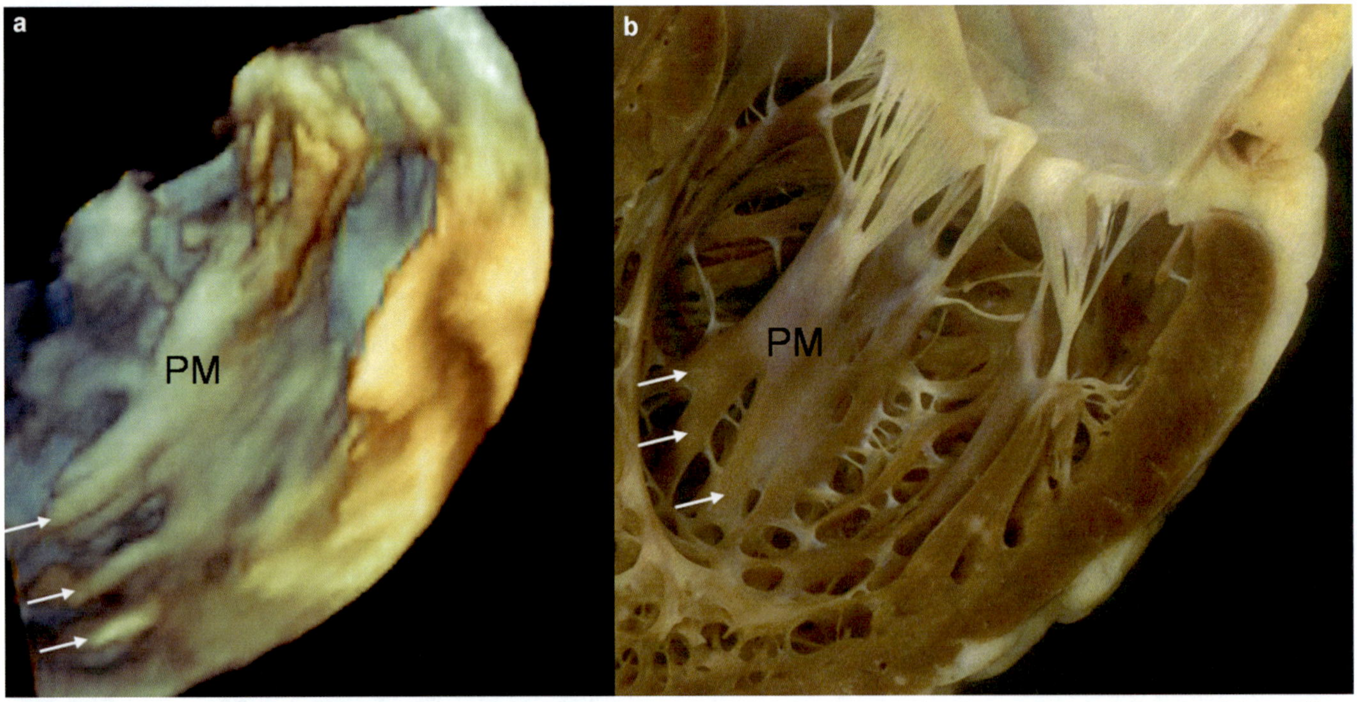

FIGURE 9.4 (a) Real-time 3D TEE in zoom modality from a transgastric viewpoint showing the characteristic architecture of the papillary muscle (PM) insertion. A network of trabeculae carneae (*arrows*) joins the base of papillary muscle to the left ventricular cavity; (b) the correspondingm orphologyi na spec imen.

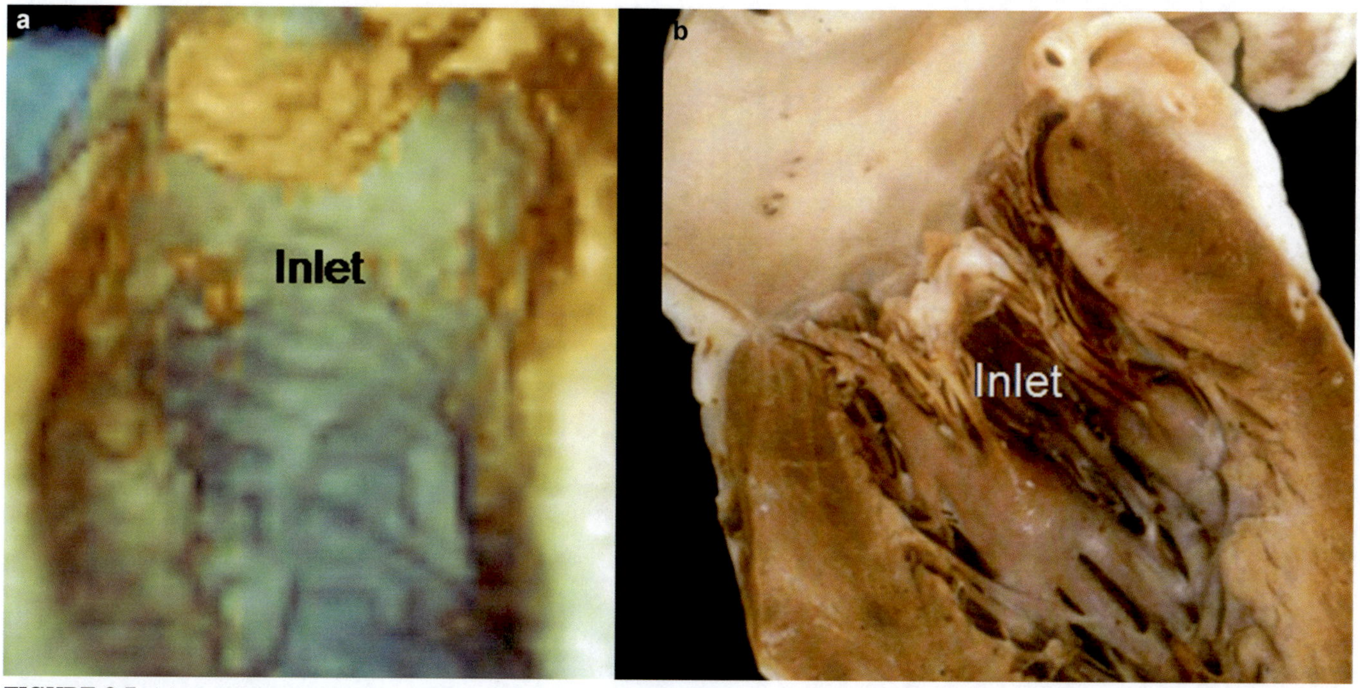

FIGURE 9.5 (a) 3D TEE in full volume modality from a lateral perspective showing the inlet component of the left ventricle; (b) a correspondinga natomicalspec imen.

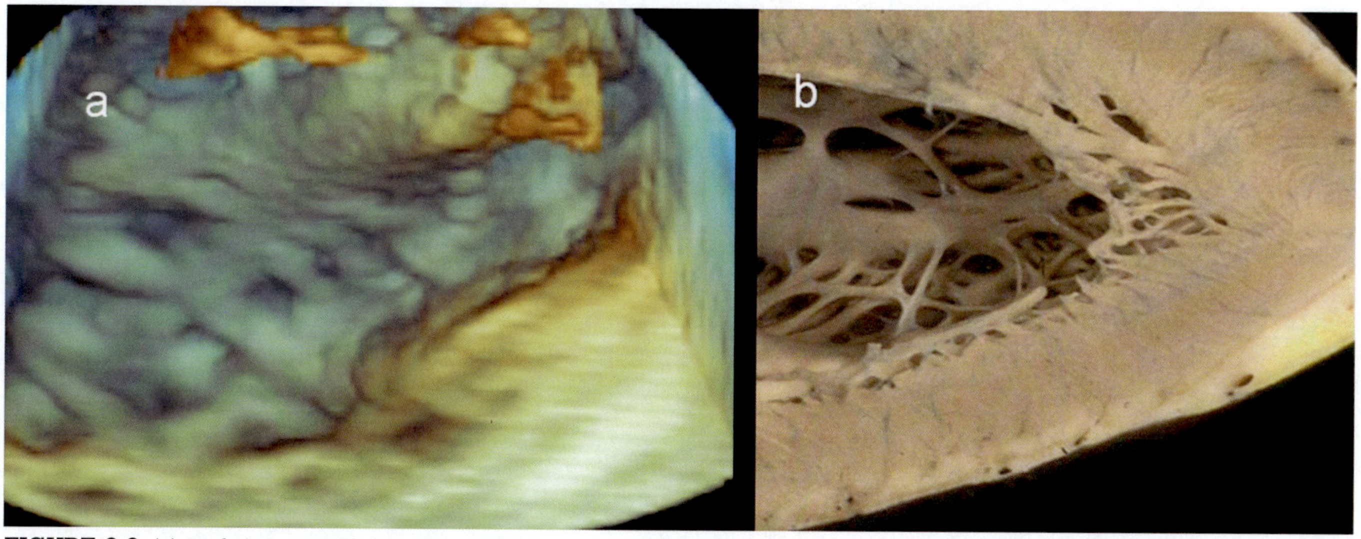

FIGURE 9.6 (a) Real-time 3D TEE in zoom modality from a transgastric viewpoint showing the fine trabeculations of the left ventricle; (b)a na natomicals pecimens howing similar architecture.

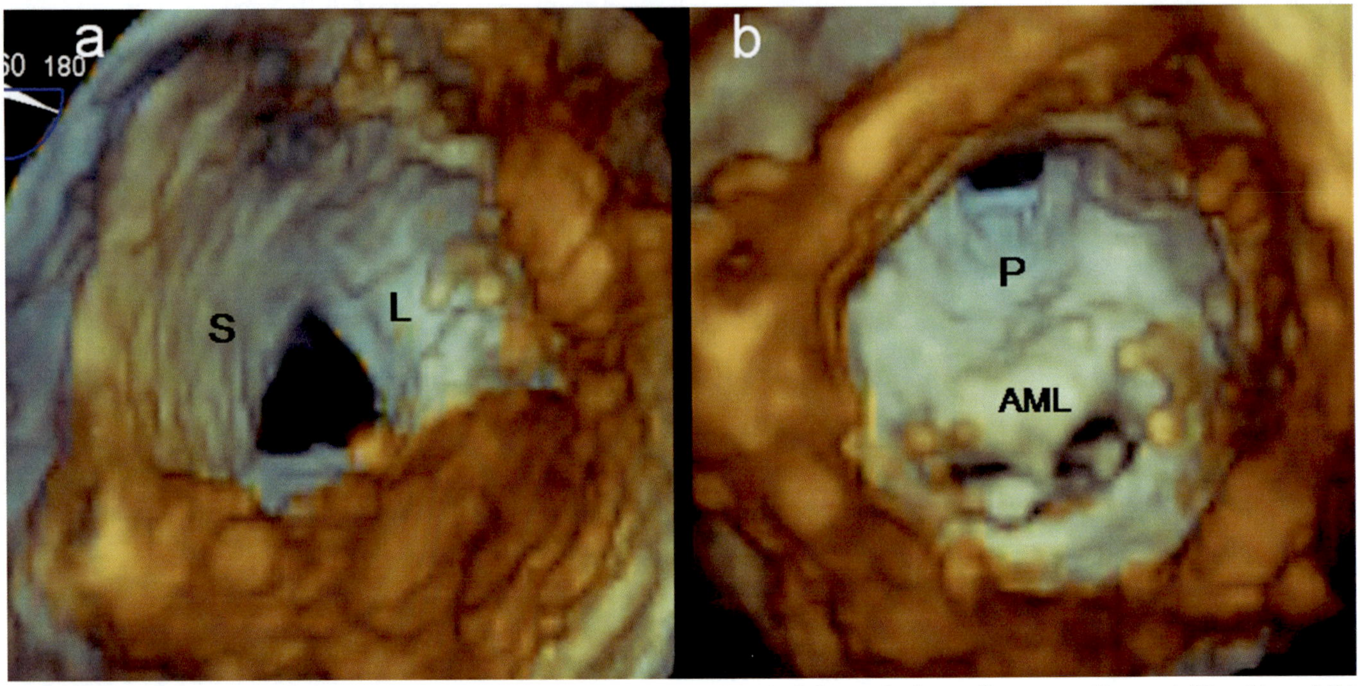

FIGURE 9.7 3D TEE in full volume modality from an apical perspective. (a) The left ventricular outflow tract with septal (S) and lateral (L) portions; (b) a slight up–down angulation reveals the posterior (P) portion. *AML* anterior mitral leaflet.

portions. This combination is in contrast to the infundibulum of the right ventricle, which is comprised entirely of muscle. It can be roughly divided into septal, posterior, and lateral portions. The septal portion, although primarily muscular, also includes the membranous portion of the ventricular septum. The posterior portion consists of an extensive fibrous curtain that extends from the fibrous skeleton of the heart across the aortic leaflet of the mitral valve. It supports the leaflets of the aortic valve in the area of aortic-mitral fibrous continuity (see Chap. 3). The lateral portion is muscular and consists of the lateral margin of the inner curvature of the heart (Fig. 9.7).

If the entire left ventricle is included in the volume data set, the left ventricular shape, as well as quantitative evaluation of volumes, and global and regional function can be measured by a 3D quantification software. This semiautomatic program requires the operators to determine reference points along the base of the left ventricle and the LV apex. An automatic endocardial border-tracking program then identifies and traces the endocardial border (Fig. 9.8). The program then calculates left end-systolic and end-diastolic volumes using a 3D deformable model without geometric assumptions, thereby enabling the determination of a true ejection fraction.

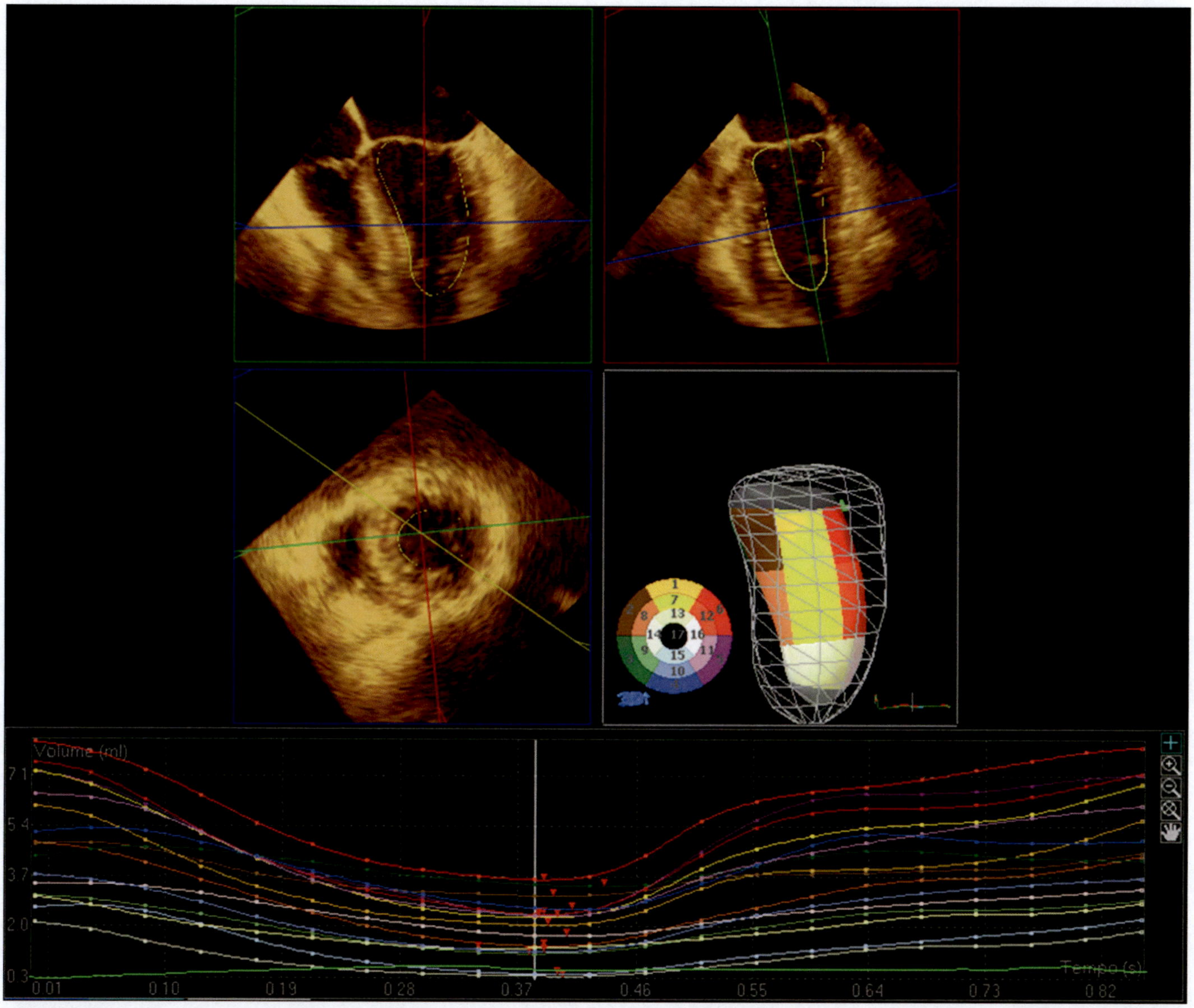

FIGURE 9.8 Left ventricular shape and global and regional function can be assessed by using an advanced software (QLAB-3DQAdv).

CHAPTER 10

Clinical Cases

CASE 1

A 45-year-old man, with a past history of endocarditis suffering from progressive shortness of breath on exertion was hospitalized. A preliminary examination revealed normal heart sounds but a grade 3 diastolic murmur along the left sternal border. 2D TEE revealed severe aortic regurgitation with two converging jets and two different flow convergence zones suggestive of two regurgitant orifices (Fig. 10.1). The aortic root was normal in size. When 3D RT TEE was performed, *en face* views of the aortic valve revealed what appeared to be perforations in all three cusps (Fig. 10.2). The main question from the surgeon was: .... "Are the aortic valve leafleats intact or are there some erosions/perforations?...." Whether the leaflets are normal or not makes a big difference in the case of this relatively young individual. If the leaflets are normal, the valve could be repaired. If not, the valve should probably be replaced. The final diagnosis from the echocardiographic study was severe aortic regurgitation caused by multiple aortic valve perforations. The diagnosis was based on an observation of at least two convergence zones in the 2D images and the features of the perforations in the valve in the real-time 3D images. It also took into account the patient's past history of endocarditis. In the operating room, the surgeon found the aortic leaflets to be redundant but without any perforation or erosion. The valve was successfully repaired (Fig. 10.3). The two flow convergence zones in the plane seen in the 2D image can be explained by the presence of redundant leaflet tissue, which might have produced small folds in the coapting surfaces of leaflets, resulting in several regurgitant orifices. Multiple perforations apparently seen on the 3D image were in fact drop-out artifacts. When very thin structures such as the aortic valve cusps are imaged by ultrasound, weak echoes are generated by the structure, particularly if the ultrasound plane intersects the structure on a parallel plane. In real-time 3D TEE, weak echoes are quite frequent during the adjustment of the image using the gain, compression, and smoothing, and are known as *leaflet drop-out artifacts*. As a general rule, the gain and the compression should be reduced so as to decrease ultrasound noise, but not the tissue signals. The reason for the apparent perforations was the fact that, in diastole, part of the body of leaflets was parallel to the ultrasound pyramid generating weak echo signals. These signals disappeared with the reduction in ultrasound gain, thus causing the drop-out artifacts.

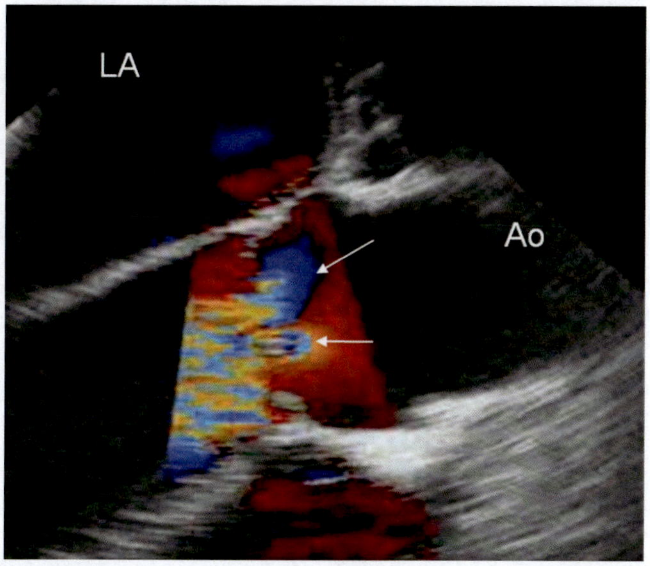

FIGURE 10.1 2D TEE image showing severe aortic regurgitation. *Arrows* indicate the two proximal flow convergence zones. The sinutubular junction and the ascending aorta appear normal.

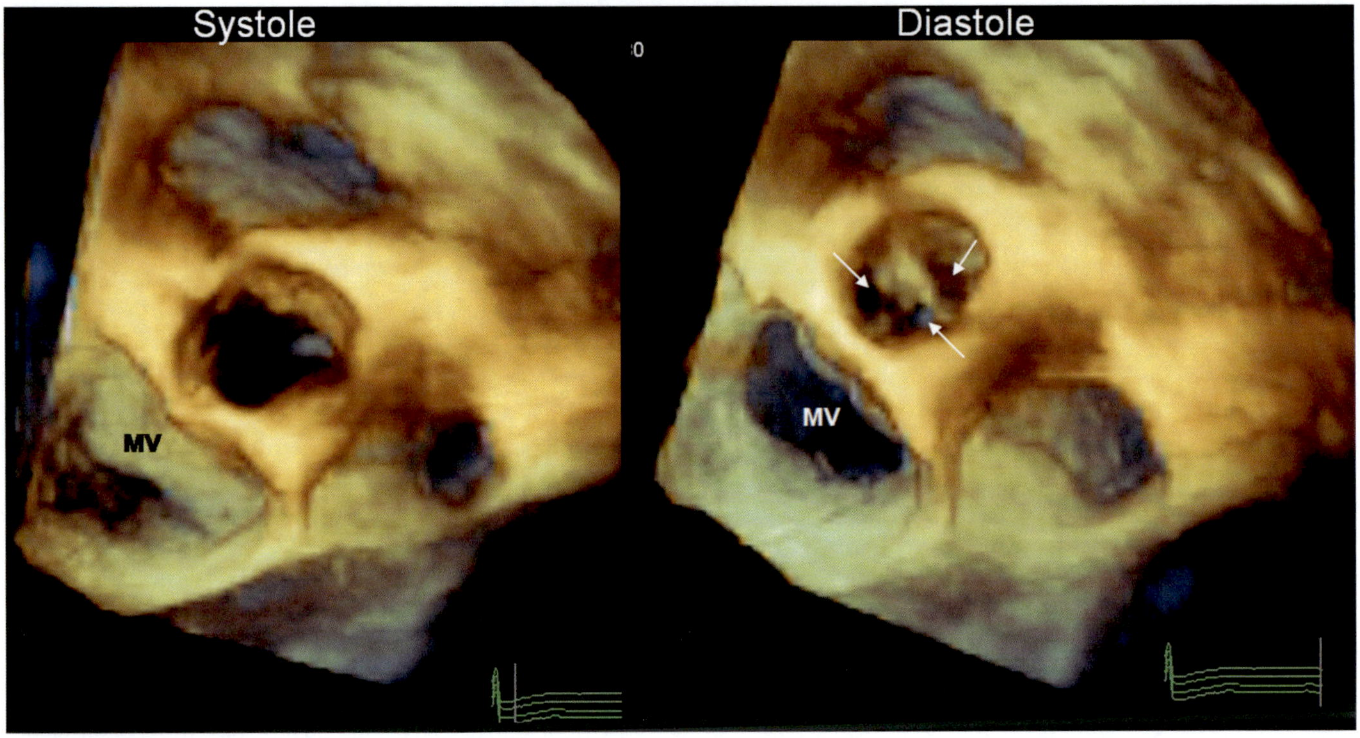

FIGURE 10.2 3D TEE of the base of the heart in full volume modality in systole and in diastole. The *arrows* indicate apparent perforations resulting from previous endocarditis. *MV*m itralv alve.

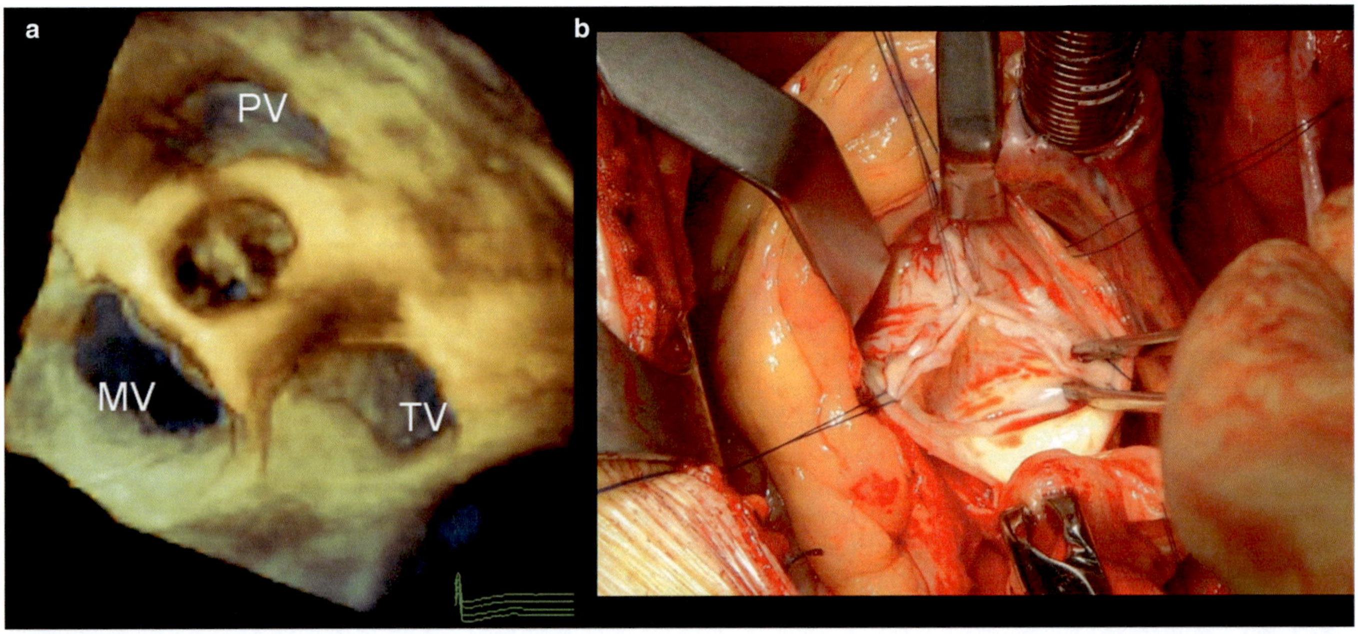

FIGURE 10.3 (a) 3D TEE image in full volume of the base of the heart and (b) the corresponding intraoperative photo of the aortic valve. No perforations were found in the aortic valve.

CASE2

An 81-year-old man with an acute inferior myocardial infarction and cardiogenic shock (blood pressure 70 mmHg; heart rate 110 b/min) was admitted to the catheterization laboratory for emergency coronary angiography. A soft systolic ejection murmur could be heard. The coronary angiography revealed an occlusion of the posterior descending artery (PDA) and severe stenosis of the circumflex artery (Cx) (Fig. 10.4). No other significant lesions were found. 2D transthoracic examinations (performed from the subcostal viewpoint) showed a large ventricular septal defect involving the para-apical area of the inferior septum (Fig. 10.5) A real-time 3D TEE was performed while the patient was awaiting an attempted surgical repair of the VSD (Fig. 10.6). The huge VSD was confirmed.

From a diagnostic point of view, no incremental data were obtained by real-time 3D TEE. However, the *en face* visualization of the VSD allowed a better evaluation of the size and the shape of the defect. In this patient, real-time 3D TEE confirmed that the defect was very large and had an irregular shape. Because of the prolonged cardiogenic shock, the poor right ventricular function, and the presence of a large defect without sufficient residual tissue on the inferior and apical borders, the surgeon's final decision was not to intervene. The patient died 3 h later.

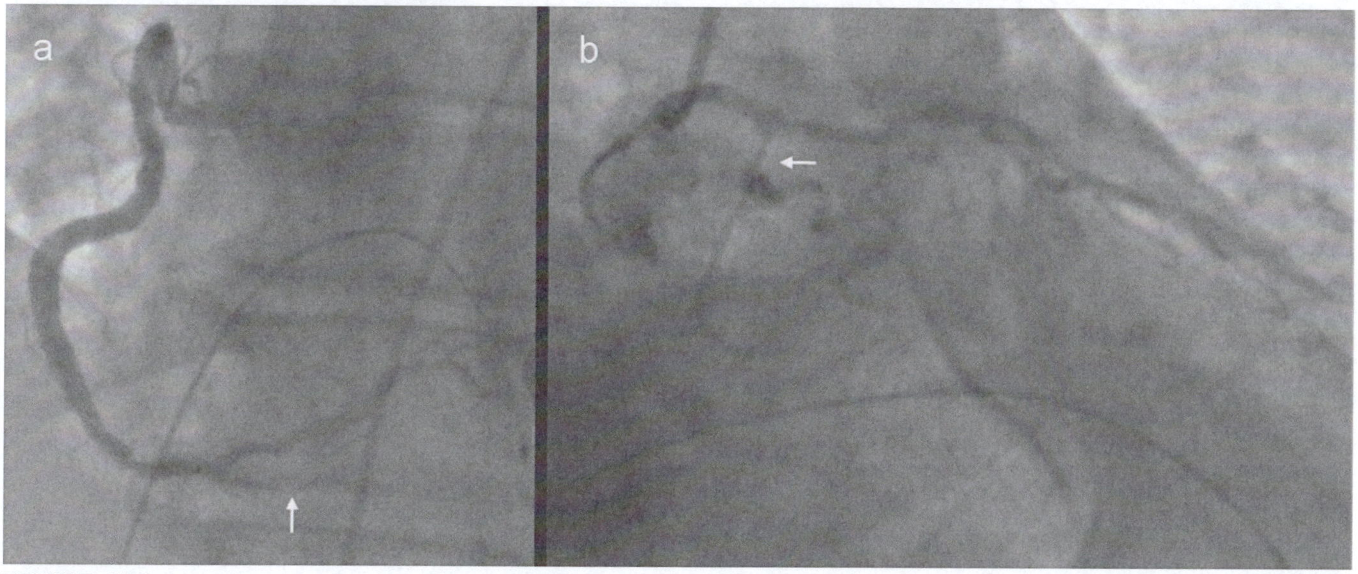

FIGURE 10.4 (a) Right coronary artery. The *arrow* indicates the occlusion of the PDA. (b) The *arrow* indicates the severe stenosis of the circumflex coronary artery.

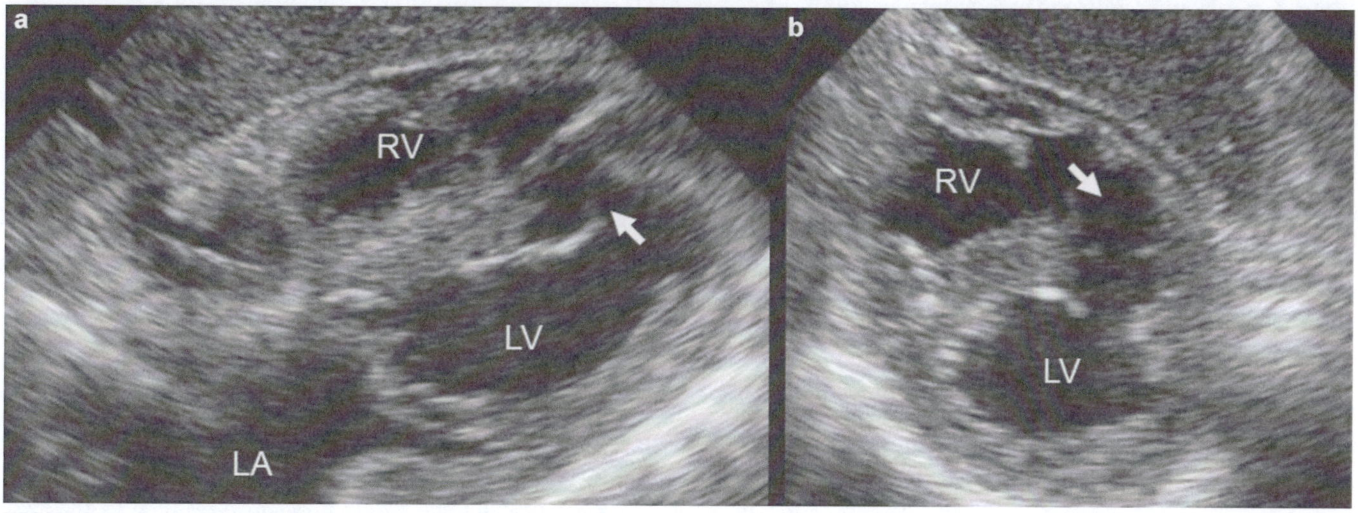

FIGURE 10.5 (a) Subcostal four chamber and (b) short axis view showing a large ventricular septal defect (*arrow*). *LA* leaft atrium; *LV* left ventricle; *RV*r ightv entricle.

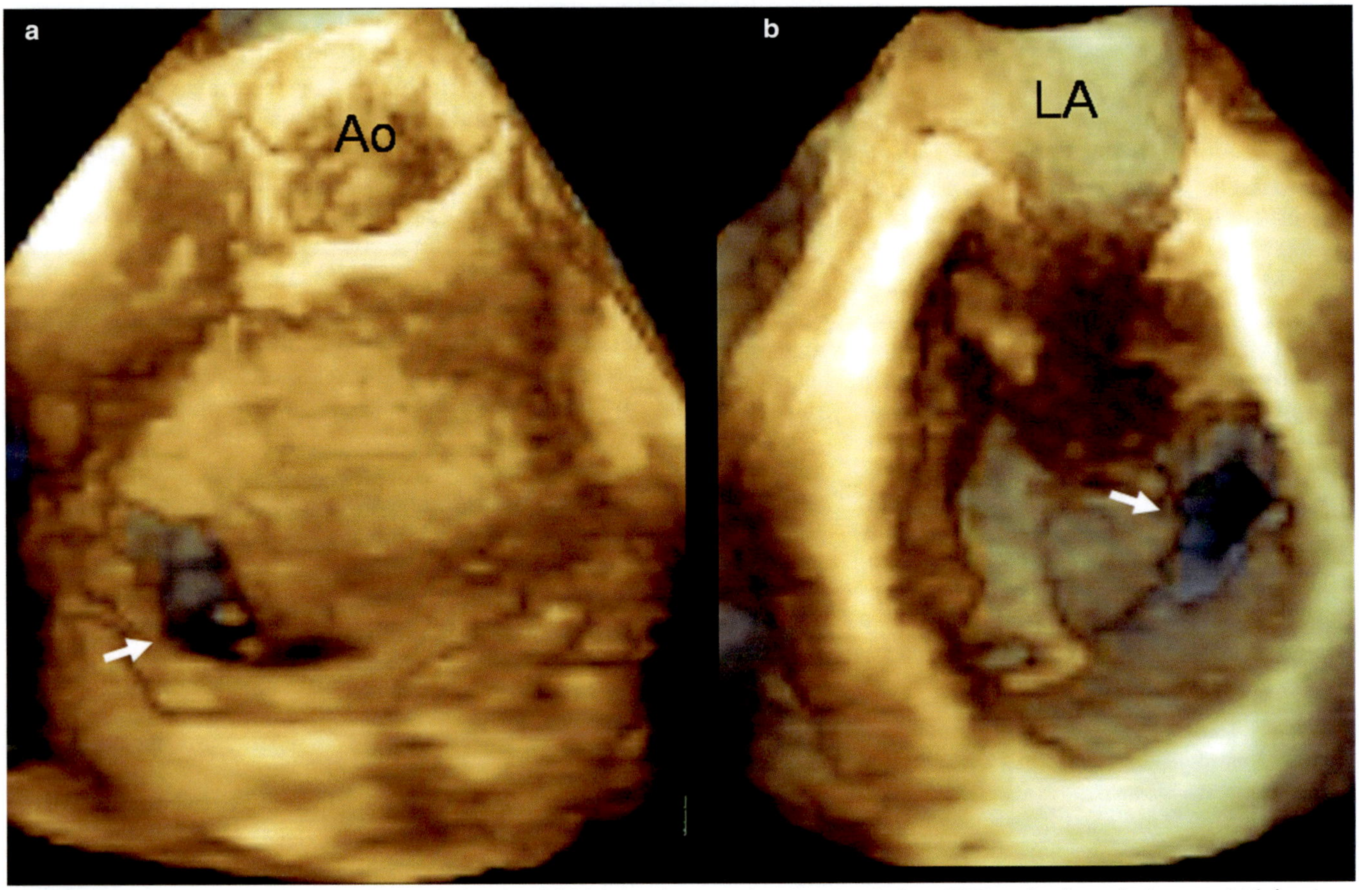

FIGURE 10.6 (a) Real-time 3D TEE from right-hand and (b) left-hand perspectives showing the large VSD *en face* (*arrow*). *Ao* aorta; *LA* left atrium.

CASE3

An 83-year-old male with a past clinical history of an inferior myocardial infarction and coronary bypass graft surgery for multi-vessel coronary artery disease followed by several angioplasty procedures, was admitted to our hospital with an acute deterioration in heart failure symptoms. He also suffered from several comorbidities such as chronic obstructive pulmonary disease, peripheral vascular disease, and chronic renal insufficiency. On admission, he showed signs of pulmonary congestion. Cardiac auscultation revealed a systolic murmur. 2D TEE demonstrated severe mitral regurgitation related to ruptured chordae tendineae of the anterior leaflet. There was also evidence of a slight tethering of the central region of the posterior leaflets owing to inferior wall remodeling (Fig. 10.7). Real-time 3D echocardiography confirmed a flail of the medial region of the anterior mitral leaflet due to a ruptured chorda tendinea (Fig. 10.8). Because of the high risk of a surgical procedure on the mitral valve in the case of this patient, it was decided to intervene by clipping the medial part of anterior leaflet (A3) edge-to-edge with the corresponding posterior part (P3), using a percutaneous procedure. The procedure was monitored using 2D and real-time 3D TEE. Figure 10.9 shows the catheter delivery system passing through the atrial septum. Figure 10.10 shows how the delivery system was curved so as to be positioned over the mitral orifice. After having positioned the delivery system over the mitral valve, the arms were opened and oriented perpendicularly to the leaflet rims (Fig. 10.11). The asterisk on the figure indicates the region of the anterior leaflet, the target of the clip delivery system. Thus, the whole system was shifted medially (Fig. 10.12). Then the clip was released and the delivery system withdrawn, leaving two asymmetrical orifices (Fig. 10.13). While the procedure reduced the regurgitation resulting from the ruptured chordae tendineae, a new regurgitation appeared, which was probably owing to tethering caused by the clip (Fig. 10.14). It was then decided to insert a second clip (Fig. 10.15). The insertion of a second clip lateral to the first one resulted in significant reduction in mitral regurgitation (Fig. 10.16). Characteristically, the whole procedure resulted in the creation of three orifices (Fig. 10.17).

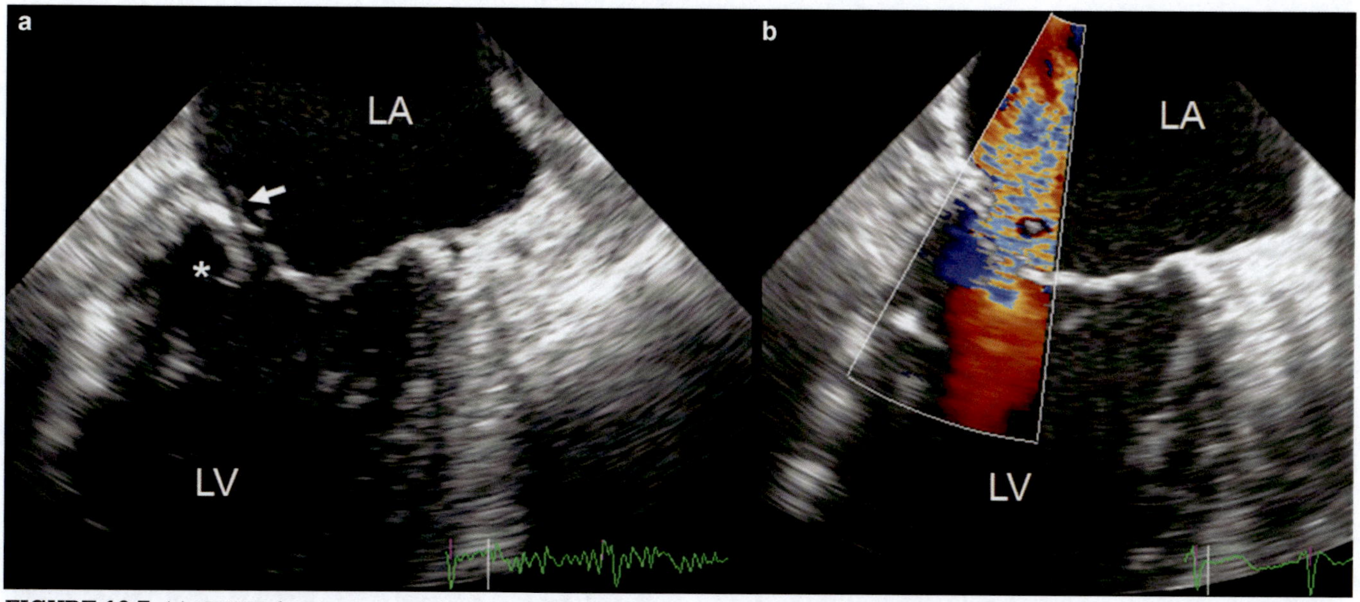

FIGURE 10.7 (a) 2D TEE shows a ruptured chordae tendineae (*arrow*) located on the medial region of anterior leaflet causing severe mitral regurgitation (b). There was also a slight tethering of the posterior leaflet (*asterisk*) due to left ventricular remodeling. *LA* left atrium; *LV* left ventricle.

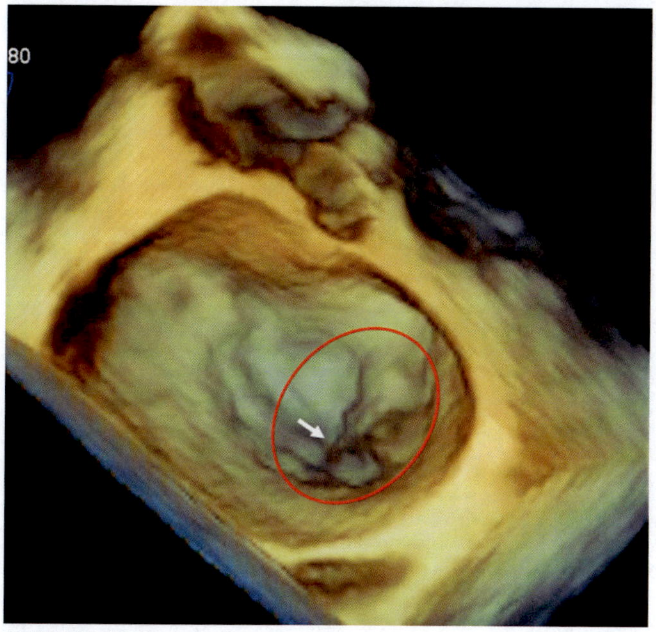

FIGURE 10.8 Real-time 3D TEE in zoom modality confirms the existence of a ruptured chordae tendineae (*arrow*) leading to flail medial segment of the anterior leaflet (*red circle*).

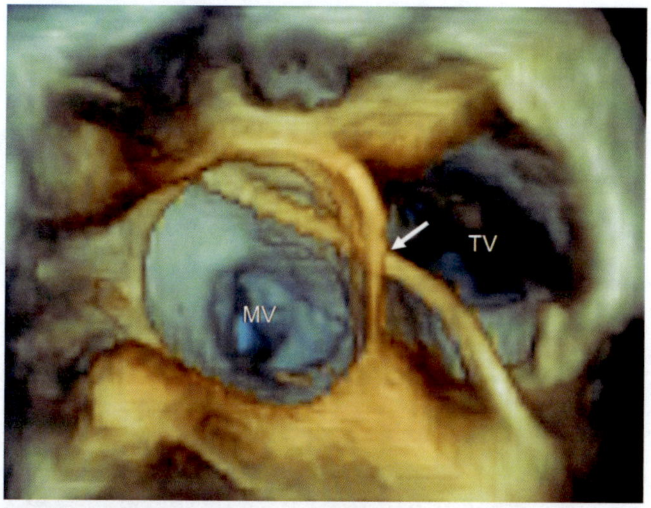

FIGURE 10.9 Real-time 3D TEE in zoom modality showing a catheter delivery system passing through the atrial septum (*arrow*). *MV* mitral valve; *TV* tricuspid valve.

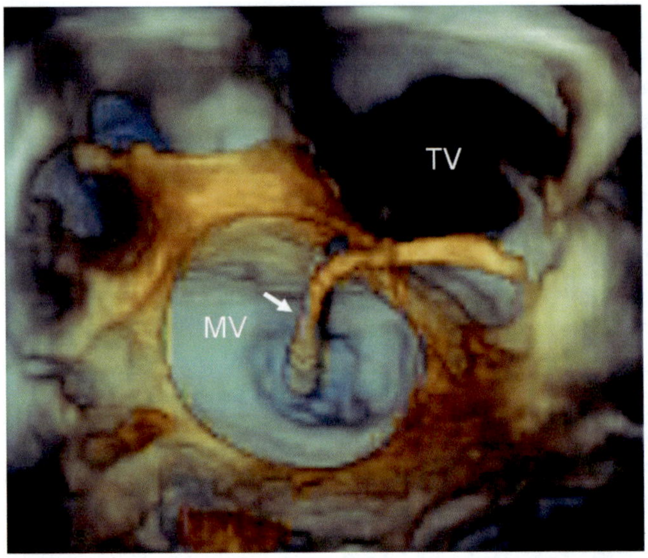

FIGURE 10.10 Real-time 3D TEE in zoom modality showing the catheter delivery system (*arrow*) curved and positioned over the mitral orifice. *MV* mitral valve; *TV*t ricuspidv alve.

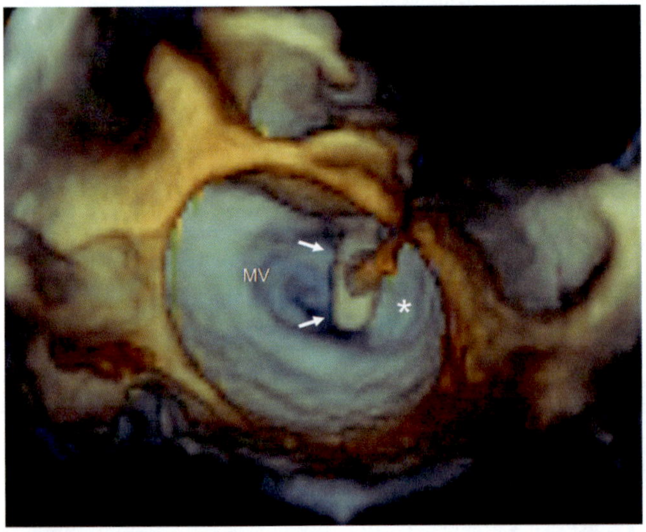

FIGURE 10.11 Real-time 3D TEE in zoom modality showing the arms of the delivery system opened (*arrows*) and oriented perpendicularly to the leaflets' rim. The *asterisk* indicates the prolapsing region of the anterior leaflet, the target of the clip delivery system. *MV*m itralv alve.

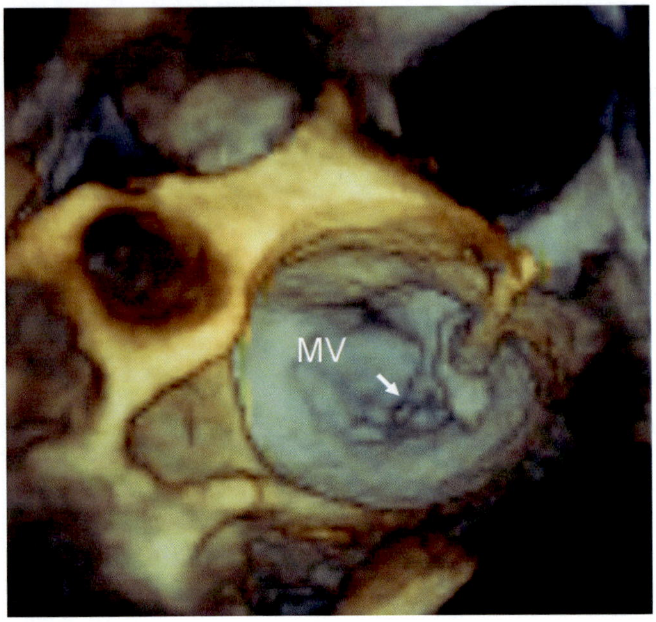

FIGURE 10.12 Real-time 3D TEE in zoom modality showing how the system is moved medially just over the flail region (*arrow*). *MV* mitral valve.

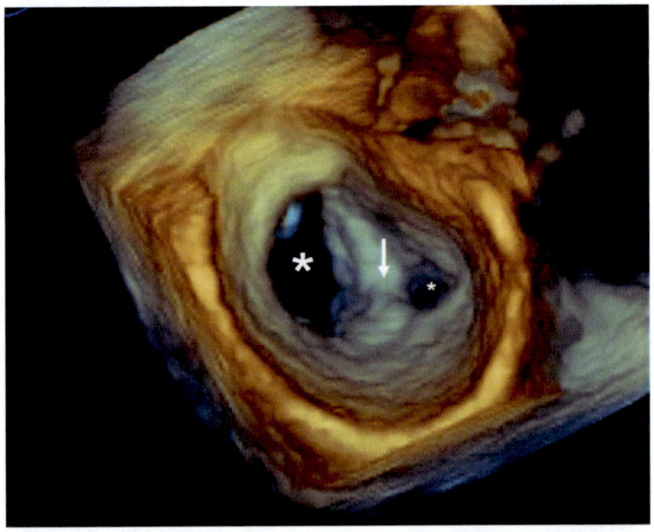

FIGURE 10.13 Real-time 3D TEE in zoom modality showing the result of the procedure. The *arrow* indicates the region where the clip has been delivered providing an edge-to-edge repair. Two asymmetric orifices (*asterisks*) were created.

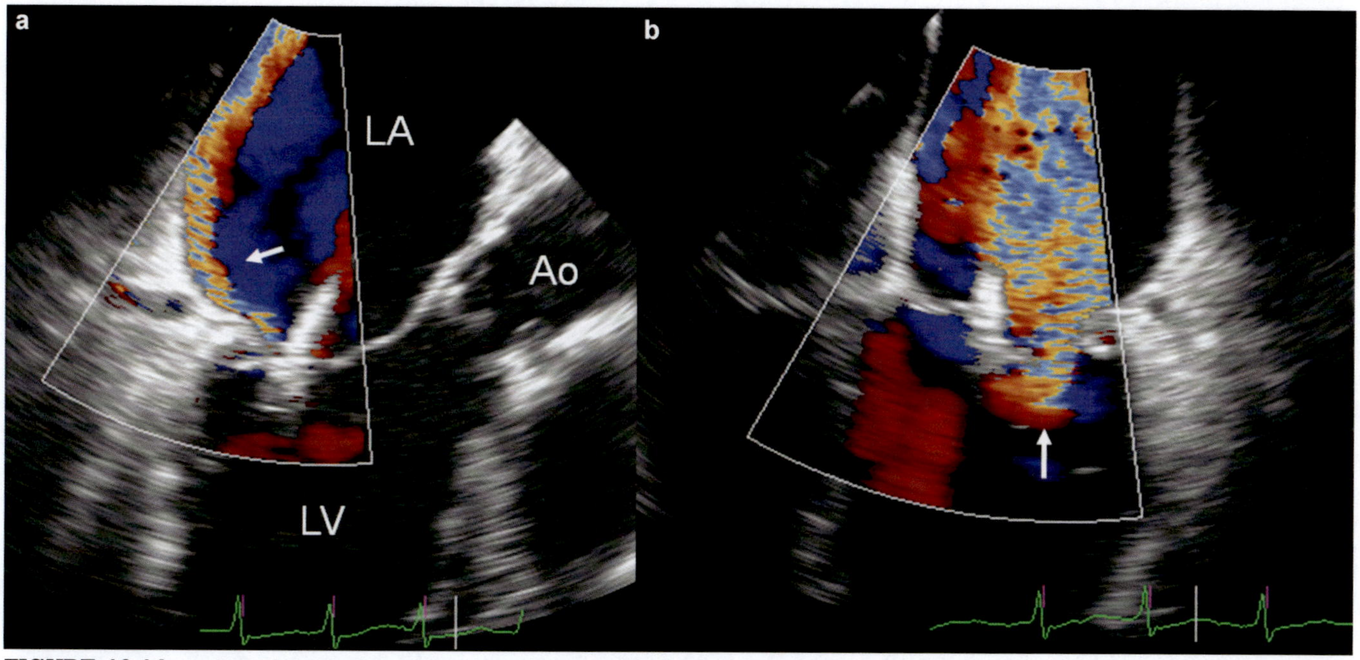

FIGURE 10.14 2D TEE showing that after positioning the clip severe regurgitation (*arrow*) located laterally to the clip appeared (a, b). This was probably due to the tethering caused by the clip. *LA* left atrium; *Ao* aorta; *LV* left ventricle.

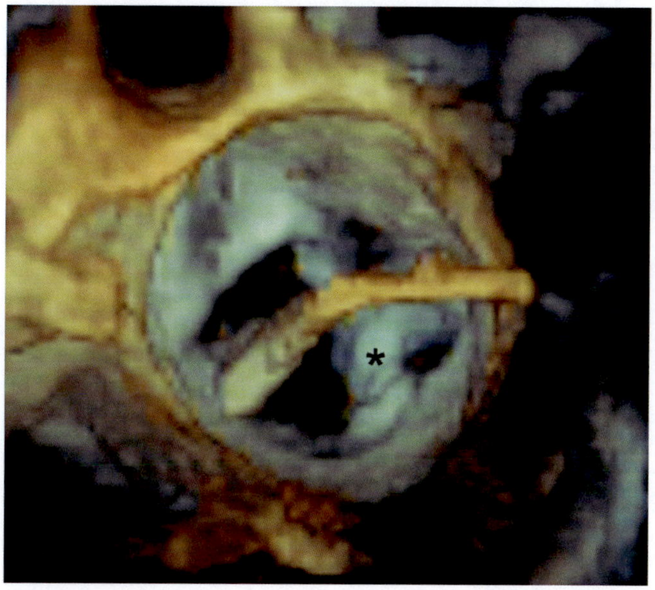

FIGURE 10.15 Real-time 3D TEE in zoom modality showing the clip system delivery being positioned laterally to the first implant (*asterisk*).

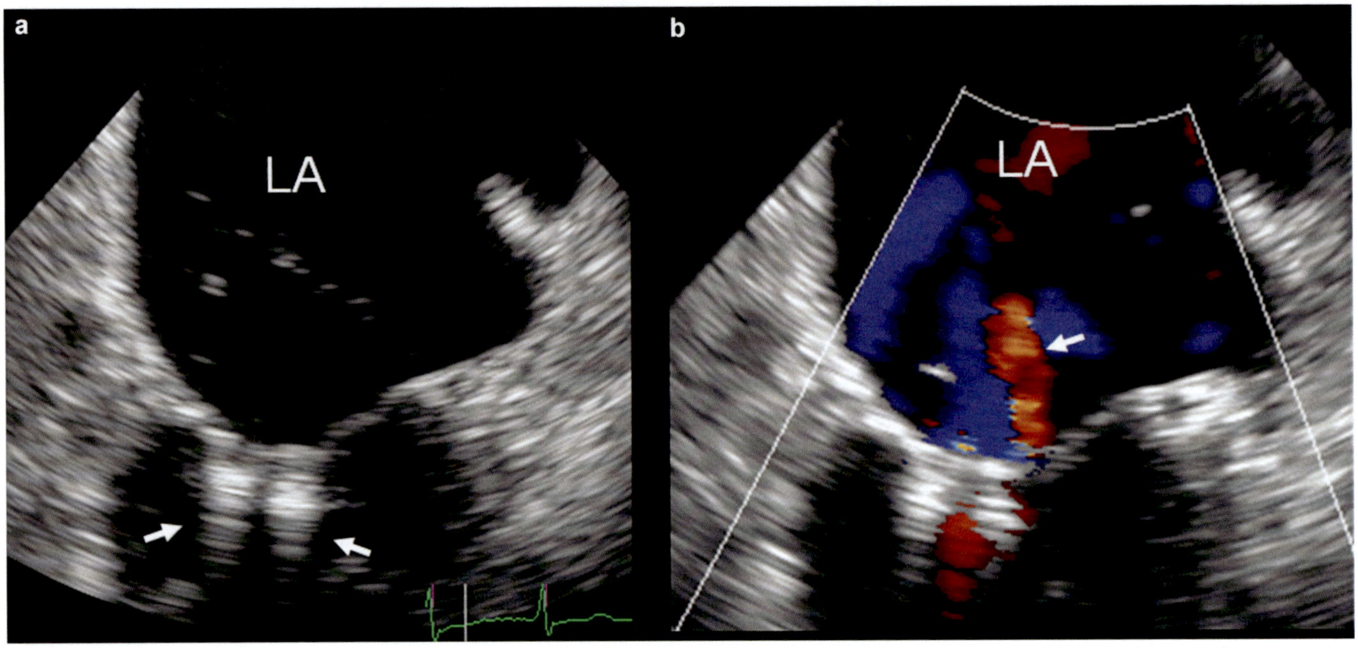

FIGURE 10.16 (a) 2D TEE in two chamber view. *Arrows* point at the two clips. Image in (b) shows the significant reduction of regurgitation (*arrow*) after positioning of the second clip. *Arrows* point to trivial residual regurgitation. *LA* left atrium.

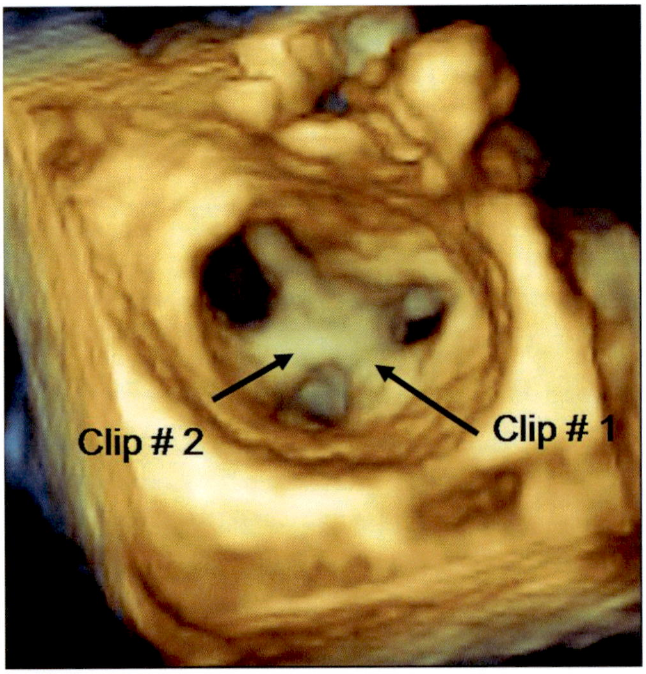

FIGURE 10.17 Real-time 3D TEE in zoom modality showing the three orificesa ndt het woc lips.

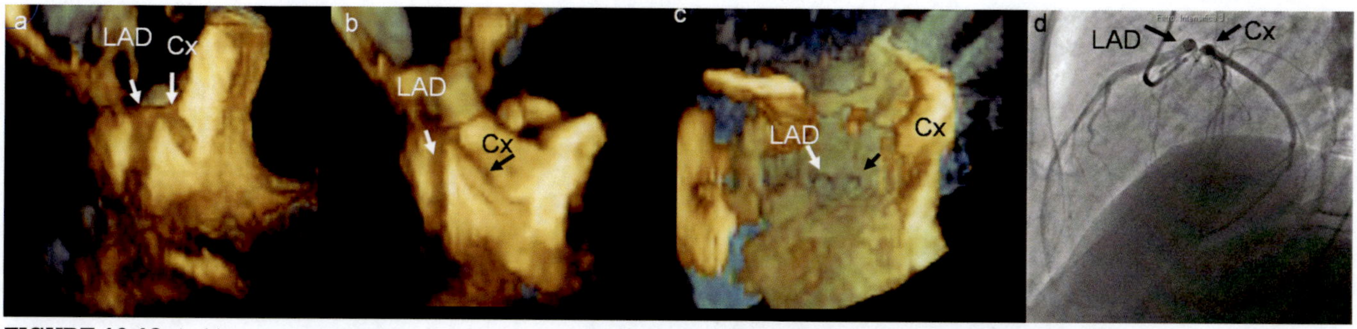

FIGURE 10.18 (a, b) A composite image showing the separate origin of the left anterior descending artery (LAD) and the circumflex artery (Cx) in a long axis view. (c) Separate ostia of the two coronary arteries. (d) The angiographic image.

CASE4

A 45-year-old female patient underwent a mitral valvuloplasty. During the monitoring of the valve repair in the operating room, the absence of a common trunk of the left coronary artery (i.e., the left descending artery and circumflex artery had separate origins) was observed (Fig. 10.18). Although images of coronary arteries are traditionally obtained with conventional coronary angiography or with multidetector computed tomography, real-time 3D TEE can also be used on occasions to observe the proximal segment of the left and right coronary artery (RCA).

CASE5

An 80-year-old man with acute coronary syndrome and a history of CABG was admitted to our institution. ECG showed ST segment elevation in II, III, and aVF leads. The patient urgently underwent coronary angiography which revealed occlusion of the venous graft to the RCA. Percutaneous coronary intervention and stenting resulted in TIMI 3 blood flow but persistent ST-elevation in the inferior leads. 2D transthoracic echocardiography (TTE) showed a LV inferior wall aneurysm without any sign of thrombus. 2D TEE confirmed the diagnosis of infero-posterior aneurysm with a thin but uninterrupted wall (Fig. 10.19).

Real-time 3D TEE made it possible to clearly define anatomic position, size, and shape of the neck of the aneurysm (Fig. 10.20). Because of the high gradient of acoustic impedance between blood and tissues, 3D reconstruction of internal structures provides high quality images. In contrast, the low difference in acoustic impedance makes it impossible to differentiate the external surface of the ventricle from the surrounding structures even with the use of high frequency broad band transducers equipped with the new generation of piezoelectric crystals. Figure 10.21 shows the difference in image quality between (a) internal structures and (d) the external surface.

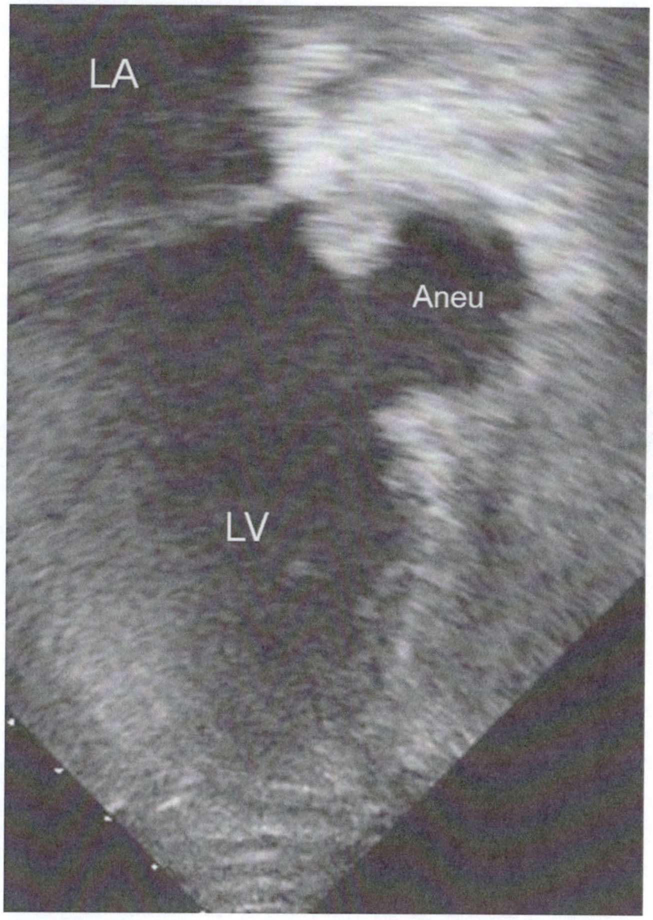

FIGURE 10.19 2D TEE showing an infero-posterior aneurysm. *LA* left atrium; *LV* left ventricle.

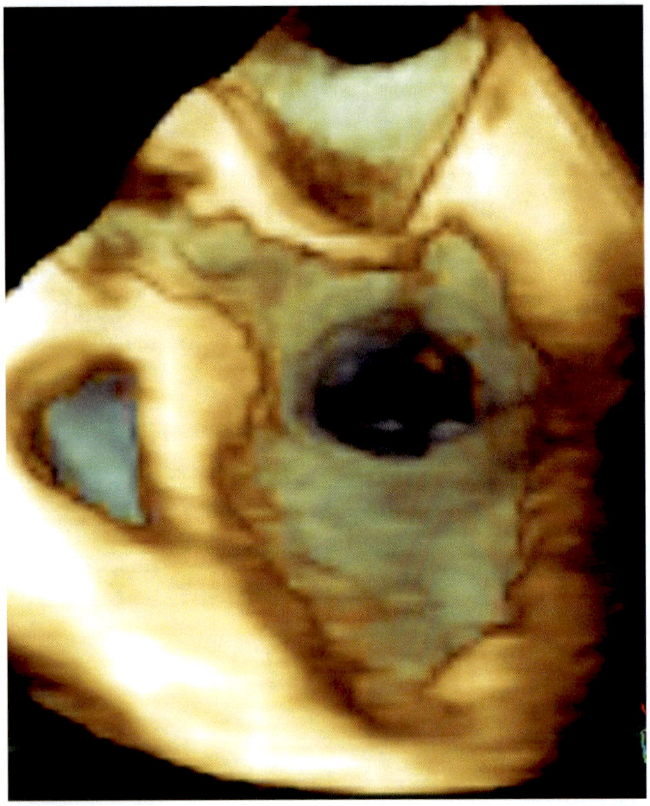

FIGURE 10.20 3D TEE in full volume modality after removing the anterior wall. The image shows the entry of the aneurysm, exactly delineating site, size, and shape of the neck of the aneurysm.

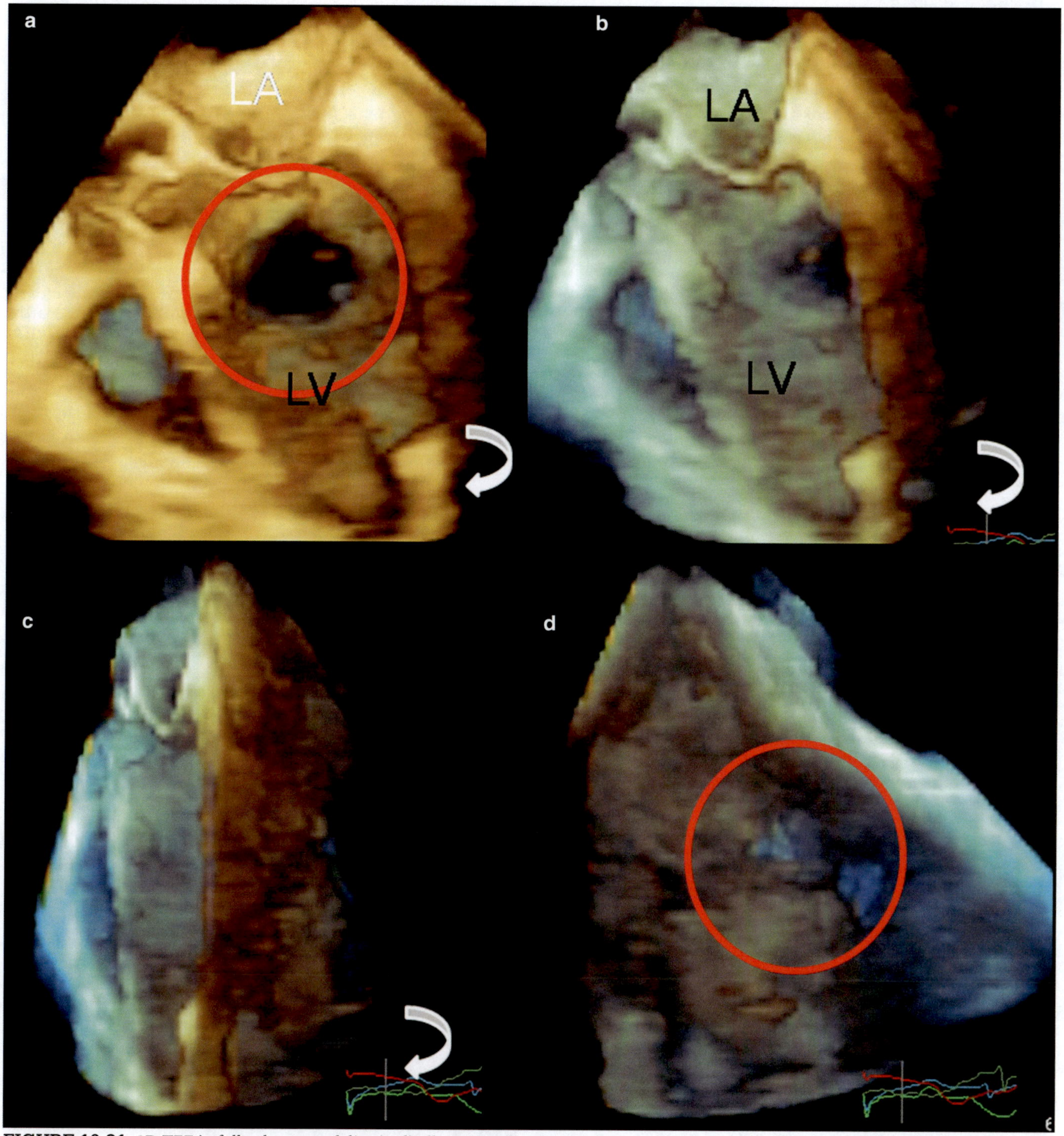

FIGURE 10.21 3D TEE in full volume modality (a-d) allows visualization of the external surface of the aneurysm by progressive right-to-left rotation (*curved arrows*) of the image (see also text). *LA* left atrium; *LV* left ventricle.

CASE6

A 75-year-old female with a subacute anterior myocardial infarction was admitted to our intensive care unit in a state of cardiogenic shock. Because a harsh systolic murmur was heard at physical examination, she was referred for an echocardiogram. A 2D transthoracic apical approach showed a left-to-right shunt near the apex, leading to the diagnosis of a ventricular septal defect (VSD) resulting from myocardial infarction. With the exception of the apical area, the remaining regions of the left ventricle had a normal wall motion, while the right ventricle was enlarged and hypokinetic. Because of the hemodynamic instability, the patient was intubated and a further transesophageal study (TEE) was performed. A TEE examination confirmed the VSD, and RT 3D TEE showed a large VSD from *en face* perspectives (Figs. 10.22 and 10.23). Due to hemodynamic instability and the large VSD, coronary angiography was urgently performed showing a severe stenosis (90% of lumen narrowing) of the left anterior descending coronary artery (LAD) and collateral vessels from the right coronary artery. It was subsequently decided to intervene surgically in an attempt to repair the VSD. Figure 10.24 shows two steps of the surgical intervention. A patch was inserted and the left mammary artery was grafted to the LAD. The patient survived and returned to the emergency care unit. The murmur disappeared and the patient improved. After 2 days, a new systolic murmur was heard and her clinical status worsened. A patch detachment was suspected. RT 3D TEE confirmed the diagnosis (Fig. 10.25). Because surgeons refused to reintervene, a percutaneous closure of the defect was attempted. The closure was monitored by RT 3D TEE (Figs. 10.26 and 10.27). The percutaneous procedure was successful and the residual left-to-right shunt was significantly reduced (Fig. 10.28). The patient was discharged after 6 days in good clinical condition. After 1 month she was still in good clinical status and the TEE showed a small residual left-to-right shunt. Even if the apical region is distant from transesophageal transducer, in some patients, RT 3D TEE can produce helpful diagnostic images and is a very useful tool as a guide for percutaneous procedures.

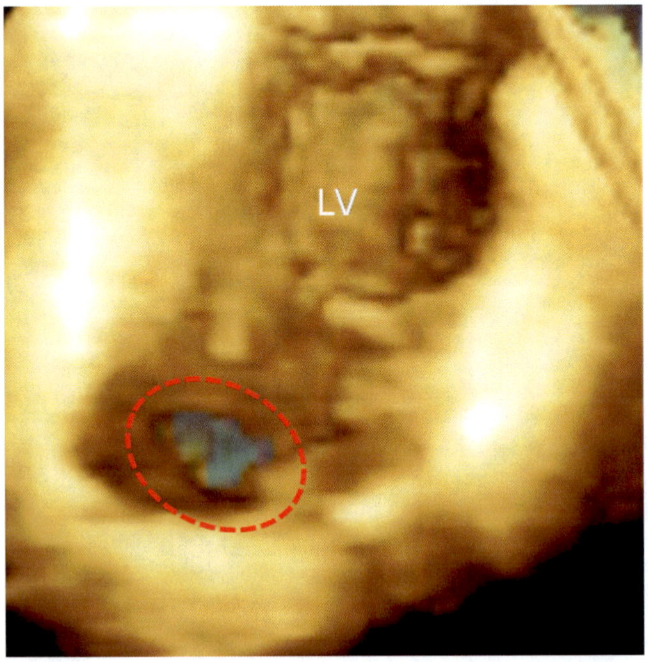

FIGURE 10.22 RT 3D TEE showing a large apical ventricular septal defect (*red dotted circle*) from the left side. *LV* leftv entricle.

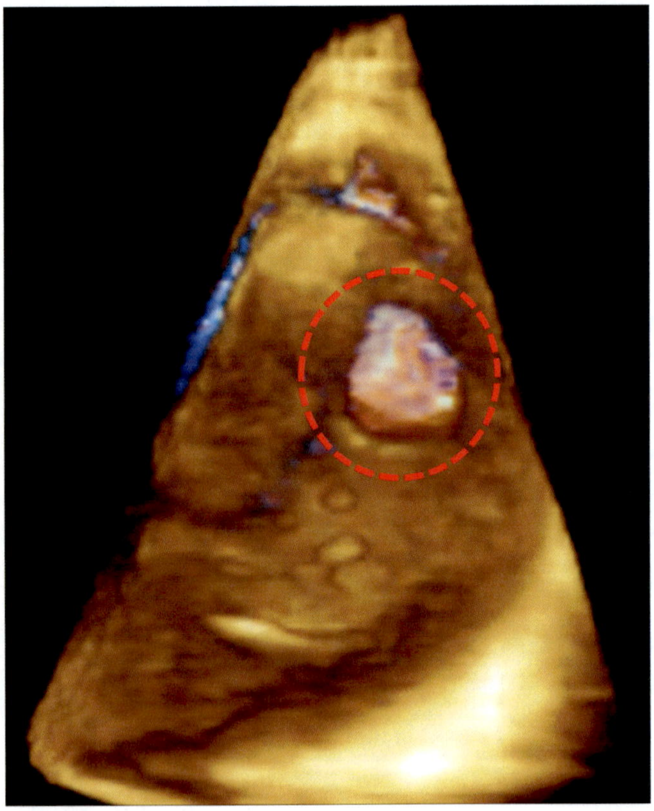

FIGURE 10.23 Color Doppler modality showing a large apical ventricular septal defect (*red dotted circle*) from the left side in a transgastric approach. A color Doppler helps to define the border of the defect.

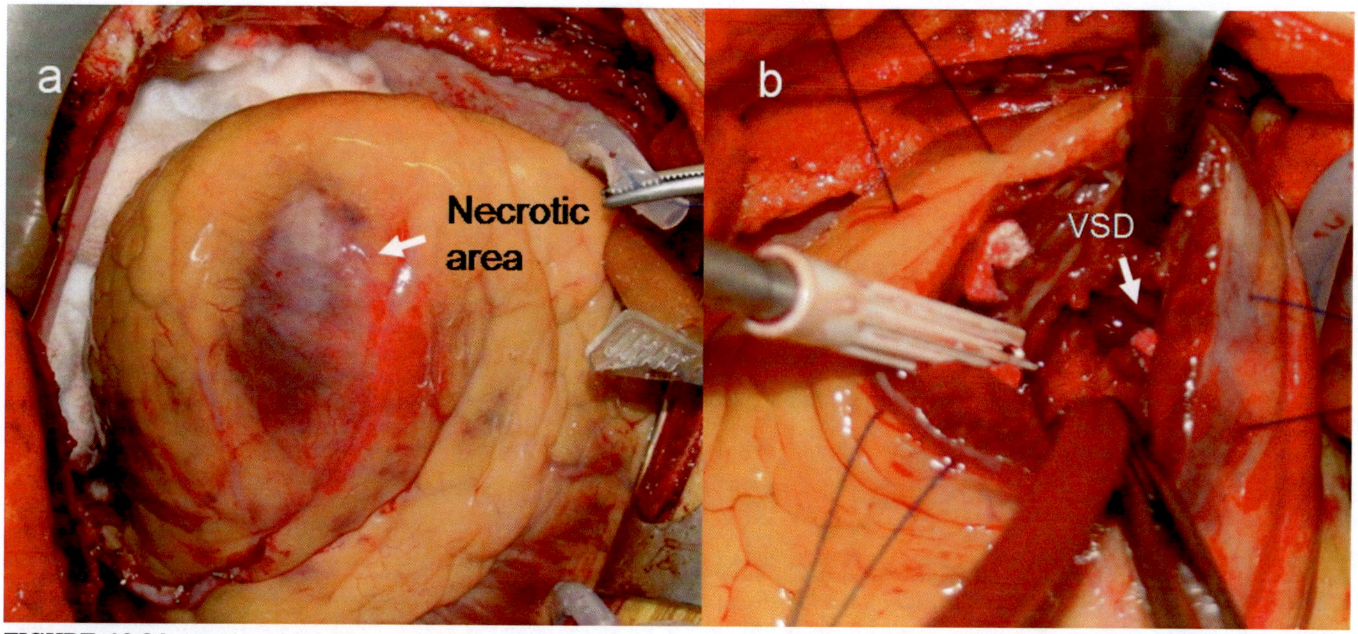

FIGURE 10.24 (a) The exposed heart and the apical infarction. (b) The ventricular septal defect (VSD) is shown through the apical incision.

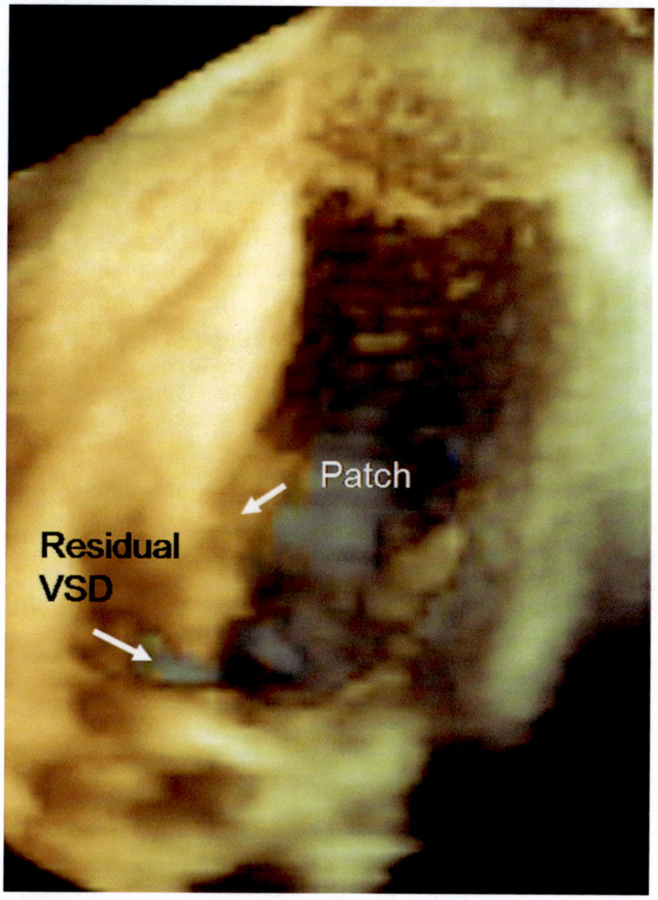

FIGURE 10.25 3D TEE shows the patch detachment of its apical border. *VSD*v entricularsept alde fect.

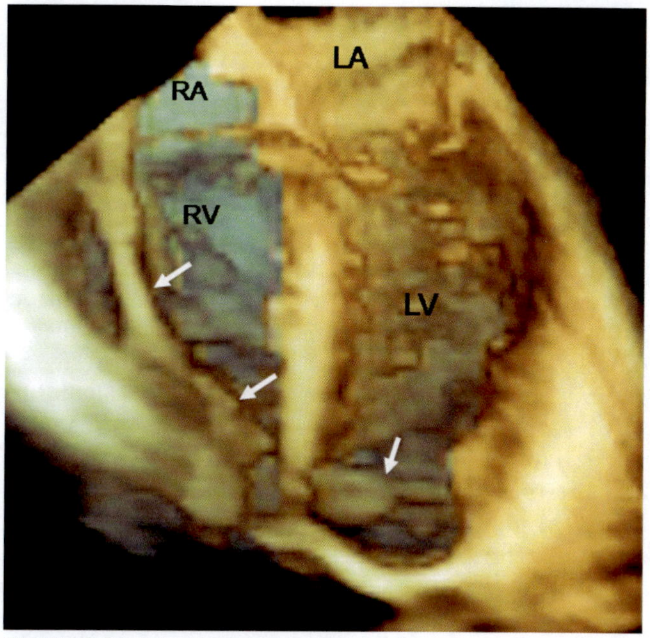

FIGURE 10.26 RT 3D TEE showing a catheter passing through the defect (*arrow*). *LV* left ventricle; *RV* right ventricle; *RA* right atrium; *LA* left atrium.

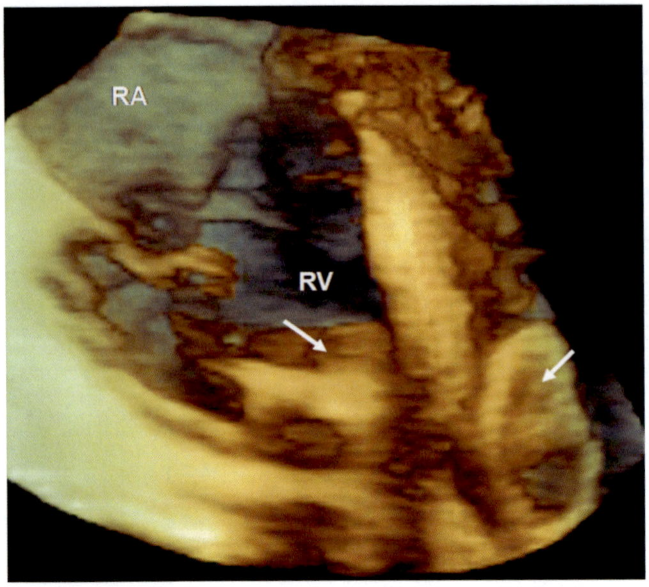

FIGURE 10.27 RT 3D TEE showing the device on both sites of the interventricular septum (*arrows*). *RV* right ventricle; *RA* right atrium.

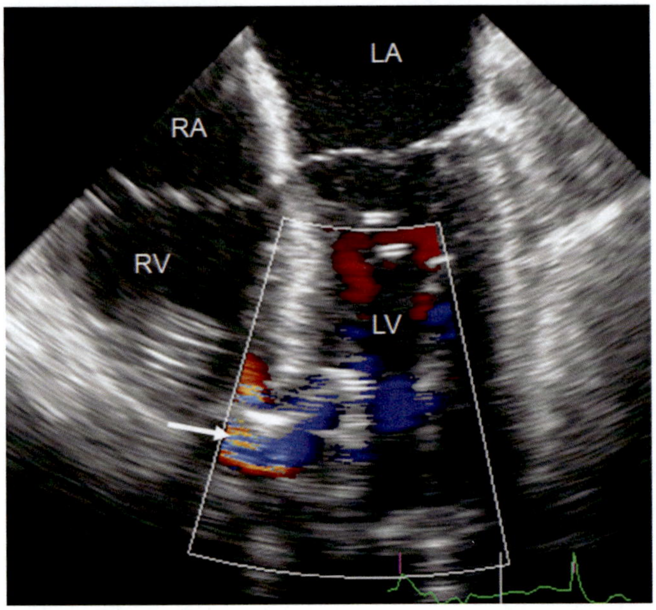

FIGURE 10.28 2D TEE showing a small residual left-to-right shunt (*arrow*). *LV* left ventricle; *RV* right ventricle; *RA* right atrium; *LA* left atrium.

CASE7

A 58-year-old woman suffered from increasing dyspnea on exertion. The patient was known with a history of rheumatic heart disease. Over the course of the previous several months, the patient described increasing dyspnea on exertion, gradually limiting her activities. She ultimately became limited even in her daily routine prompting further evaluation. A transthoracic echocardiogram demonstrated moderate to severe mitral stenosis and minimal mitral regurgitation with a favorable valve score for percutaneous valvuloplasty. She was referred to our institution for the treatment. Under general anesthesia and RT 3D TEE guidance, percutaneous balloon mitral valvuloplasty was performed via a transseptal puncture. On the preprocedure examination, the valve was noted to be thickened with restricted motion and clear commissural fusion (Fig. 10.29). The mitral valve area was 1.1 cm^2. RT 3D TEE was used to guide the operator during the transseptal puncture, and for placing the Inoue balloon in the mitral orifice, prior to balloon inflation (Fig. 10.30). The balloon was inflated under direct visualization (Fig. 10.31). The valve was inspected immediately following the balloon inflation to assess for success and/or complications. Commissural tear was confirmed using RT 3D imaging, as well as an increase in the mitral valve orifice area to 1.7 cm^2 (Fig. 10.32). This was accompanied by a significant drop in left atrial pressure, as measured directly during the procedure. There was no leaflet tear, nor significant residual mitral regurgitation. The patient was discharged to return home the next day and has been doing well, with marked increase in her exercise tolerance since the procedure.

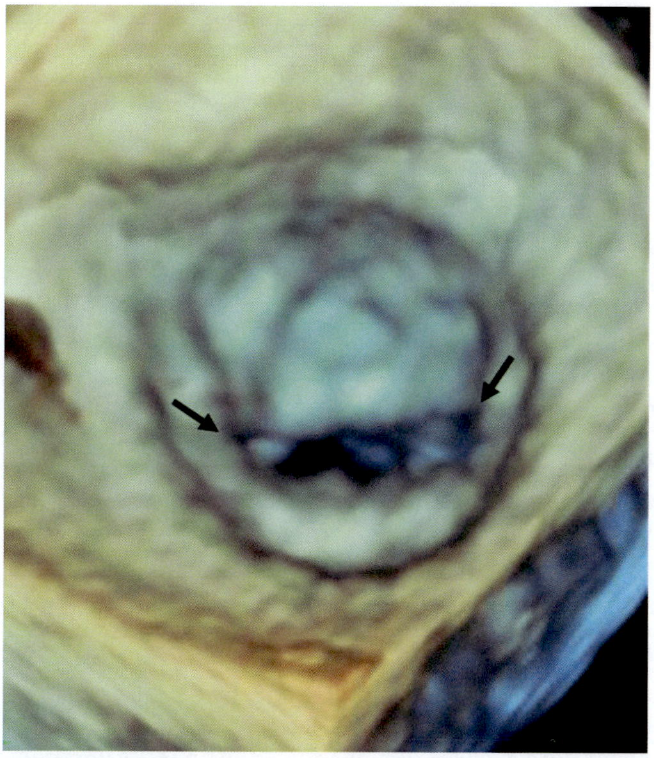

FIGURE 10.29 Real-time 3D TEE of mitral valve orifice seen from the atrial perspective. The valve is thickened with a clear commissural fusion (*arrows*).

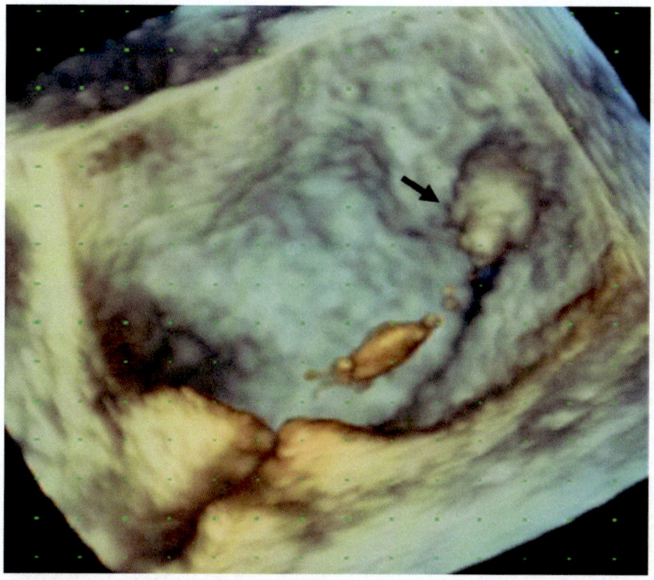

FIGURE 10.30 Real-time 3D TEE showing the deflated balloon (*arrow*)c rossingt hea trials eptum.

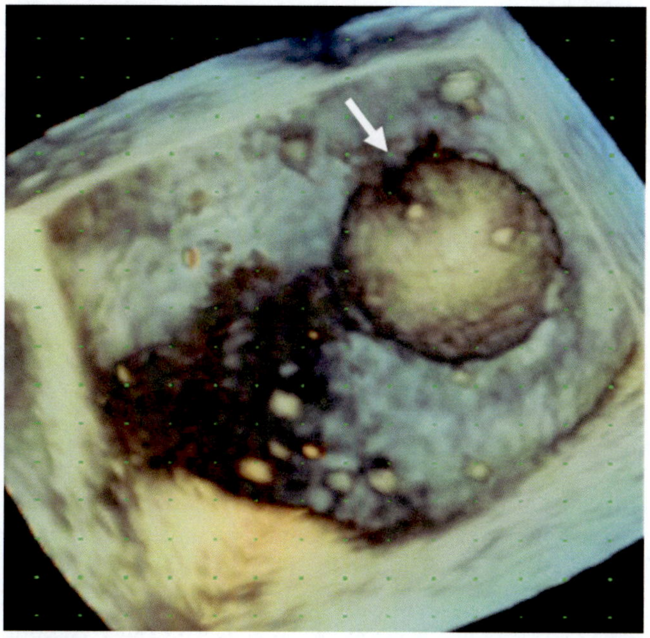

FIGURE 10.31 Real-time 3D TEE showing the balloon inflated (*arrow*).

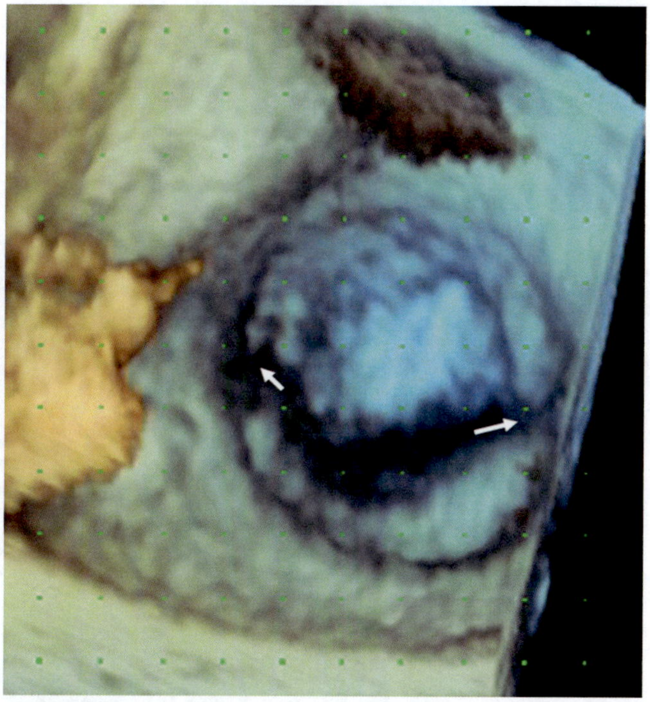

FIGURE 10.32 Real-time 3D TEE showing commissural tears (*arrows*) after the procedure.

PROLOGUE TO CASE 8

Prosthetic mitral valve or mitral valve ring dehiscence is a potential complication of mitral valve surgery. Dehiscence has been reported to occur in as many as 3–4% of all mitral valve procedures. Valve or ring dehiscence can be accompanied with signs and symptoms of congestive heart failure (due to significant paravalvular mitral regurgitation) or with hemolysis, which can be severe and result in blood transfusion requirements as well as heart failure. Traditionally the treatment includes surgical correction. However, since all of these cases involve a reoperation, the surgical risk is elevated and the complication rate is high. More recently, a percutaneous approach to correct these dehiscences has been developed, sparing patients the need for a repeat open heart surgery. One of the key elements for successful percutaneous correction is appropriate selection of the patients, as well as guidance during the procedure. RT 3D TEE is essential for these tasks. RT 3D TEE is used to identify the site of dehiscence. The mitral ring or prosthesis is clearly visualized both from the atrial and ventricular perspective, and the dehisced segment can be visualized from both aspects (Fig. 10.33a). This can help differentiate between a focal, distinct area of dehiscence (which may be amenable to percutaneous closure) and a more diffuse, slit-like dehiscence (which will require surgical replacement). The exact site, shape, and size of the dehisced segment is clearly delineated. 3D TEE imaging is used to guide the percutaneous closure procedure, which can be done via a transseptal approach. Correct placement of the guiding catheter through the dehisced segment is confirmed by RT 3D TEE imaging. Once the catheter is passed through the dehisced segment, an occlusion device is placed. Correct placement, as well as assessment of any residual regurgitation is performed immediately, allowing repositioning if necessary (Fig 10.33b).

CASE 8

A 58-year-old woman, a member of the Jehovah's Witnesses community, was hospitalized due to progressive dyspnea and jaundice. She had undergone mitral valvuloplasty in 1997 for rheumatic mitral stenosis. Following this procedure in 1998 the mitral valve replacement with mechanical bi-leaflet prosthesis was performed due to severe valvular regurgitation.

On admission, the patient revealed the signs of heart failure, anemia, and jaundice. She had a chronic atrial fibrillation and was on warfarin and digoxin therapy. Laboratory analyses demonstrated the presence of hemolytic hyperregenerative anemia (LDH > 2,000 U/L; hemoglobin 7 g/dL with reactive reticulocitosis). TEE demonstrated a slightly decreased left ventricular ejection

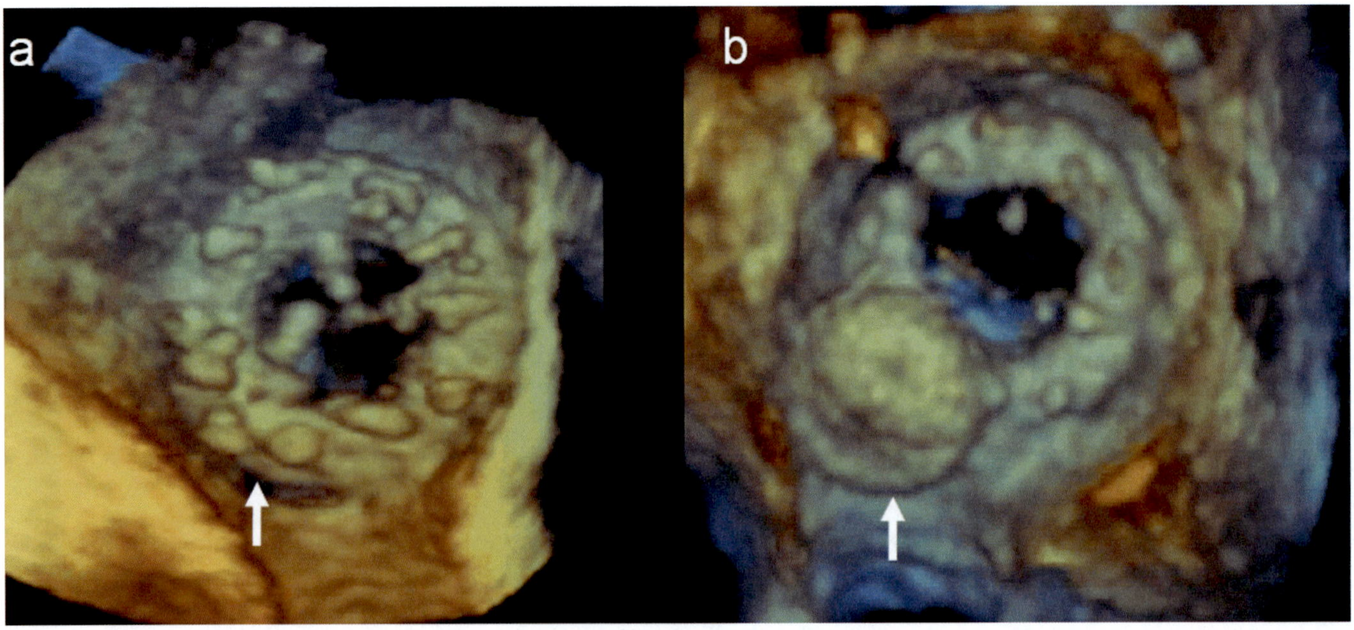

FIGURE 10.33 RT 3D TEE. (a) Dehisced mitral ring as seen from the left atrial perspective. (b) The closure device is in place, completely occludingt hed ehiscedseg ment.

fraction, atriomegaly, mechanical mitral valve prosthesis with normal excursion of hemidiscs, and a medially-located severe para-prosthetic leak. For precise evaluation of the location and relevance of the para-prosthetic leak, 3D TEE was performed. A large para-valvular leak was documented on the postero-medial quadrant (Fig. 10.34). The diagnosis and possible treatment options were thoroughly discussed with the patient. The situation was complicated by the patient's membership of the Jehovah's Witnesses community which does not allow blood transfusions. She had, therefore, an increased risk of surgical intervention. Finally, with the consent of the patient, percutaneous closure of para-prosthetic leak was performed (Fig. 10.35). Postprocedural 3D TEE demonstrated that the Amplatzer Vascular Plug device was well positioned with a moderate residual para-prosthetic leak (Fig. 10.36). The postprocedural period has not revealed complications.

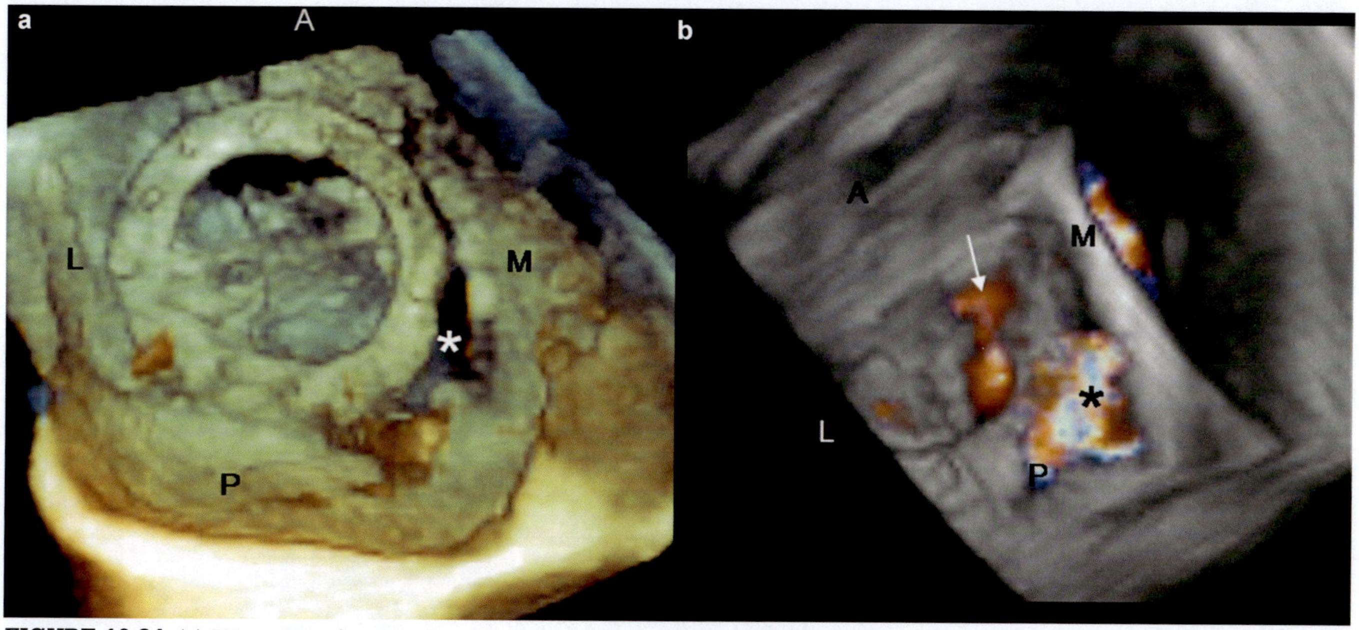

FIGURE 10.34 (a) RT 3D TEE showing the site and size of the dehiscence (*asterisk*). (b) 3D TEE color Doppler showing the paravalvular regurgitant jet (*asterisk*). The *arrow* points to a minor jet of intraprosthetic regurgitation. *A* anterior; *M* medial; *P* posterior; *L* lateral.

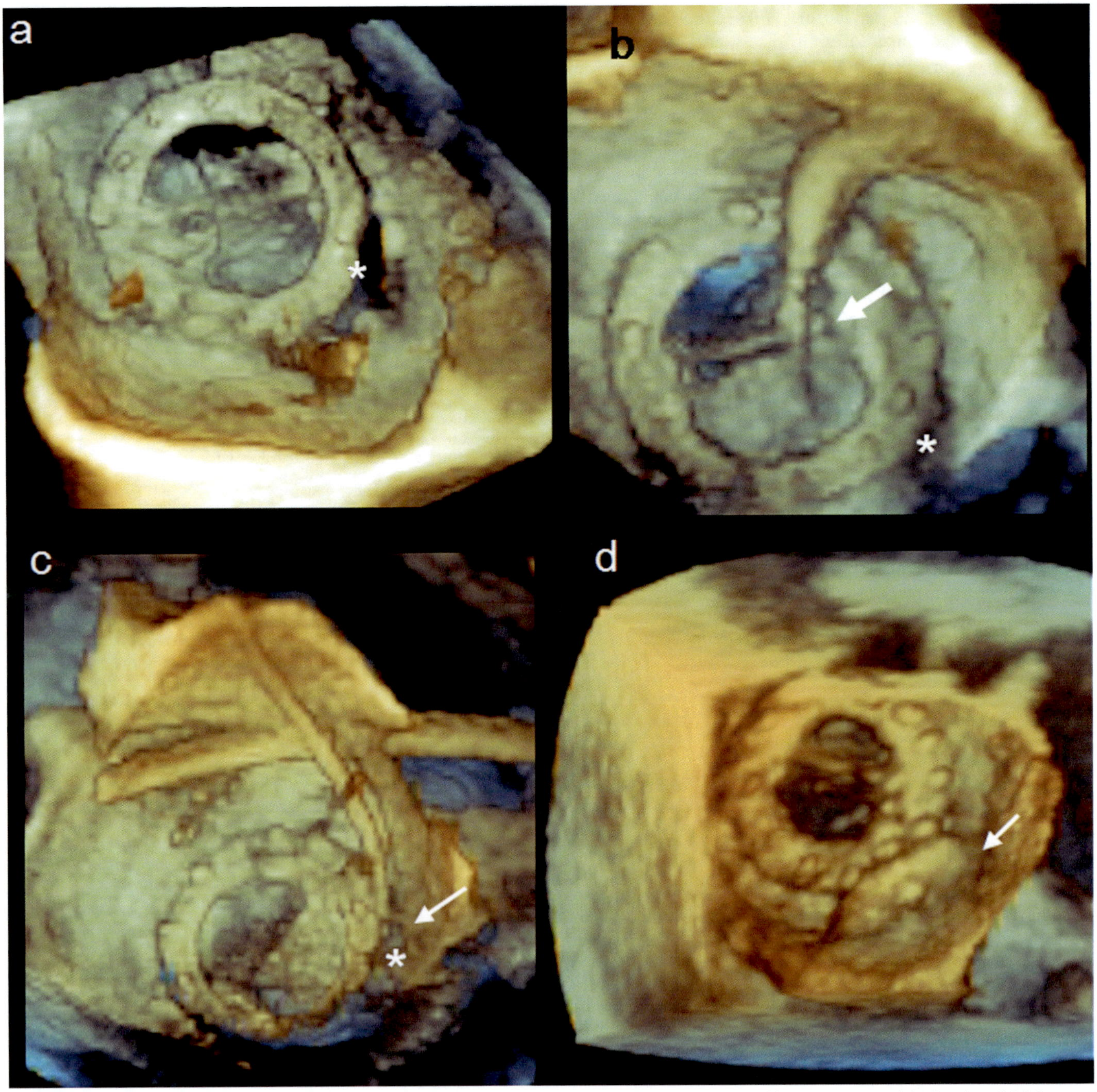

FIGURE 10.35 Steps of the percutaneous closure of the para-prosthetic leak (*asterisk*) monitored by RT 3D TEE. (a) The site of dehiscence. (b) The first attempt to pass a guiding catheter through the dehisced segment: the catheter was wrongly located through the prosthesis orifice (*arrow*). (c) Upon second attempt, the catheter was successfully inserted through the dehiscence (*arrow*). (d) The closure device was deployed correctly (*arrow*).

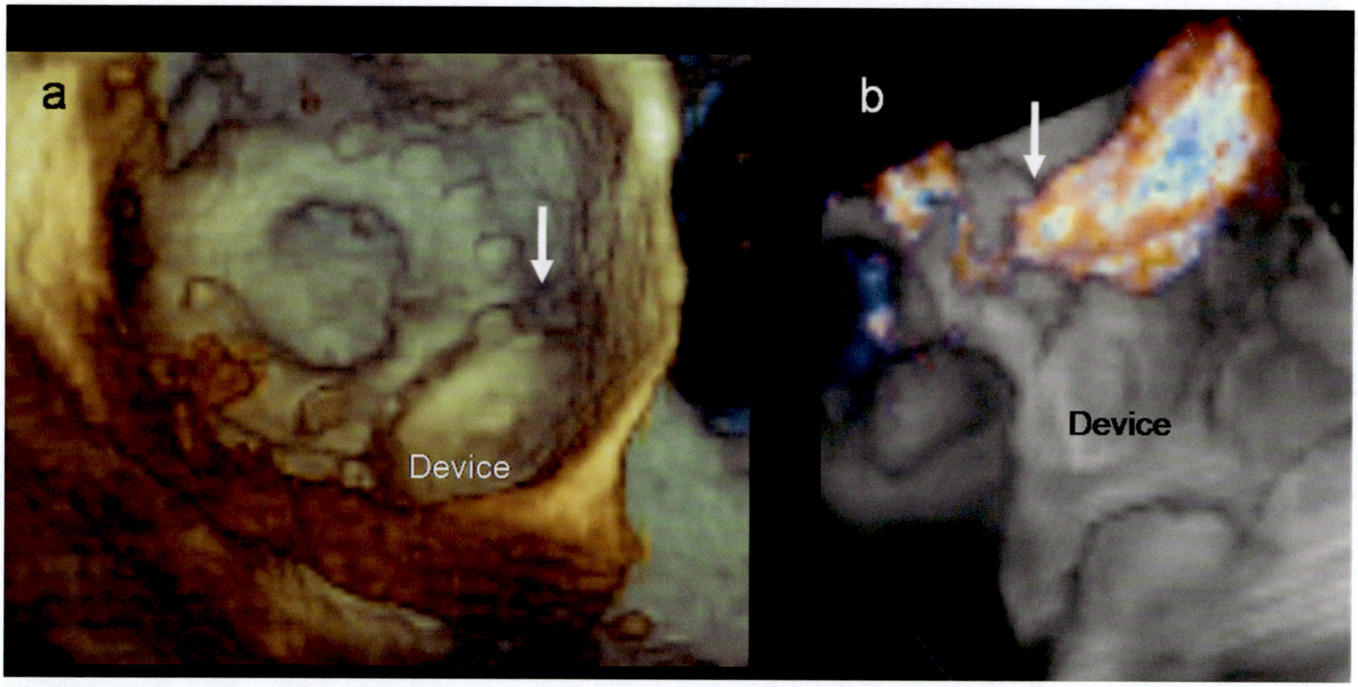

FIGURE 10.36 (a) RT 3D TEE showing the device and a residual leak (*arrow*). (b) The full volume 3D TEE color Doppler shows a residual moderate para-prosthetic regurgitation (*arrow*).

CASE 9

A 64-year-old male patient with a history of severe coronary artery disease (multiple myocardial infarctions and coronary bypass graft surgery), dyslipidemia, diabetes mellitus, and chronic obstructive pulmonary disease, was referred to our center with worsening heart failure symptoms.

TEE showed left ventricular enlargement with severe dysfunction (ejection fraction <0.30), multiple wall motion abnormalities including akinesis with thin and hyperechogenic walls (presumably scar tissue) at the apex, septum, and inferior segments. There was pronounced pulmonary hypertension (65 mmHg) and severe mitral regurgitation. For a better understanding of the valve morphology and regurgitation mechanism, RT 3D TEE was performed. The examination revealed dilatation of the mitral annulus with a loss of coaptation between the mitral leaflets, predominantly located in the medial region (Figs. 10.37 and 10.38).

The possible treatment options were discussed with the cardiac surgeons and the patient. For primary prevention of sudden cardiac death, an ICD was implanted. Then taking into account the high operative risk (EUROSCORE 26%) and with the consent of the patient, a percutaneous edge-to-edge MitraClip procedure was performed. Figs. 10.38–10.48, show the procedure step-by-step.

The postprocedural period was free of complications. RT 3D TEE showed mild residual regurgitation without signs of mitral flow obstruction (Fig 10.49). The patient was discharged from the hospital 2 days after the procedure in improved clinical status.

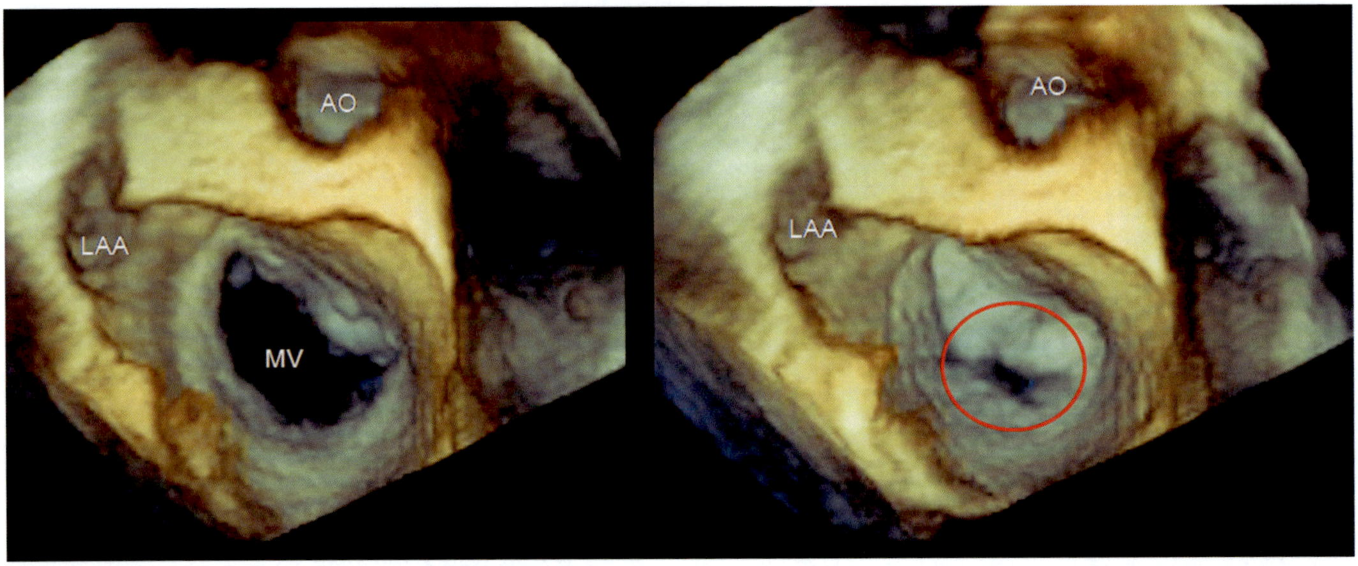

FIGURE 10.37 3D TEE in full volume modality showing the mitral valve (MV) (a) in diastole and (b) in systole. An evident regurgitant orifice is marked with a red circle. *Ao* aorta; *LAA*l efta triala ppendage.

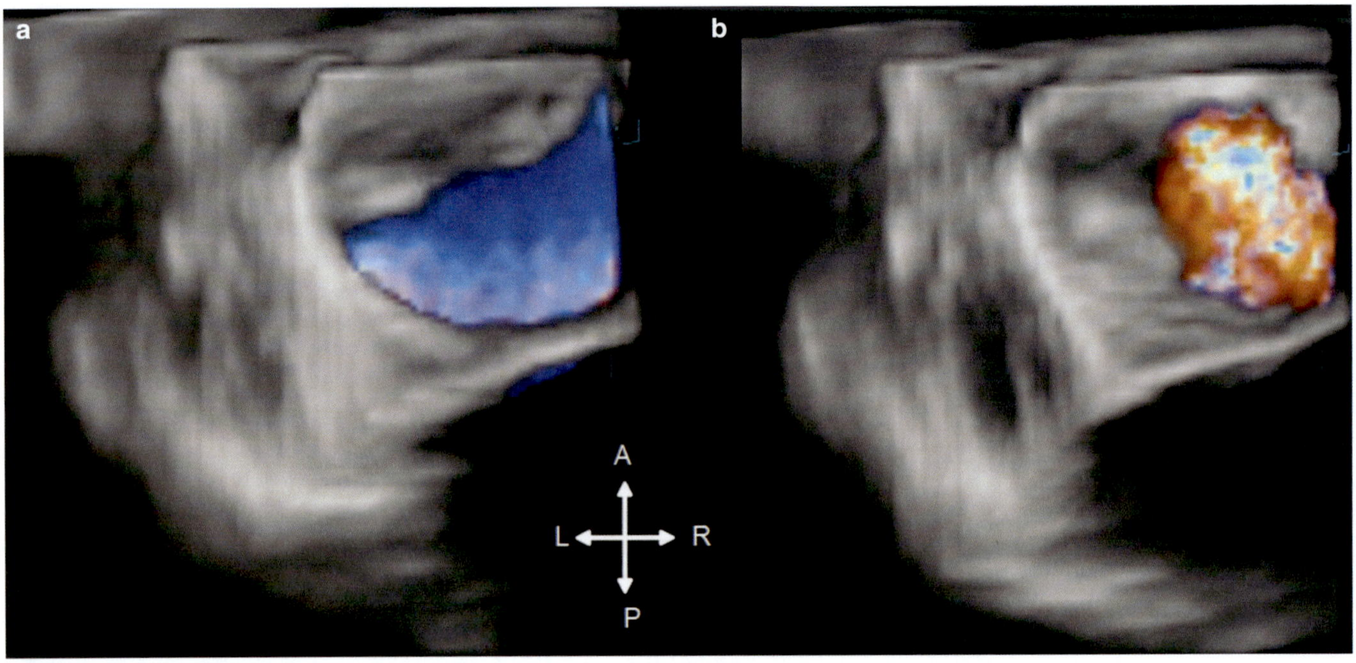

FIGURE 10.38 Full volume 3D TEE in color Doppler modality showing the mitral valve (a) in diastole and (b) in systole. The regurgitant jet is emerging from the medial region of the coaptation line.

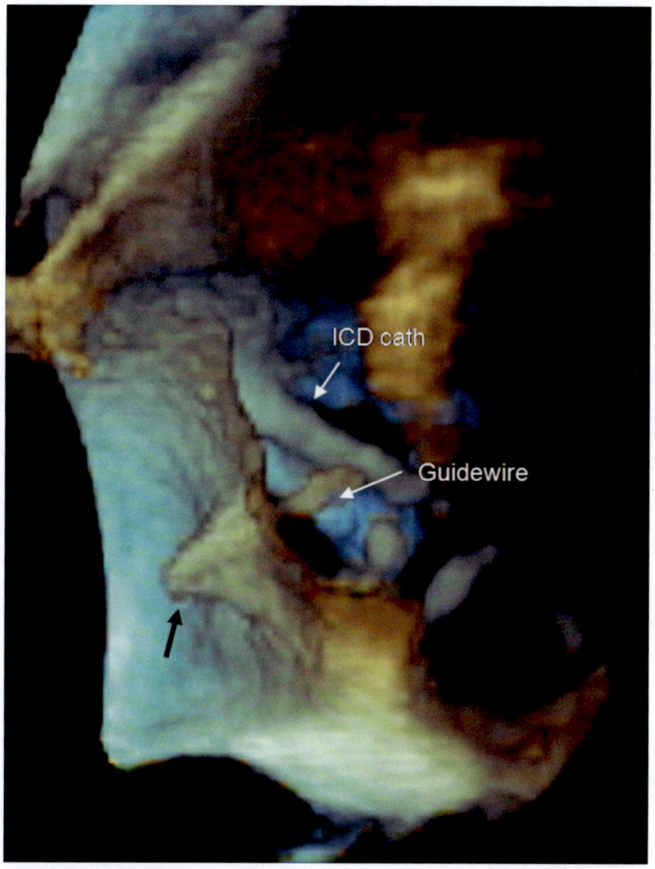

FIGURE 10.39 Step 1. The correct puncture site on the atrial septum was identified through recognition of the tenting (*black arrow*).

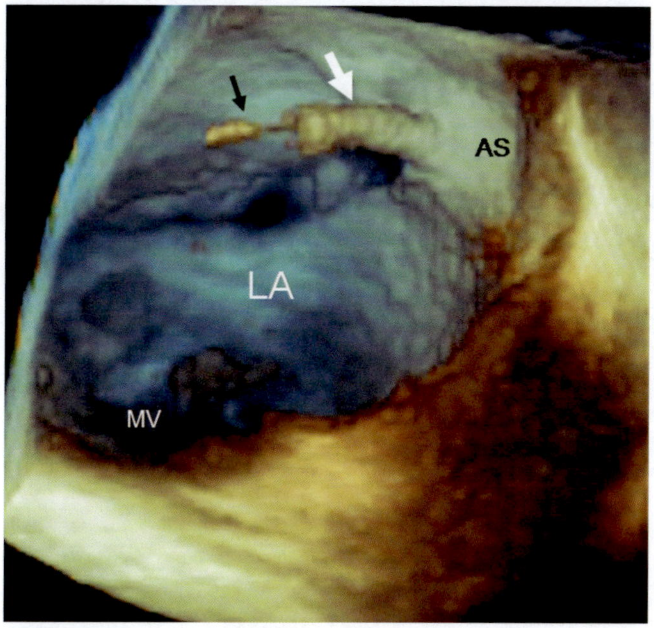

FIGURE 10.40 Step 2. A transseptal apparatus (*black arrow*) was exchanged for a guide catheter (*white arrow*). *LA* left atrium; *MV* mitral valve; *AS*a trialsept um.

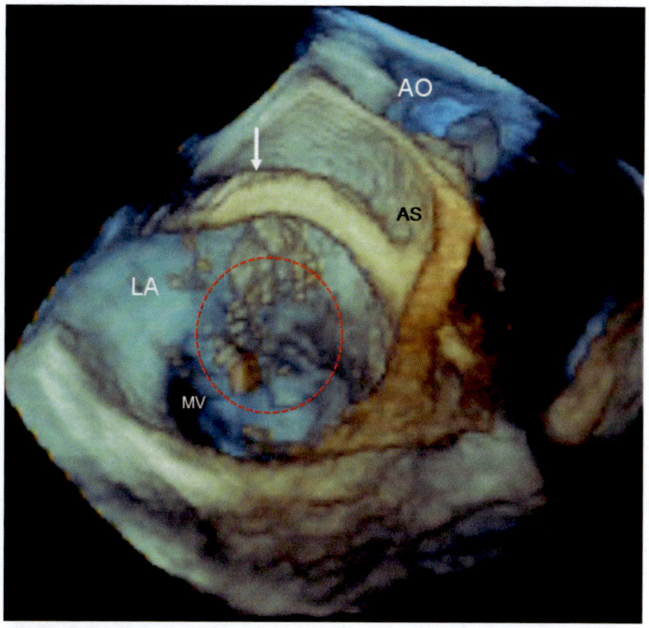

FIGURE 10.41 Step 3. The guide (*arrow*) was positioned in the mid left atrium (LA) de-aired and flushed (bubbles in the atrium are indicated by the *red dotted circle*). *LA* left atrium; *MV* mitral valve; *AS* atrial septum; *AO* aorta.

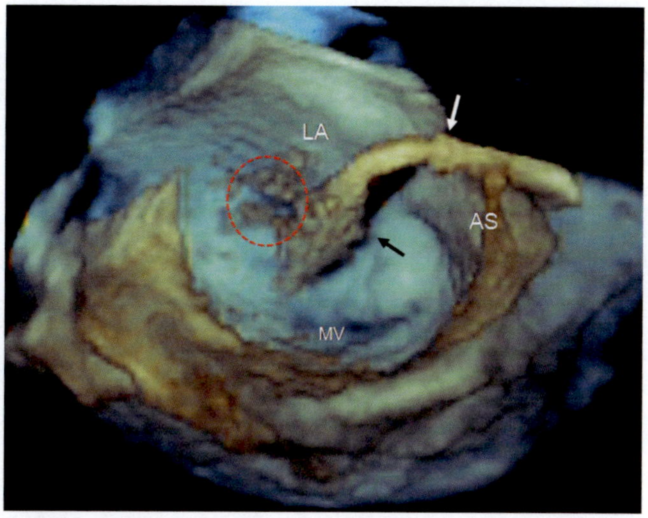

FIGURE 10.42 Step 4. The clip delivery system (*black arrow*) was introduced into the guide catheter (*white arrow*) and advanced into the left atrium (LA). Bubbles in the atrium are indicated by the *red dotted circle*. The clip was moved in small iterations until it was centered over the mitral orifice. *MV* mitral valve; *AS* atrial septum.

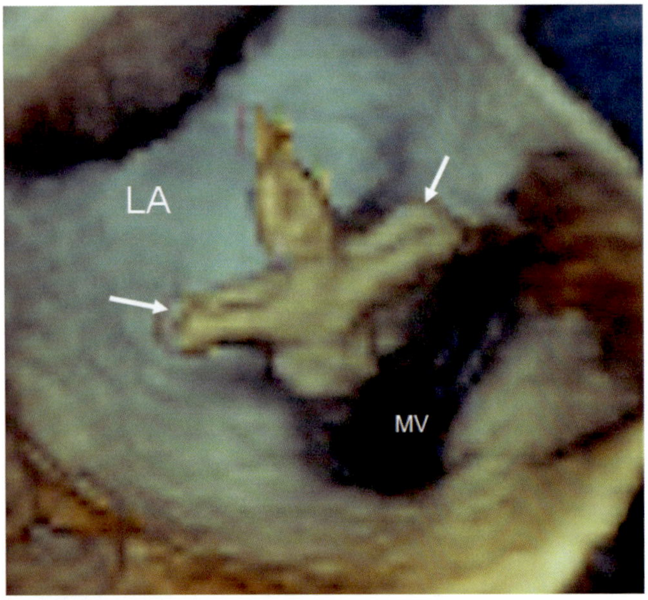

FIGURE 10.43 Step 5. The arms of the clip were opened (*arrows*). *LA* left atrium; *MV*m itralv alve.

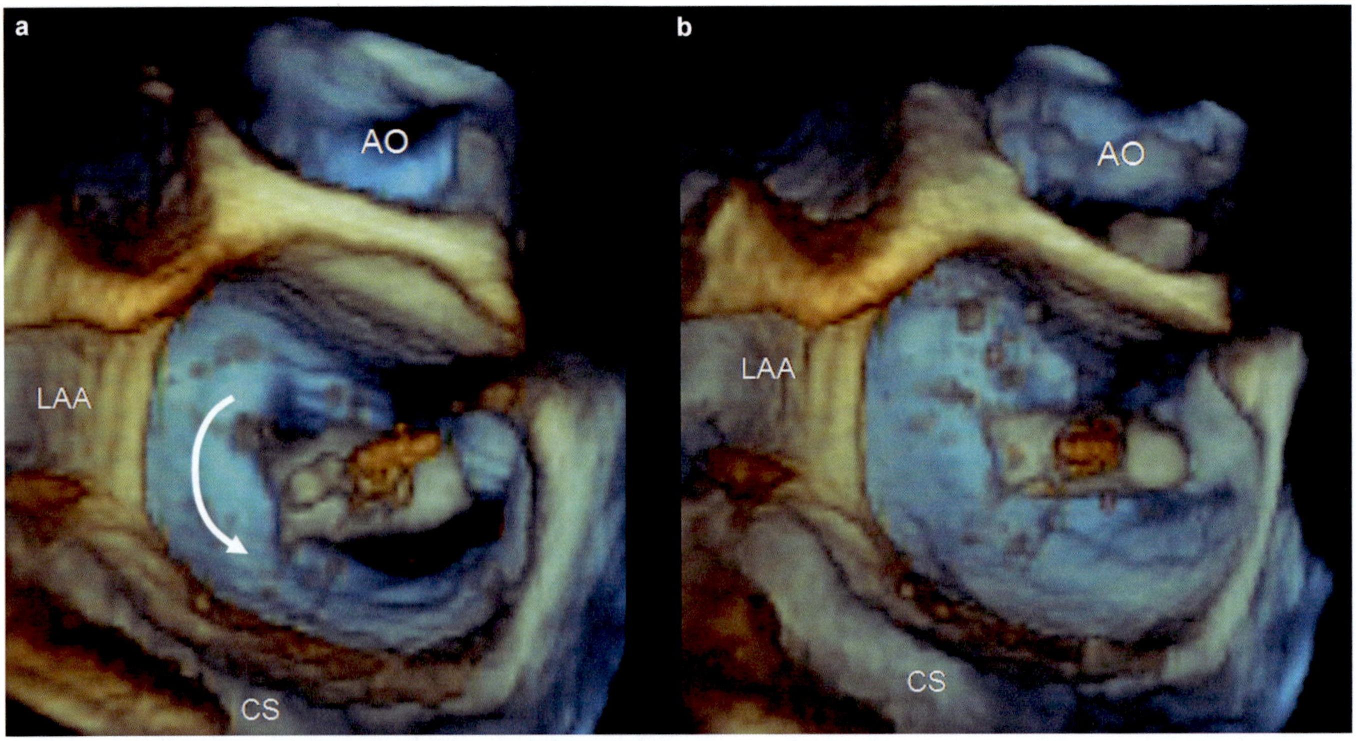

FIGURE 10.44 Step 6. The arms were not aligned perpendicular to the line of coaptation. Thus, a counter-clockwise rotation (*curved arrow*) was necessary. Images (a) in diastole and (b) in systole. *LAA* left atrial appendage; *AO* aorta; *CS* coronary sinus.

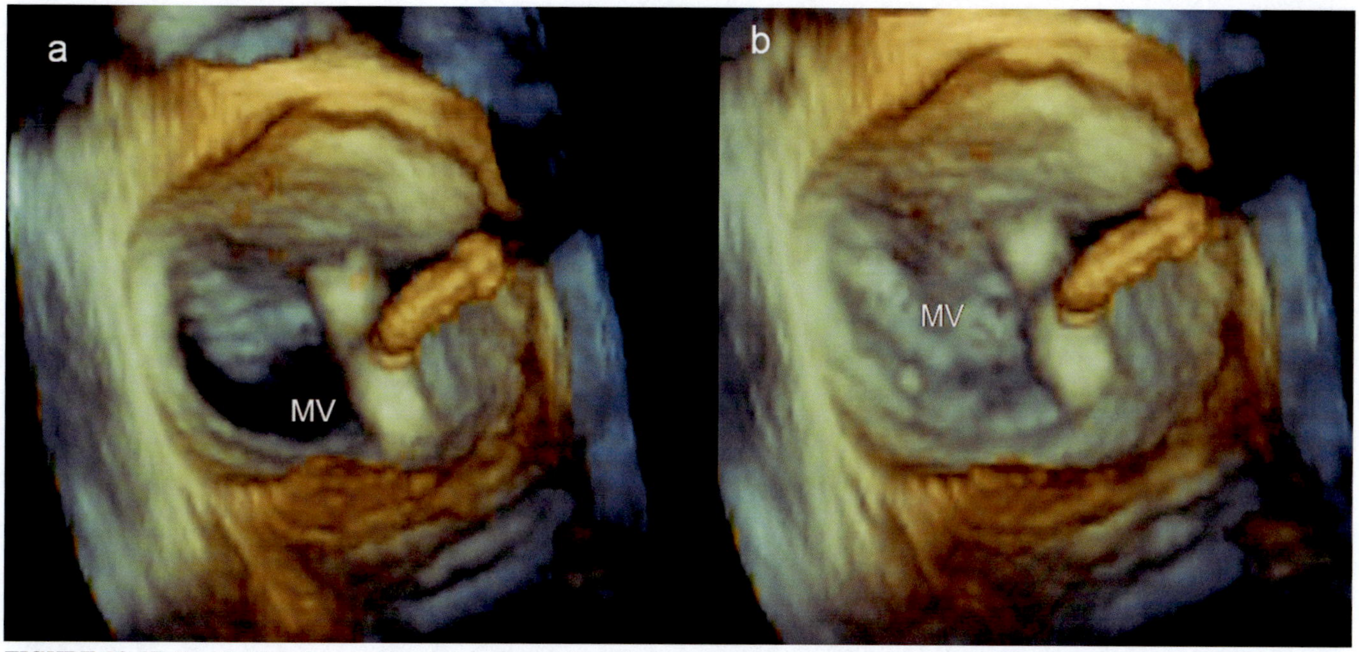

FIGURE 10.45 Step 7. After the rotation, the arms were aligned perpendicular to the line of coaptation of the mitral leaflets and positioned over the medial region (the target region). Images (a) in diastole and (b) in systole. *MV* mitral valve.

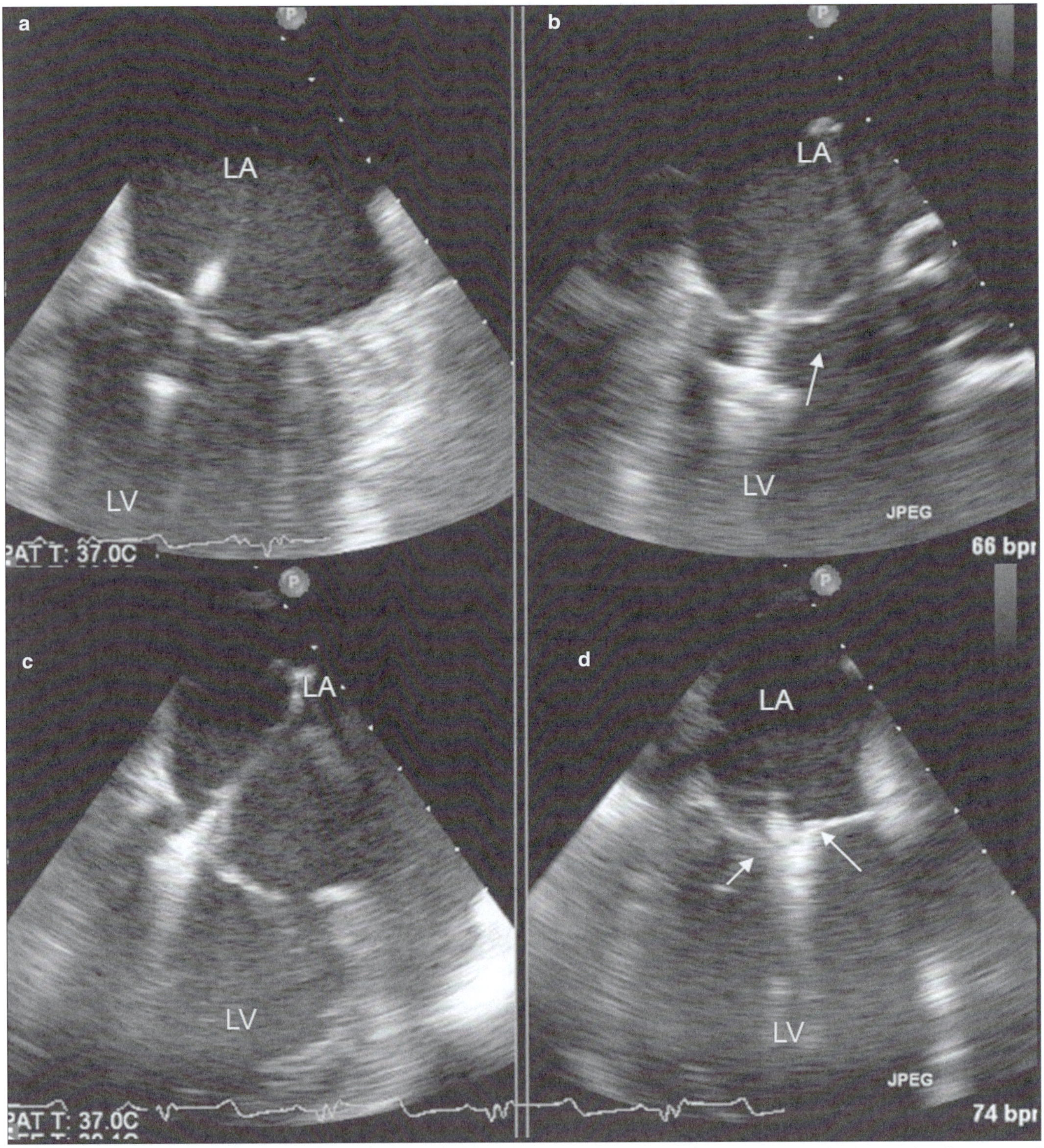

FIGURE 10.46 Step 8. (a, b) The clip was advanced into the left ventricle just below the mitral leaflet edges. Then it was closed to 120° and pulled back (*arrow*). (c, d) Mitral leaflets were captured in the arms of the clip (*arrows*). These maneuvers are usually better monitored with 2D TEE. *LA* left atrium; *LV* leftv entricle.

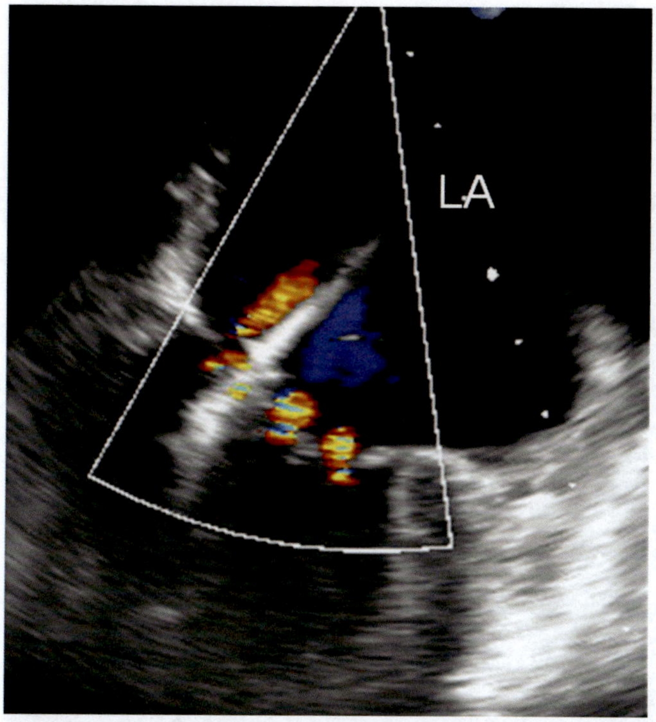

FIGURE 10.47 Step 9. The clip was incrementally closed under the guidance of 2D TEE. The adequacy of the grasp, degree of regurgitation, and diastolic transmitral gradients were assessed before the clip was released. *LA*l efta trium.

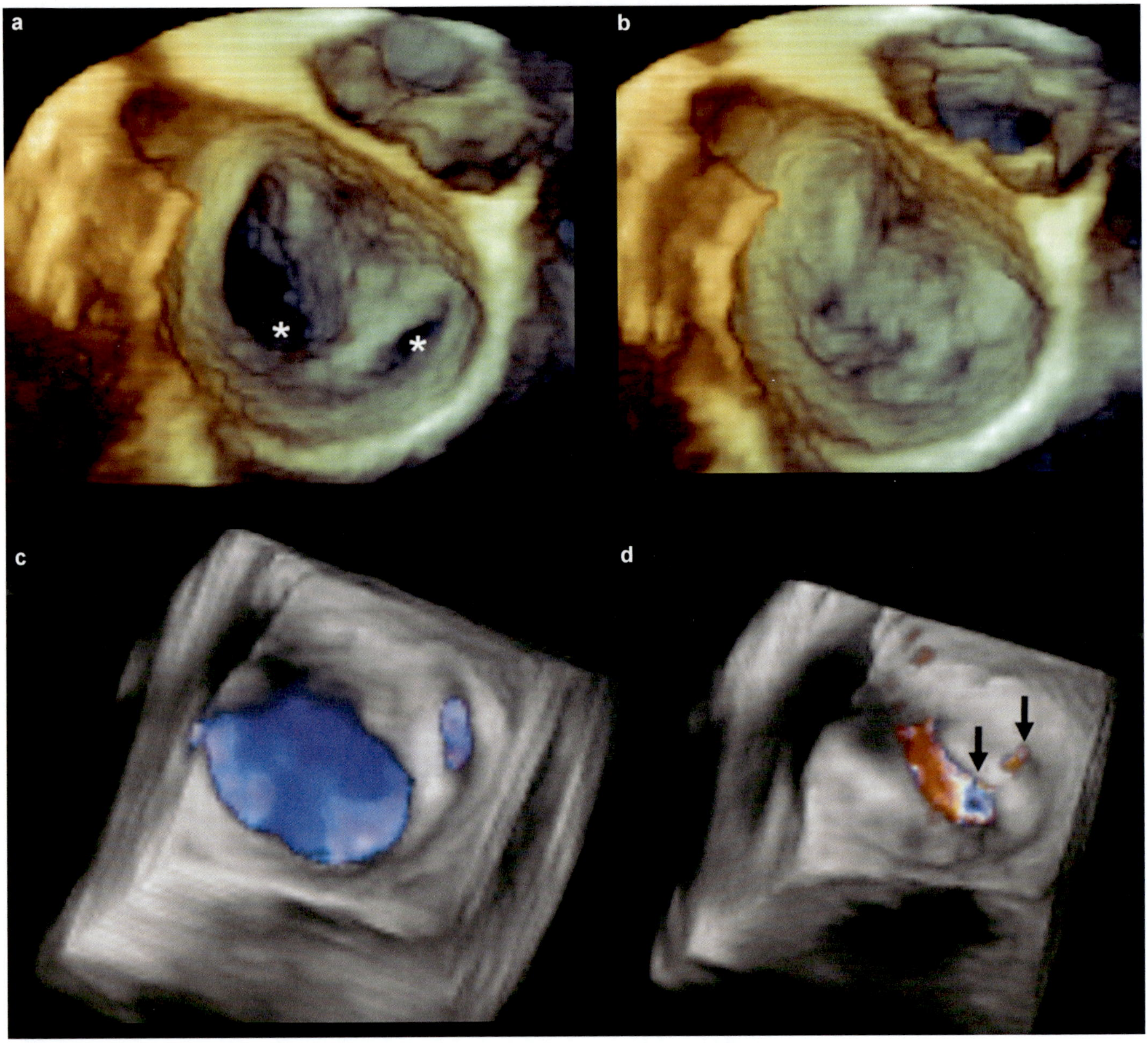

FIGURE 10.48 Real-time 3D TEE in zoom modality from the atrial perspective (a) in diastole and (b) in systole. A double orifice is shown (*asterisks*). (c,d) 3D TEE in color Doppler modality from the atrial perspective: (c) diastolic frame showing the absence of turbulence flow (which means the absence of significant gradient); (d) systolic frame showing a residual mild mitral regurgitation (*arrows*).

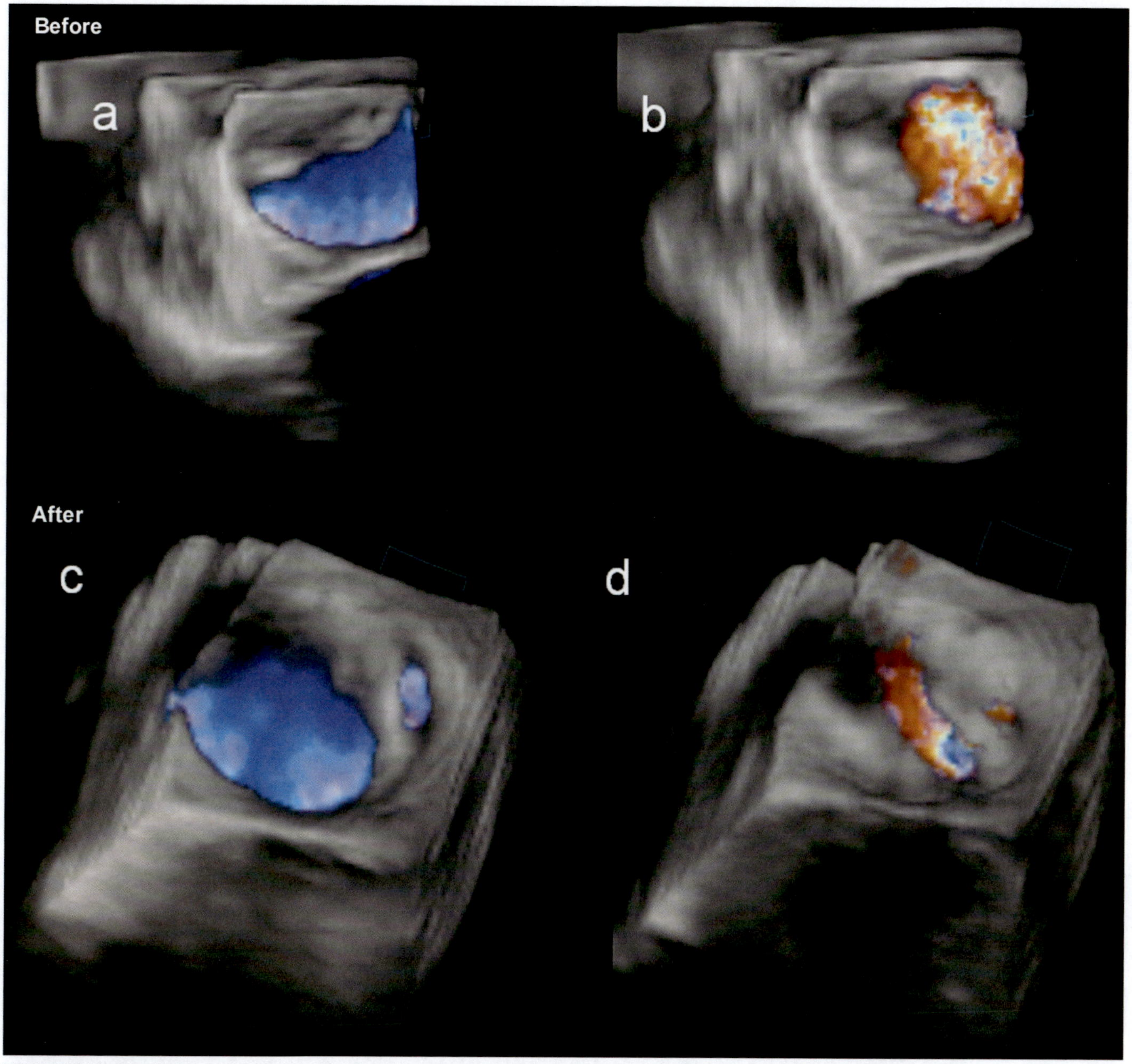

FIGURE 10.49 3D TEE (a, b) before and (c, d) after the procedure showing the significant reduction in mitral regurgitation.

CASE 10

A 59-year-old male was admitted due to progressive shortness of breath, nocturnal dyspnea, increase of weight, and peripheral edemas. He had a history of myxomatous mitral valve disease with prolapse of both leaflets with mild regurgitation. Antibiotics prophylaxis for endocarditis had been recommended. The patient did not claim fever, recent infections, or surgical interventions. No comorbidities were found. Physical examination revealed a harsh systolic murmur at the apex, mild hepatomegaly, and leg edema. Both 2D and 3D TEE demonstrated anterior leaflet perforation with small elongated mobile vegetations (Figs. 10.50 and 10.51). With real-time 3D TEE, the perforation was precisely localized centrally on the body of the anterior leaflet (Fig. 10.51). Surgical inspection before valve replacement confirmed 3D TEE findings (Fig. 10.52).

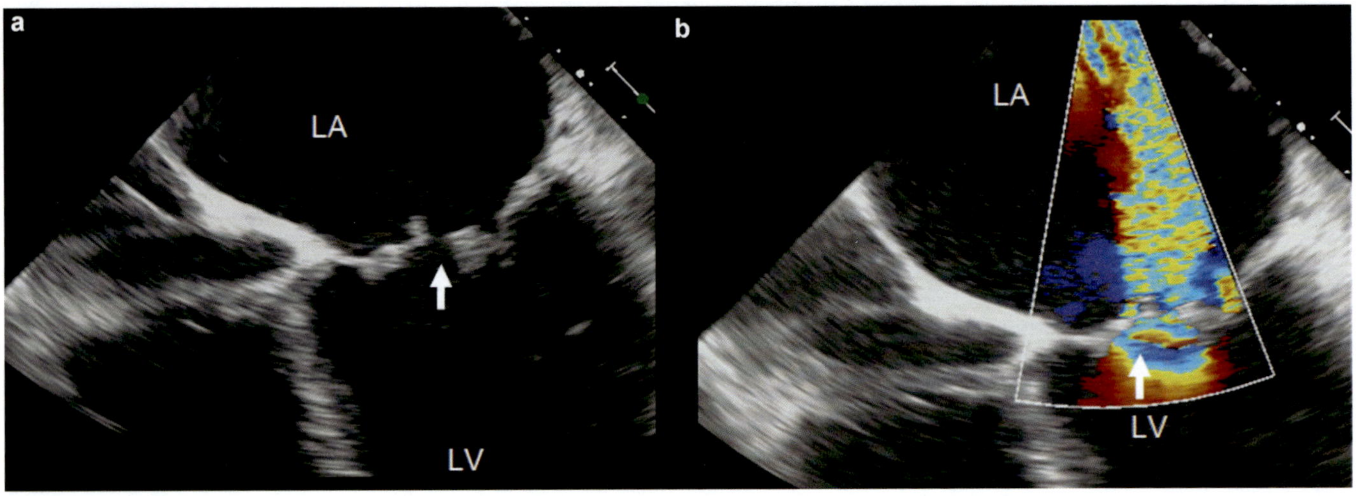

FIGURE 10.50 2D TEE in systole showing (a) the perforation (*arrow*) and (b) the severe mitral regurgitation through the hole (*arrow*). *LA* left atrium; *LV*l eftv entricle.

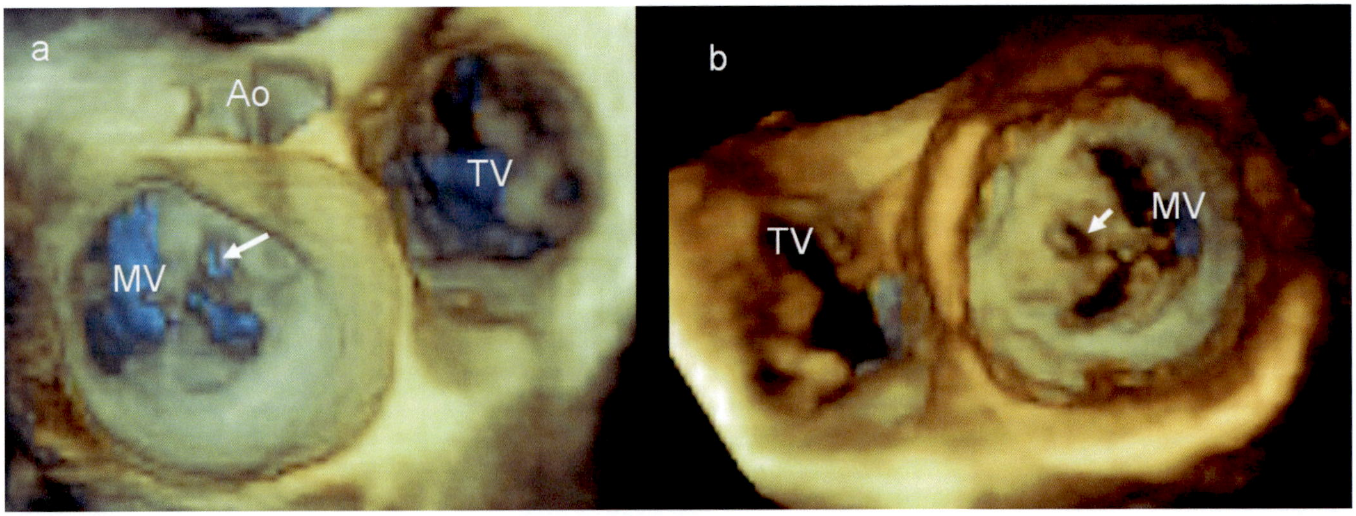

FIGURE 10.51 3D TEE in full volume modality showing the hole on the anterior leaflet (*arrow*) from (a) the left atrial and (b) the left ventricular perspectives. *MV* mitral valve; *TV* tricuspid valve; *Ao* aortic valve.

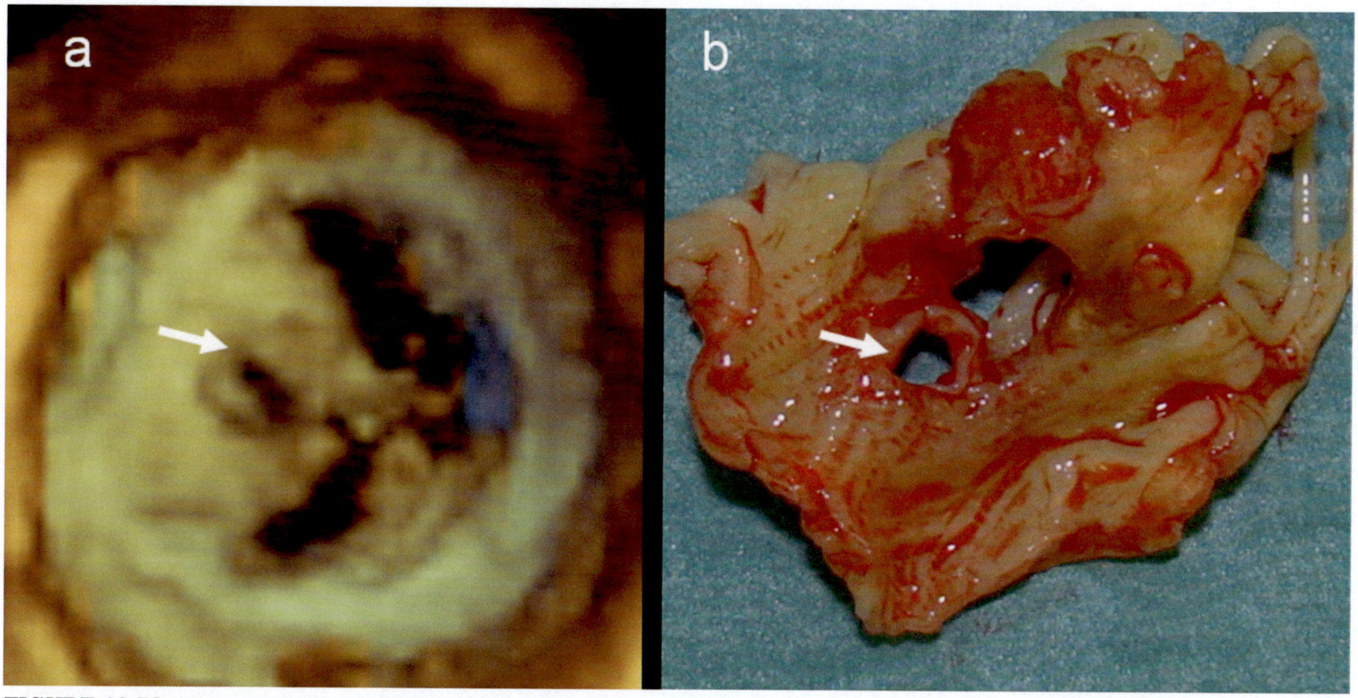

FIGURE 10.52 (a) Details of the 3D TEE image showing the hole in the body of the anterior leaflet (*arrow*) from a ventricular perspective and(b)t hec orrespondinga natomical specimen.

SUGGESTEDR EADINGS

General

American Heart Association, American College of Cardiology, and Society of Nuclear Medicine. Standardization of cardiac tomographic imaging. *Circulation*. 1992;86:338–339.

Anderson RH, Becker AE. *Cardiac Anatomy*. Edinburgh: Churchill Livingstone; 1980.

Anderson RH, Ho SY, Brecker SJ. Anatomic basis of cross–sectional echocardiography. *Heart*. 2001;85:716–720.

Anderson RH, Razavi R, Taylor AM. Cardiac anatomy revisited. *J Anat*.2004; 205:159–177.

Cook AC, Anderson RH. Attitudinally correct nomenclature. *Heart*.2002; 87:503–506.

Lang RM, Mor–Avi V, Sugeng L, Nieman PS, Sahn DJ. Three–dimensional echocardiography: the benefits of the additional dimension. *J Am Coll Cardiol*. 2006;48:2053–2069.

Waller BF, Taliercio CP, Slack JD, et al. Tomographic views of normal and abnormal hearts: the anatomic basis for various cardiac imaging techniques, Part I. *Clin Cardiol*. 1990;13:804–812.

Mitral Valve

de Castro S, Salandin V, Cartoni D, et al. Qualitative and quantitative evaluation of mitral valve morphology by intraoperative volume–rendered three–dimensional echocardiography. *J Heart Valve Dis*.2 002;11:173–180.

Ho SY. Anatomy of the mitral valve. *Heart*. 2002;88:5–10.

Kahlert P, Plicht B, Schenk IM, Janosi RA, Erbel R, Buck T. Direct assessment of size and shape of noncircular vena contracta area in functional versus organic mitral regurgitation using real–time three–dimensional echocardiography. *J Am Soc Echocardiogr*.2008 ;21:912–921.

Kronzon I, Sugeng L, Perk G, Hirsh D, Weinert L, Garcia Fernandez MA, Lang RM. Real–time 3–dimensional transesophageal echocardiography in the evaluation of post–operative mitral annuloplasty ring and prosthetic valve dehiscence. *J Am Coll Cardiol*. 2009;53(17):1543–1547.

O'Gara P, Sugeng L, Lang R, Sarano M, Hung J, Raman S, Fischer G, Carabello B, Adams D, Vannan M. The role of imaging in chronic degenerative mitral regurgitation. *JACC Cardiovasc Imaging*. 2008;1(2):221–237; review.

Perloff JK, Roberts WC. The mitral valve apparatus. Functional anatomy of mitral regurgitation. *Circulation*. 1972;46:227–239.

Sugeng L, Shernan SK, Weinert L, Shook D, Raman J, Jeevanandam V, DuPont F, Fox J, Mor–Avi V, Lang RM. Real–time three–dimensional transesophageal echocardiography in valve disease: comparison with surgical findings and evaluation of prosthetic valve. *J Am Soc Echocardiogr*. 2008;21(12):1347–1354.

Tsukiji M, Watanabe N, Yamaura Y, et al. Three–dimensional quantitation of mitral valve coaptation by a novel software system with transthoracic real–time three–dimensional echocardiography. *J Am Soc Echocardiogr*. 2008;21:43–46.

Yosefy C, Levine RA, Solis J, Vaturi M, Handschumacher MD, Hung J. Proximal flow convergence region as assessed by real–time 3–dimensional echocardiography: challenging the hemispheric assumption. *J Am Soc Echocardiogr*. 2007;20:389–396.

Zamorano J, Cordeiro P, Sugeng L, et al. Real–time three–dimensional echocardiography for rheumatic mitral valve stenosis evaluation: an accurate and novel approach. *J Am Coll Cardiol*. 2004;43:2091–2096.

Tricuspid Valve

Anwar AM, Soliman OI, Nemes A, van Geuns RJ, Geleijnse ML, ten Cate FJ. Value of assessment of tricuspid annulus: real–time three–dimensional echocardiography and magnetic resonance imaging. *Int J Cardiovasc Imaging*. 2007;23:701–705.

Faletra F, La Marchesina U, Bragato R, De Chiara F. Three dimensional transthoracic echocardiography images of tricuspid stenosis. *Heart*. 2005;91:499.

Kwan J, Kim GC, Jeon MJ, et al. 3D geometry of a normal tricuspid annulus during systole: a comparison study with the mitral annulus using real–time 3D echocardiography. *Eur J Echocardiogr*.2007; 8:375–383.

Park YH, Song JM, Lee EY, Kim YJ, Kang DH, Song JK. Geometric and hemodynamic determinants of functional tricuspid regurgitation: a real–time three–dimensional echocardiography study. *Int J Cardiol*. 2008;124:160–165.

Aortic Valve

Anderson RH. Clinical anatomy of aortic root. *Heart*. 2000; 84:670–673.

Gutierrez–Chico JL, Zamorano JL, Prieto–Moriche E, et al. Real–time three–dimensional echocardiography in aortic stenosis: a novel, simple, and reliable method to improve accuracy in area calculation. *Eur Heart J*. 2008;29:1296–1306.

Ho SY. Structure and anatomy of the aortic root. *Eur J Echocardiogr*.2009; 10:i3–10.

Underwood M, Khoury GE, Deronck D, et al. *The aortic root: structure, function and surgical reconstruction. Heart*. 2000;83:376–380.

Yacoub MH, Kilner PJ, Birks EJ, Misfeld M. The aortic outflow and root: a tale of dynamism and crosstalk. *Ann Thorac Surg*.1 999;68(3su ppl):S37–S43.

Leftan dR ight Atrium

Anwar AM, Soliman OI, Geleijnse ML, Nemes A, Vletter WB, ten Cate FJ. Assessment of left atrial volume and function by real–time three–dimensional echocardiography. *Int J Cardiol*.2008; 123:155–161.

Asirvatham SJ. Correlative anatomy and electrophysiology for interventional electrophysiologist: right atrial flutter. *J Cardiovasc Electrophysiol*. 2009;20:113–122.

Cabrera JA, Sanchez–Quintana D, Farre J, Rubio JA, Ho SY. The inferior right atrial isthmus: further architectural insights for current and coming ablation technologies. *J Cardiovasc Electrophysiol*.2005 ;16:402–408.

de Castro S, Caselli S, Di Angelantonio E, et al. Relation of left atrial maximal volume measured by real–time 3D echocardiography to demographic, clinical, and Doppler variables. *Am J Cardiol*.2008; 101:1347–1352.

Ernst G, Stollberger C, Abzieher F, et al. Morphology of the left atrial appendage. *Anat Rec*. 1995;242:553–561.

Ho SY, Anderson RH, Sanchez–Quintana D. Atrial structure and fibres: morphological basis of atrial conduction. *Cardiovasc Res*.2002; 54:325–336.

Shah SJ, Bardo DM, Sugeng L, Weinert L, Lodato JA, Knight BP, Lopez JJ, Lang RM. Real–time three–dimensional transesophageal echocardiography in the left atrial appendage: initial experience in the clinical setting. *J Am Soc Echocardiogr*. 2008;21(12):1362–1368.

Left and Right Ventricle

Gopal AS, Chukwu EO, Iwuchukwu CJ, et al. Normal values of right ventricular size and function by real–time 3–dimensional echocardiography: comparison with cardiac magnetic resonance imaging. *J Am Soc Echocardiogr*. 2007; 20:445–455.

Ho S Y, Nihoyannopoulos P. Anatomy, echocardiography, and normal right ventricular dimensions. *Heart*. 2006;92:2–13.

Merrick AF, Yacoub MH, Ho SY, Anderson RH. Anatomy of the muscular subpulmonary infundibulum with regard to the Ross procedure. *Ann Thorac Surg*. 2000;69:556–561.

Mor–Avi V, Jenkins C, Kuhl HP, et al. Real–time 3D echocardiographic quantification of left ventricular volumes: multicenter study for validation with magnetic resonance imaging and investigation of sources of error. *J Am Coll Cardiol Imaging*. 2008;1:413–423.

Nesser HJ, Sugeng L, Corsi C, et al. Volumetric analysis of regional left ventricular function with real–time three–dimensional echocardiography: validation by magnetic resonance and clinical utility testing. *Heart*. 2007;93:572–578.

Sugeng L, Mor–Avi V, Weinert L, et al. Quantitative assessment of left ventricular size and function: side–by–side comparison of real–time three–dimensional echocardiography and computed tomography with magnetic resonance reference. *Circulation*. 2006;114:654–661.

Catheter-Based Percutaneous Procedures

Acar P, Abadir S, Aggoun Y. Transcatheter closure of perimembranous ventricular septal defects with Amplatzer occluder assessed by real–time three–dimensional echocardiography. *Eur J Echocardiogr*. 2007;8:110–115.

Faletra FF, Grimaldi A, Pasotti E, et al. Real–time 3–Dimensional transesophageal echocardiography during double percutaneous mitral edge–to–edge procedure. *J Am Coll Cardiol Imaging*. 2009;8:1031–1033.

Morgan GJ, Casey F, Craig B, Sands A. Assessing ASDs prior to device closure using 3D echocardiography: just pretty pictures or a useful clinical tool? *Eur J Echocardiogr*. 2008; 9:478–482.

Perk G, Lang R, Garcia–fernandez MA, et al. Use of real time three dimensional transesophageal echocardiography in intracardiac catheter based Interventions. *J Am Soc Echocardiogr*. 2009;22:865–882.

APPENDIX

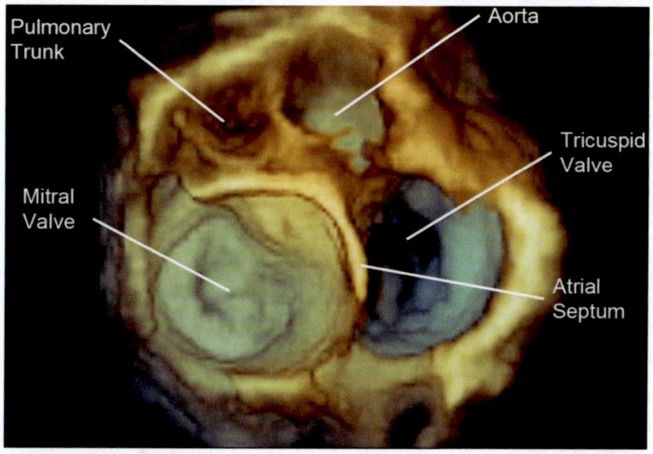

FIGURE 1 Image of the base of the heart viewed from above. Mitral and tricuspid valves, aorta, and pulmonary trunk are visualized in a single image.

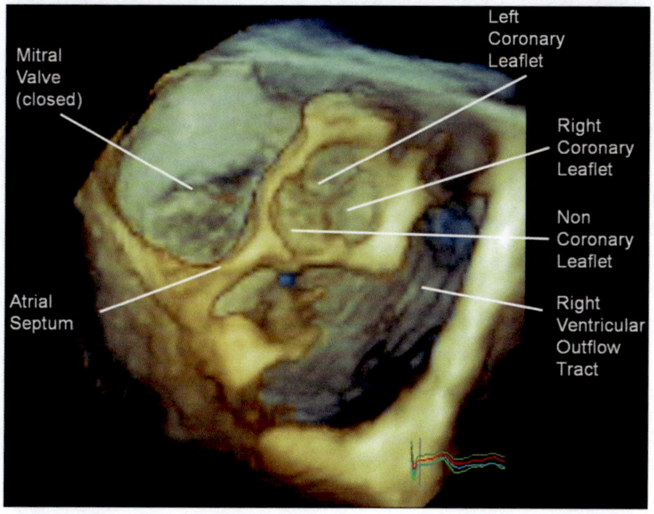

FIGURE 2 Aortic leaflets imaged from above. Atrial septum, mitral valve, and right ventricle outflow tract can be recognized.

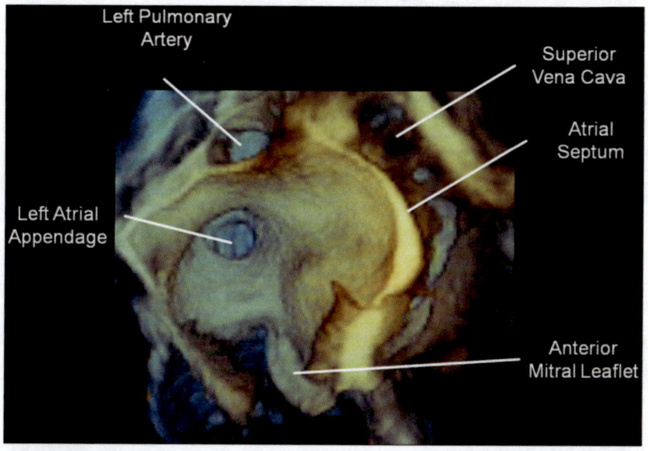

FIGURE 3 Image showing the left atrium viewed from above. Left atrial appendage, left pulmonary artery, superior vena cava, atrial septum, and anterior mitral leaflet are also visualized.

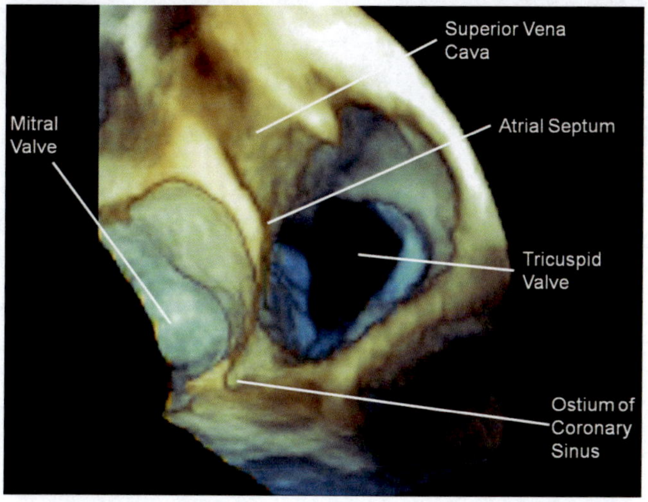

FIGURE 4 Image showing the tricuspid valve (open) and (partially) the mitral valve viewed from atrial perspective. Superior vena cava, atrial septum, and ostium of coronary sinus are also visualized.

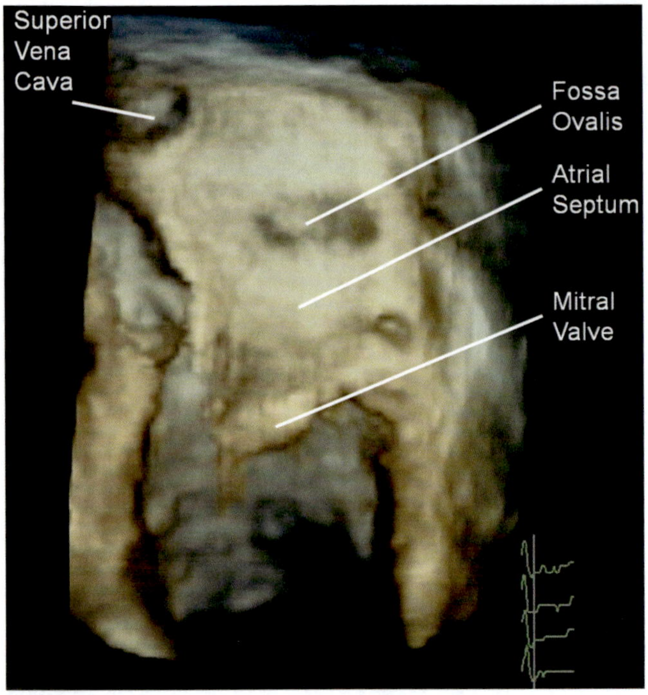

FIGURE 5 The atrial septum "en face" from left atrial perspective. Superior vena cava is seen in cross-section. The anterior mitral leaflet is imaged from an "en face" view.

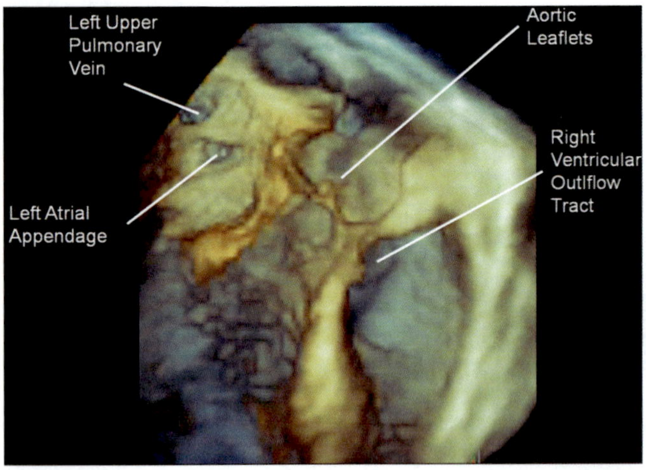

FIGURE 6 Aortic root in long axis section viewed from posteriorly and inferiorly toward the front of the chest. Left atrial appendage and left upper pulmonary vein are seen from above. Right ventricular outflow tract is partially depicted in an oblique plane.

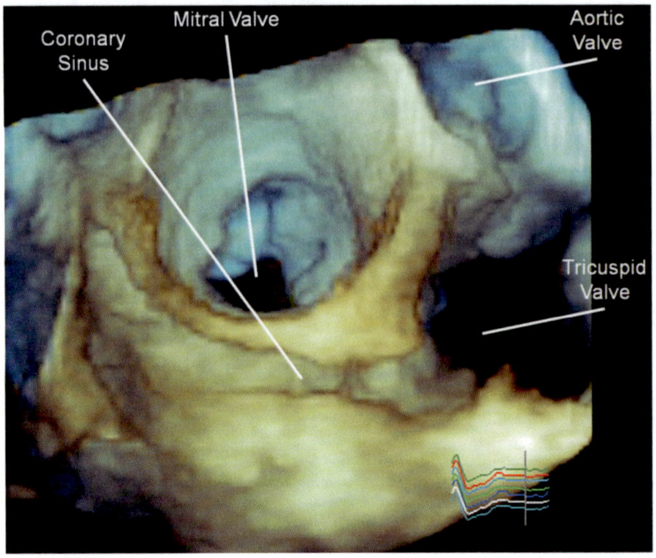

FIGURE 7 A view of a large portion of coronary sinus seen in the atrio-ventricular groove from a superior-posterior perspective. Mitral valve, aortic valve, and tricuspid orifice are also visualized.

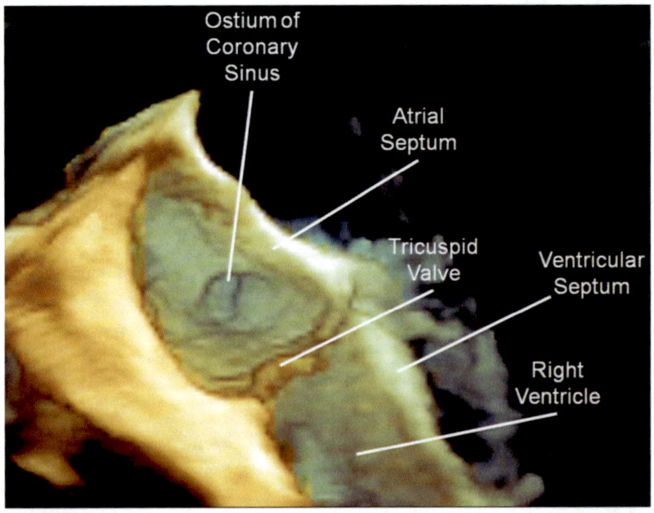

FIGURE 8 Image showing the postero-medial wall of the right atrium with the ostium of coronary sinus, the atrial septum. Tricuspid valve, right ventricle, and ventricular septum are partially depicted.

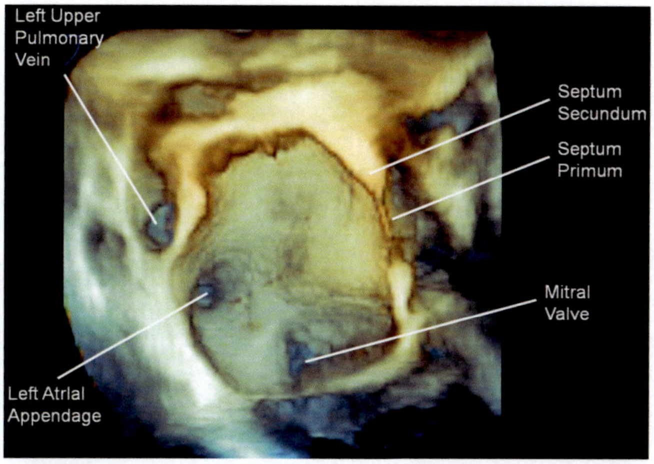

FIGURE 9 Left atrium viewed from above with the left atrial appendage, left upper pulmonary vein, atrial septum, and mitral valve.

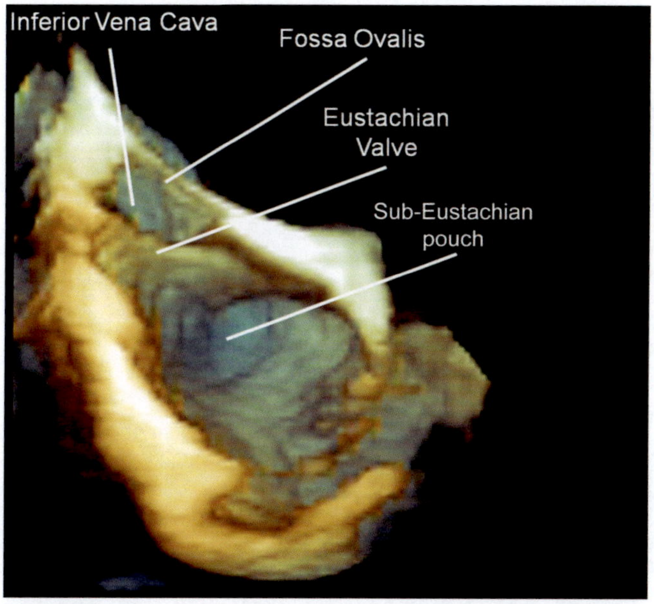

FIGURE 10 Right atrium from above. Inferior vena cava, Eustachian valve, atrial septum (fossa ovalis), tricuspid valve, and right atrial appendage are also visualized.

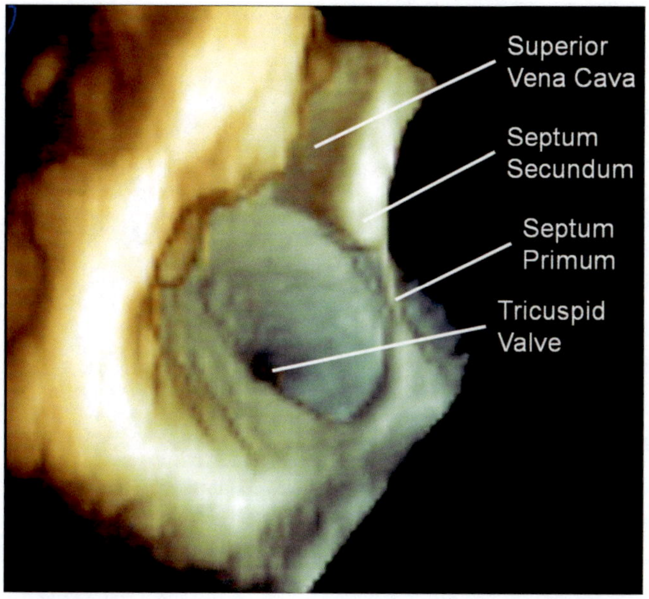

FIGURE 11 Right atrium viewed from an anterior perspective. Note the superior vena cava imaged in its long axis view. Atrial septum and tricuspid valve are partially visualized.

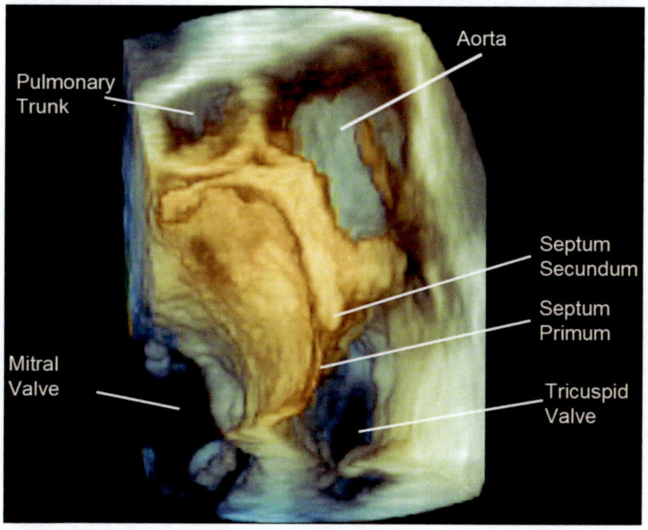

FIGURE 12 View showing both septum secundum and septum primum (fossa ovalis) in an "oblique" perspective. Tricuspid and mitral valve are partially shown. Pulmonary trunk is imaged in cross-section.

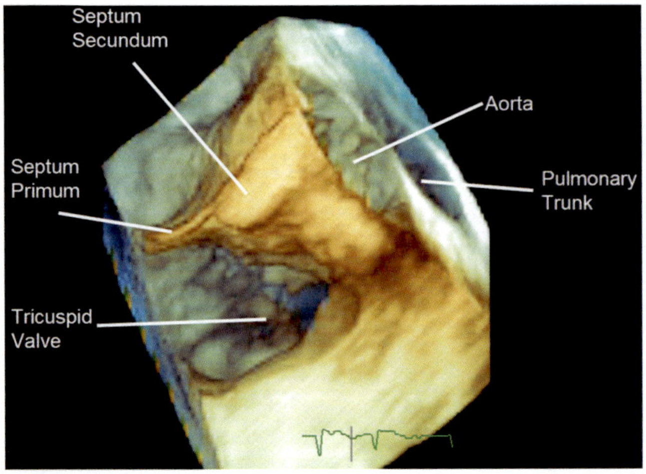

FIGURE 13 View showing the aorta and pulmonary trunk (cross-section) from a lateral perspective. Tricuspid valve is partially visualized from above. Septum secundum and septum primum (fossa ovalis) are partially imaged.

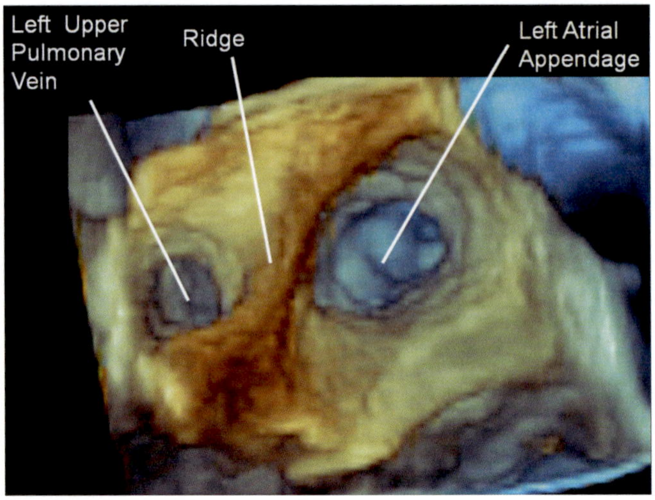

FIGURE 15 Magnified image of left atrial appendage and left upper pulmonary vein with the ridge in between viewed from a superior perspective.

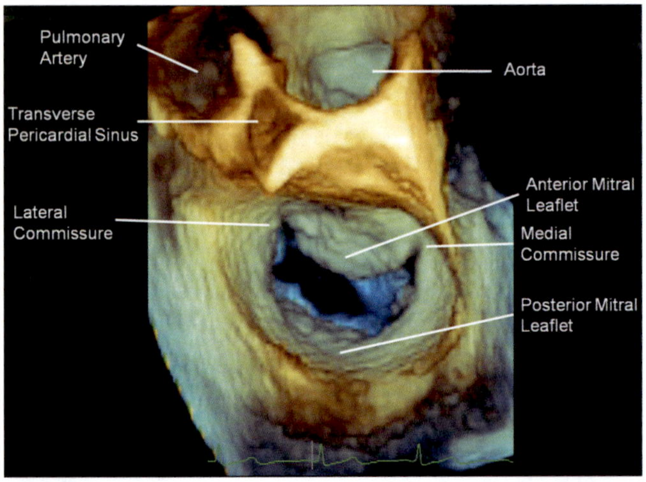

FIGURE 14 A "classic" view of mitral valve seen from atrial perspective. The lateral and medial commissures are well imaged. Aorta and pulmonary artery are visualized in cross-sectional view from an "oblique" perspective. The triangular area in between the aorta, pulmonary trunk, and mitral valve is the transverse pericardial sinus.

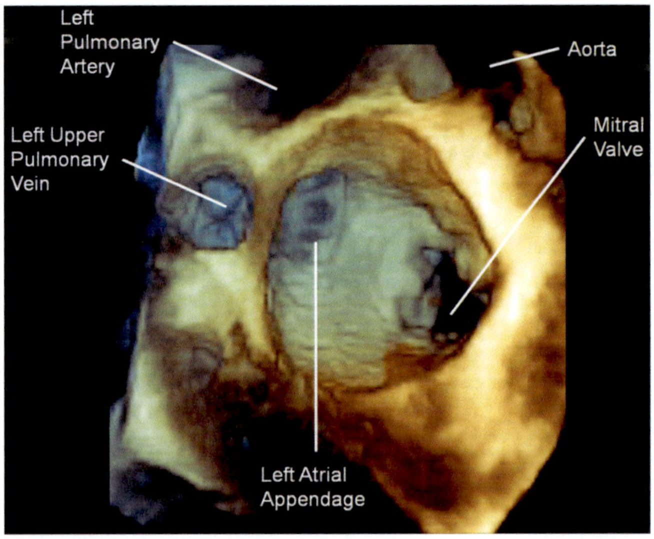

FIGURE 16 View from the left atrium with the left atrial appendage (seen pectinate muscles inside) and the left upper pulmonary vein. The left pulmonary artery and the aorta are partially shown.

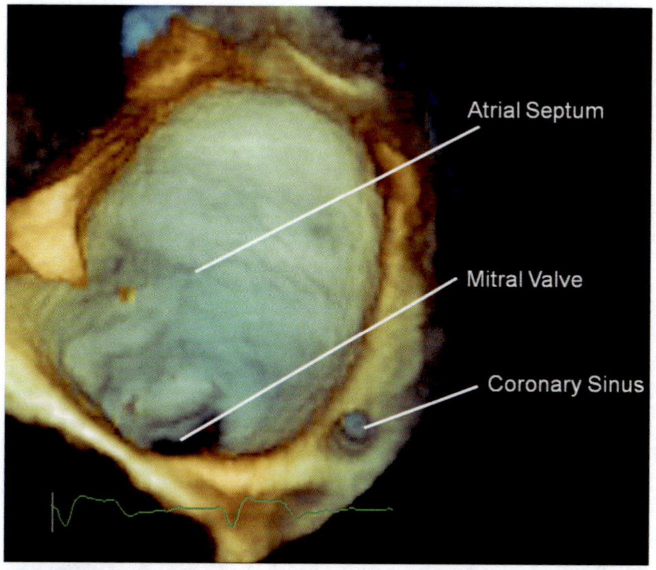

FIGURE 17 A view from above of the left atrium. The atrial septum (en face), the mitral valve (from above), and coronary sinus (cross-section) are visualized.

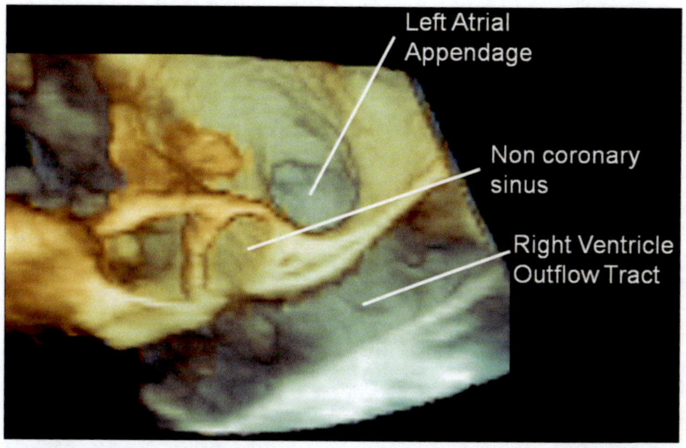

FIGURE 19 A longitudinal cut of the right ventricle outflow tract. The left atrial appendage and the noncoronary aortic sinus are visualized from an "oblique" perspective.

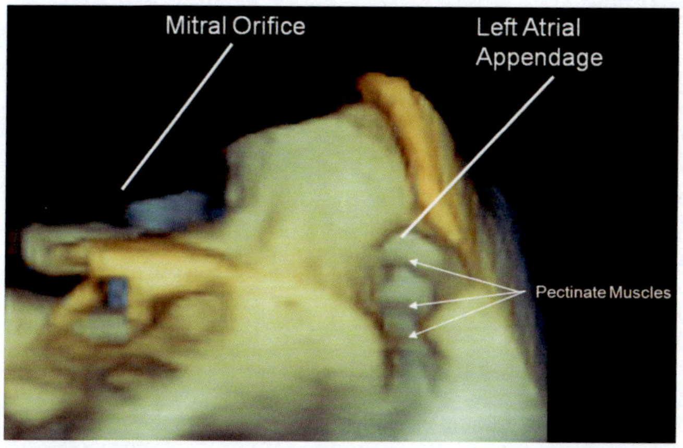

FIGURE 18 A magnified image of the left atrial appendage and pectinate muscles. The mitral orifice is partially shown.

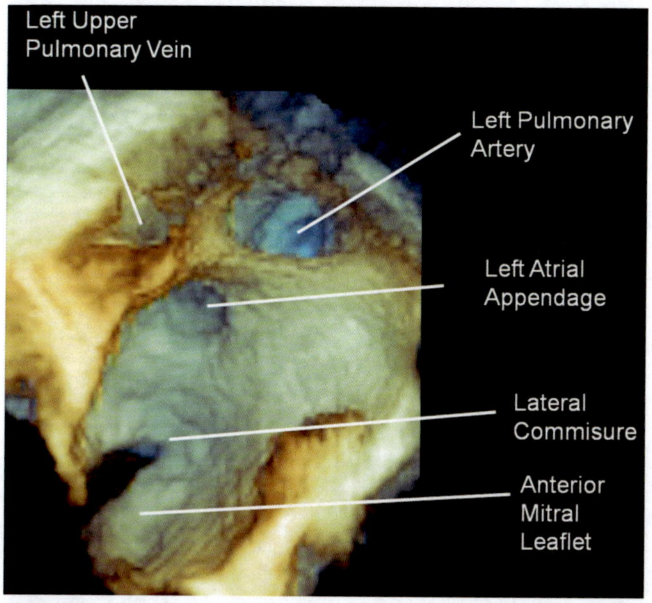

FIGURE 20 Image showing the left atrial appendage, the left pulmonary artery, the left upper pulmonary vein, and the antero-lateral commissure of mitral valve.

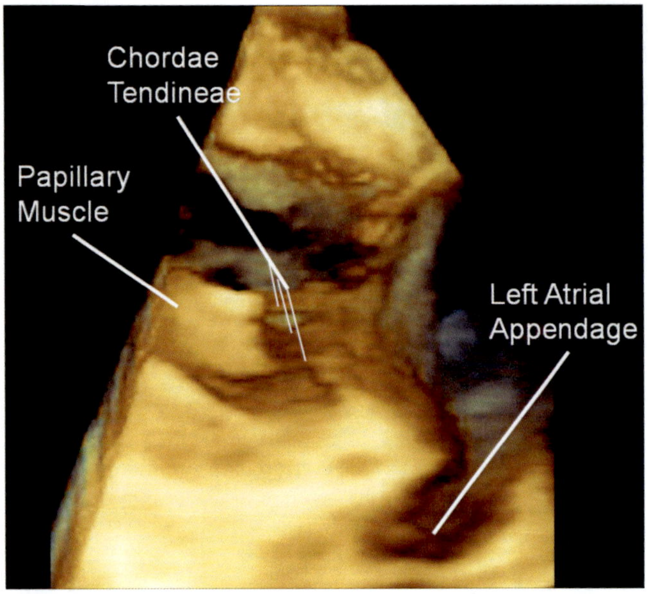

FIGURE 21 A longitudinal section of the left ventricle from transgastric approach showing the antero-lateral papillary muscle and chordae tendineae. The left atrial appendage is also visualized.

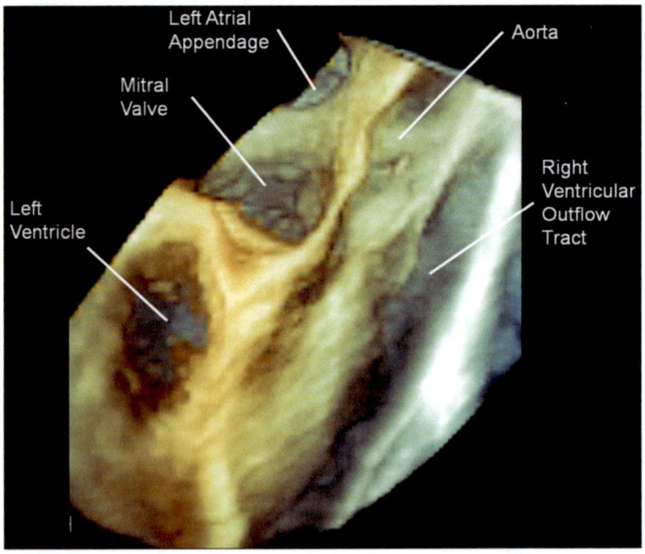

FIGURE 22 A longitudinal view of the aortic root and the right ventricle outflow tract. An "oblique" section of the left ventricle cavity, the mitral valve, and (partially) the left atrial appendage are imaged from lateral-superior perspective.

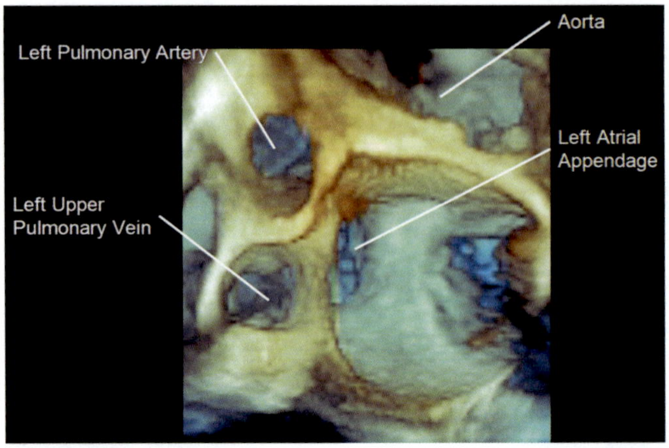

FIGURE 23 Image showing left atrial appendage, left pulmonary artery, and left upper pulmonary vein from a superior perspective.

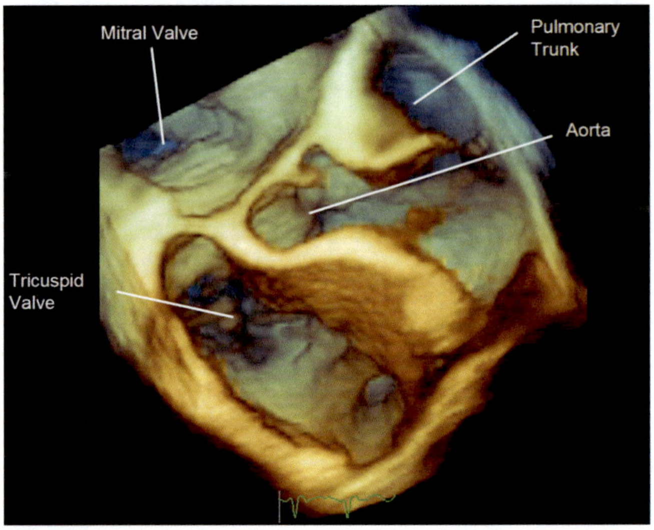

FIGURE 24 Image showing the tricuspid valve from above, the aorta (oblique cut), the mitral valve (only partially imaged from above), and the pulmonary trunk (cross-section).

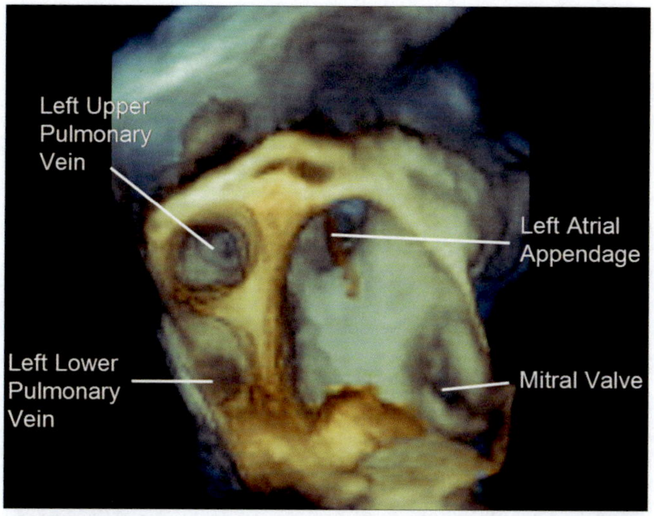

FIGURE 25 A view from above showing the left upper and lower pulmonary veins, left atrial appendage, and (partially) the mitral valve.

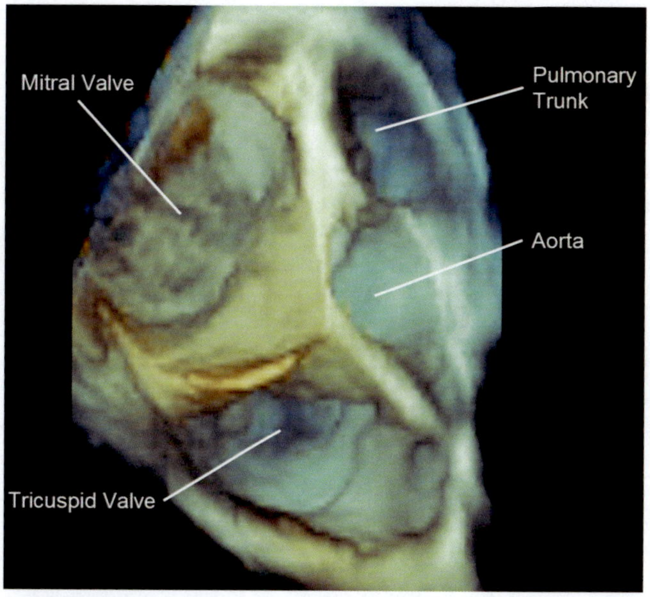

FIGURE 27 Image showing mitral valve (seen partially and in close position), and tricuspid valve from above. Aorta and pulmonary trunk are imaged side by side.

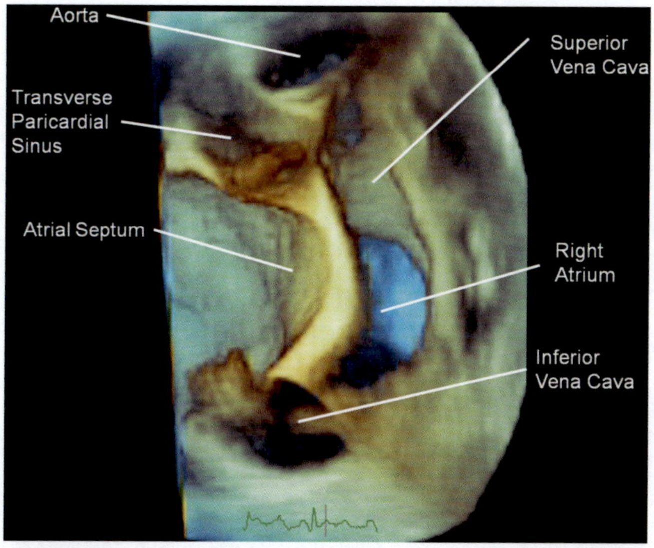

FIGURE 26 A view from a left perspective showing the superior vena cava (longitudinal cut), the inferior vena cava (cross-section), the atrial septum, the transverse pericardial sinus, and the aorta (cross-section).

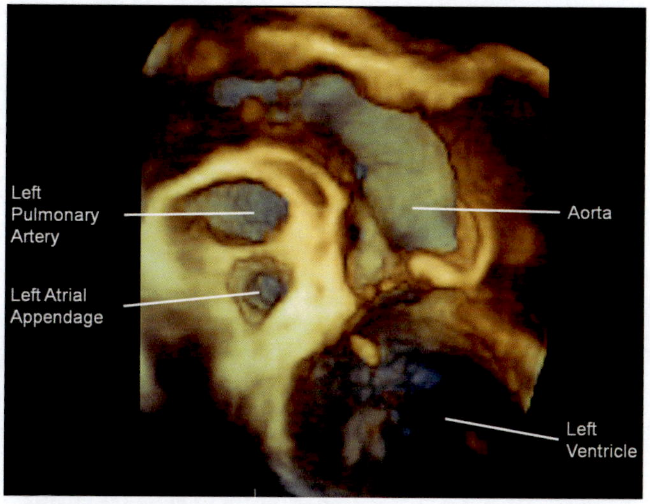

FIGURE 28 Image showing left pulmonary artery in a cross-section, left atrial appendage from above, and aorta in long axis view.

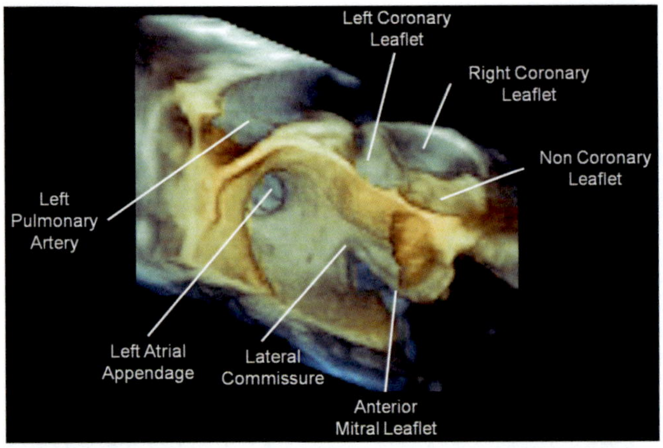

FIGURE 29 Image showing all the three aortic leaflets in closed position from an "oblique" perspective, left atrial appendage and the lateral commissure of mitral valve. The left pulmonary artery is cut longitudinally.

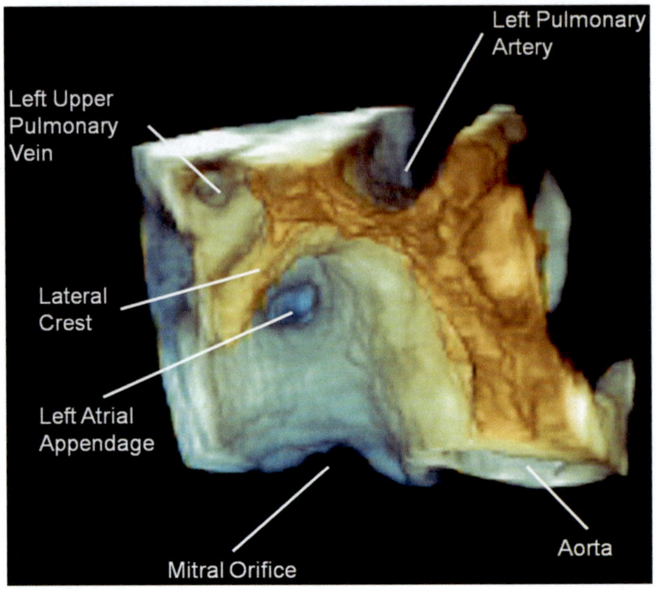

FIGURE 30 Image showing the left atrial appendage and the left upper pulmonary vein with the ridge from above. The left pulmonary artery is cut longitudinally.

INDEX

Kolibri 360 GmbH
Ferdinand-Jühlke-Straße 7
99095 Erfurt, Deutschland
produktsicherheit@kolibri360.de